PROGRESS IN DIGITAL ANGIOCARDIOGRAPHY

DEVELOPMENTS IN CARDIOVASCULAR MEDICINE

Recent volumes

PROGRESS IN DIGITAL ANGIOCARDIOGRAPHY

edited by

P.H. HEINTZEN and J.H. BÜRSCH
*Department of Pediatric Cardiology and Biomedical Engineering,
Kiel University, F.R.G.*

1988 **KLUWER ACADEMIC PUBLISHERS**
DORDRECHT / BOSTON / LONDON

Distributors

for the United States and Canada: Kluwer Academic Publishers, 101 Philip Drive, Norwell, MA 02061, USA
for all other countries: Kluwer Academic Publishers Group, P.O. Box 322, 3300 AH Dordrecht, The Netherlands

Library of Congress Cataloging in Publication Data

Progress in digital angiocardiography.

  (Developments in cardiovascular medicine)
  Includes index
  1. Angiocardiography--Digital techniques.
I. Heintzen, Paul H. II. Bürsch, J. H. III. Series.
[DNLM: 1. Angiocardiography--trends. 2. Coronary
Disease--radiography. 3. Radiographic Image Enhancement.
4. Subtraction Technic. W1 DE997VME / WG 300 P9645]
RC683.5.A5P76 1987   616.1'20757   87-20270

ISBN-13: 978-94-010-7093-5   e-ISBN-13: 978-94-009-1331-8
DOI: 10.1007/978-94-009-1331-8

Copyright

Table of Contents

VIII

**PART IV: TECHNICAL CONSIDERATIONS ON
DIGITAL SYSTEMS**

Preface

According to Schopenhauer *problems* are usually passing through three stages:
- in the first stage they are ignored or just smiled at,
- in the second stage they are fought, and
- in the third stage they are considered to be self-evident, just taken for granted.

Whereas digital subtraction *angio*graphy (DSA) has obviously reached stage three of that scale, i.e. routine use in radiology, digital angiocardiography, in particular imaging the heart and coronary circulation, is still on its way to the final goal: the filmless heart catheterization laboratory for all invasive and interventional procedures.

A few pioneers have already completely abandoned the conventional cine-coronary and angiocardiographic technique, others – as we do – still combine both digital and conventional methods in clinical routine, but most cardiologists up till now stay sceptically aside.

We hope that at least some of the articles published in this volume may convince more and more cardiologists that digital imaging procedures are the method of choice, in particular if quantitative assessment of the anatomical or functional status of the cardiovascular system is required (pre- and post-operations or pre- and post-interventions).

Such a critical control of all therapeutic procedures, be it by surgical, catheter- or medical 'interventions', is indeed an urgent and widely under-estimated or neglected requirement.

In this context digital electronic angiocardiographic imaging of the beating heart might even be more important for straightforward *quantifying* cardiac dynamics, valvular regurgitation, the coronary circulation, in particular coronary flow reserve, and myocardial perfusion, than just imaging the malformed heart or coronary arteries. Examples of the potential of digital angiocardiography with or without subtraction and digital functional angiocardiography are given in this volume.

X

Although the saying by Shakespeare that *dreams are the stuff that progress is made of* might be true, it is our experience that one needs much hard work and some luck *to convert such dreams into reality!* This is certainly true for the dream of an all-digital catheterization and cardiovascular imaging laboratory acceptable to almost all cardiologists.

The need is obvious, the technology is available and the roentgen-industry is capable and willing to cooperate, if we give them the 'right' message. Even if progress might be slow, it will be – as predicted – irresistible. We hope that these proceedings of the fourth Kiel conference will help to speed up this progress.

The editors are grateful to all those who have helped in many different ways to make this meeting and publication possible, in particular Dr. Onnasch and the staff of our department. We are again greatly indebted to Pharma Schwarz and in particular to Mr. Gücker, who – without any direct relationship to this field – sponsored the meeting in the usual generous way. Finally, Mr. Commandeur and Kluwer Academic Publishers deserve special acknowledgement for the pleasant cooperation.

Kiel, January 1988
                                      Paul H. Heintzen
                                      Joachim H. Bürsch

List of Major Contributors

H. Abe, M.D. Division of Cardiovascular Diagnostic and Interventional Medicine, Faculty of Medicine, Nihon University, 30-1 Ohyaguchi, Itabashi-ku, Tokyo 173, Japan

K. Bachmann, M.D. Medizinische Poliklinik der Universität Erlangen, Ostliche Stadtmauerstr. 29, D-8520 Erlangen, FRG

K. Barth, Ph.D. Siemens AG, Unternehmensbereich Med. Technik, Henkestr. 127, D-8520 Erlangen, FRG

R. Brennecke, Ph.D. 2. Medizinische Klinik der Universität Mainz, Langenbeckstr. 1, D-6500 Mainz, FRG

J.H. Bürsch, M.D. Abt. Kinderkardiologie und Biomedizinische Technik, Universitäts-Kinderklinik, Schwanenweg 20, D-2300 Kiel, FRG

H.L. Chernoff, M.D. The Boston Floating Hospital, 750 Washington Street, Boston, MA 02111, USA

P.-A. Doriot, Ph.D. Centre de Cardiologie, Hôpital Cantonal Universitaire de Genève, 24 Rue Micheli du Crest, CH-1211 Genève 4, Switzerland

N.L. Eigler, M.D. Division of Cardiology, Cedars-Sinai Medical Center, 8700 Deverly Blvd, Los Angeles, CA 90048, USA

J.L. Elion, M.D. Division of Cardiology, Department of Medicine, University of Kentucky College of Medicine, 800 Rose Street, MN-670, Lexington, KG 40536-0084, USA

K.L. Gould, M.D. Positron Diagnostic and Research Center, University of Texas Medical School at Houston, P.O. Box 20708, Houston, TX 77225, USA

P.A. Grayburn, M.D. Division of Cardiology, Department of Medicine, University of Kentucky College of Medicine, 800 Rose Street, MN-670, Lexington, KY 40536-0084, USA

P.H. Heintzen, M.D. Abt. Kinderkardiologie und Biomedizinische Technik, Universitäts-Kinderklinik Schwanenweg 20, D-2300 Kiel, FRG

O.M. Hess, M.D. Medizinische Poliklinik, Kardiologie, Universitäts-Klinik, Rämistrasse 100, CH-8091 Zürich, Switzerland

P.E. Lange, M.D. Abt. Kinderkardiologie und Biomedizinische Technik, Universitäts-Kinderklinik, Schwanenweg 20, D-2300 Kiel, FRG

G.B.J. Mancini, M.D. Cardiology Section, Veterans Administration Medical Center, Department of Internal Medicine, University of Michigan Medical School, 2215 Fuller Road, Ann Arbor, MI 48105, USA

M.L. Marcus, M.D. Department of Internal Medicine, E318-2 GH, University of Iowa, Iowa City, IA 52242, USA

S.E. Nissen, M.D. Division of Cardiology, Department of Medicine, University of Kentucky College of Medicine, 800 Rose Street, MN-670, Lexington, KY 40536-0084, USA

D.G.W. Onnasch, Ph.D. Abt. Kinderkardiologie und Biomedizinische Technik, Universitäts-Kinderklinik, Schwanenweg 20, D-2300 Kiel, FRG

D.L. Parker, Ph.D. Department of Medical Informatics, LDS Hospital/University of Utah, 325 Eighth Avenue, Salt Lake City, UT 84143, USA

J.H.C. Reiber, Ph.D. Erasmus University Rotterdam, Postbus 1738, 3000 DR Rotterdam, The Netherlands

W. Rutishauser, M.D. Centre de Cardiologie, Hôpital Cantonal Universitaire de Genève, 24 Rue Micheli du Crest, CH-1211 Genève 4, Switzerland

R. Simon, M.D. Abteilung Kardiologie, Medizinische Hochschule Hannover, Karl-Wiechert Allee, 3000 Hannover, FRG

R.A. Vogel, M.D. Cardiology Section, Veterans Administration Medical Center, Department of Internal Medicine, University of Michigan Medical School, 2215 Fuller Road, Ann Arbor, MI 48105, USA

T. van der Werf, M.D. Department of Cardiology, Catholic University, Geert Grooteplein zuid 8, 6500 HB Nijmegen, The Netherlands

H. Wollschläger, M.D. Medizinische Universitätsklinik, Abteilung Kardiologie, Hugstetterstr. 55, D-7800 Freiburg, FRG

E. Zeitler, M.D. Radiologisches Zentrum, Abteilung Diagnostik, D-8500 Nürnberg, FRG

Part I: Digital Angiocardiography for Diagnostic Routine

1. Results with Digital Angiography

E. ZEITLER & W. SEYFERTH

Radiological Center, Diagnostic Department, Klinikum Nuremberg, Nuremberg, FRG

The symposium on Digital Imaging in Cardiovascular Radiology in April 1982 made two matters clear:

1. For clinical application, digital subtraction angiography and computed tomography as photo-electronic-digital radiographic systems are of comparable value;
2. Real-time subtraction involving multiple cine images with a digital computer system can be used in addition to single image evaluation studies of the heart and peripheral vascular system.

The majority of systems in use today combine digital and analog systems. They permit a continuous observation of the course of the contrast medium bolus on the screen, and subsequent processing by a great number of software manipulations [1]. Though the principle of digital subtraction angiography is accepted and widely used in radiological departments, the general application of an intravenous contrast medium to document the central (heart and coronary vessels) and systemic arterial circulation is yet to be realized. (Table 1A, B).

Though many publications and symposia document the efforts to reduce the

Table 1A. Potential use of DSA in the heart.

1. I.v. contrast medium application for *Left ventriculography* at rest and after work
2. Intra-aortic contrast medium application for control of *ACBP*
3. Intracoronary contrast medium application for selective *Coronary arteriography*

Table 1B. Advantages of cardiac DSA.

ad 1. No catheter in the heart, repeatable
ad 2. Avoiding selective coronary bypass-catheterization, 5-Fr. pigtail catheter
ad 3. Reduction of contrast medium per injection, quantitative digital determination of coronary stenoses

P.H. Heintzen and J.H. Bürsch (eds), Progress in Digital Angiocardiography. ISBN 978-94-010-7093-5
© 1988, Kluwer Academic Publishers, Dordrecht

4

risks and the costs of angiographic studies by means of this new technology, we have chosen to reference only two [2, 3].

In 1985 at the Central Radiodiagnostic Department of Nuremberg, DSA was used in 1400 studies of the peripheral vascular system, 1800 studies of the cerebrovascular system (extra- and intracerebral) and 160 studies of the central vascular system.

As the number of DSA studies rises, the conventional cut-film technique and cine-angiographic numbers remain stable.

In addition, DSA plays a special role in the documentation of diseases of the inferior and superior vena cavae, as well as of the thoracic and abdominal aorta.

DSA is the preferred diagnostic procedure in 90% of patients in whom the question of pulmonary embolization arises. Only in patients in shock we start with cine-technique combined with video-tape recording.

Left ventriculography (Fig. 1) offers a good diagnostic possibility, but we use left ventriculography in combination with coronary arteriography via DSA only in patients that require additional studies of the cerebrovascular, peripheral or renal vascular systems.

Thus DSA of the coronary circulation (Fig. 2) employs selective application of the contrast medium in the coronary arteries and is not an intravenous study [4]. In this way, documentation of coronary anatomy is achieved with high contrast resolution and diagnostic information in 80% of our studies. In the others, problems result in non-diagnostic images, and cine-coronary arteriography is necessary.

The use of intravenous contrast medium application for documentation of the arterial vascular system has had a significant impact on clinical decision-making broadening the indications for use of this technique. It has also led to an increase in postoperative examinations. The vascular surgeons are pleased that arterial access is less frequently required now for these evaluations. Thus,

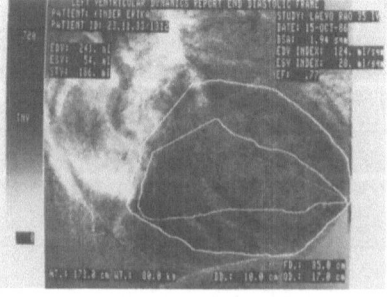 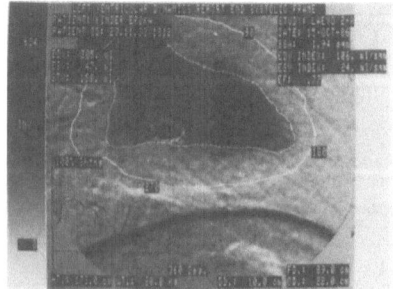

Fig. 1. Left ventriculography after intravenous (left) contrast medium application and selective (right) contrast medium injection in the left ventricle of a patient with coronary heart disease.

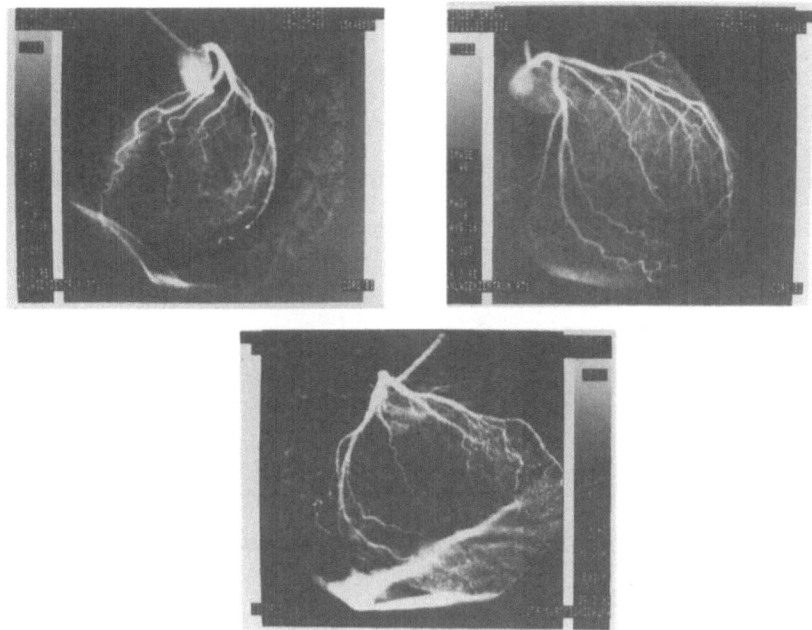

Fig. 2. Selective coronary arteriogrphy with biplane DSA of the left coronary arterial system in three different projections.

peri-arterial hematomas which might cause infections of prostheses can be avoided. But the more common use of intravenous DSA has revealed the limitations of anatomic resolution in certain cases so that today intravenous and arterial contrast media are applied selectively, depending on the problem.

In preparing this symposium, the organizing committee asked three questions:

First question: what can digital techniques offer the clinical cardiologist today and in the future? There are, in addition to nuclear medicine, two other digital techniques:
- Digital Subtraction Angiography (DSA),
- Magnetic Resonance Imaging (MRI).

There is no doubt that digital image processing improves contrast resolution with real-time information at the monitor. In contrast to cinematography, it is possible to produce a hard copy image within a very short time, providing almost immediate information for the surgeon. Due to considerably improved contrast resolution, the reduced spatial resolution is hardly significant. In selective coronary angiography and left ventriculography, using DSA techniques, the investigation time depends on the immediately available storage capacity. If it is limited, complete coronary angiography and left ventriculo-

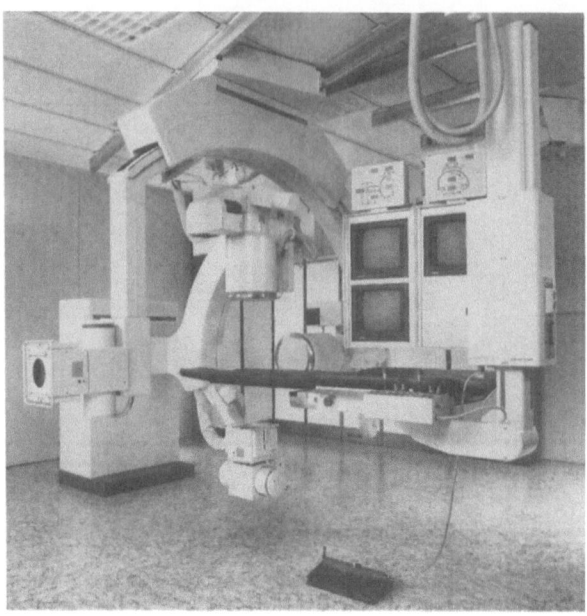

Fig. 3. Biplane DSA-System Bicor.

graphy may require a longer investigation time thus increasing the risk. This higher risk is only partially compensated for by a lower amount of contrast medium necessary for the investigation. Therefore, it must be decided in principle, whether to perform angiocardiography of the heart cavities, in- or outflow of main vessels, or to assess the coronary system only.

However, there is no doubt that DSA permits the assessment of
– inflow of the heart,
– outflow of the heart,
– pulmonary circulation,
– thoracic aorta,
– left ventricle.

Our DSA equipment includes the Angiotron, the Digitron II and the Digitron III with the Bicor system for angiocardiography and coronary studies (Fig. 3). The newer equipment allows geometric, densitometric and flow analysis of contrast medium distribution curves, depending on the available software. In patients who are able to cooperate, important diagnostic-clinical results may be obtained in 85–90% of the investigations of the heart, the pulmonary circulation and the thoracic aorta. The clear diagnostic definitions are determined to a great extent by the technical equipment, including the X-ray tube, image intensifier, DSA system, storage capacity as well as the site of contrast medium application.

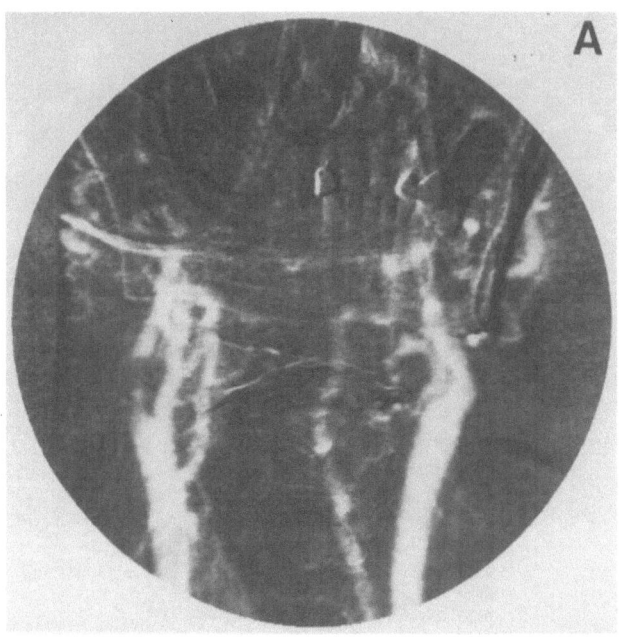

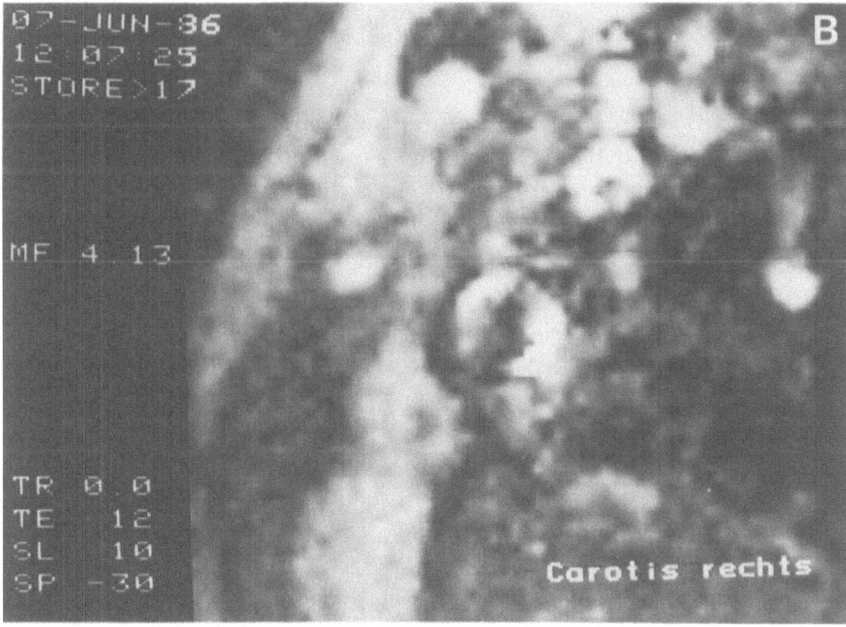

Fig. 4. A: sagittal iv. DSA of neck arteries demonstrating highgrade internal carotid artery stenosis on the right. B: functional study of the right carotid artery with MRJ-FISP-technique, demonstrating a transverse scan through right carotid artery stenosis with signals demonstrating blood flow.

8

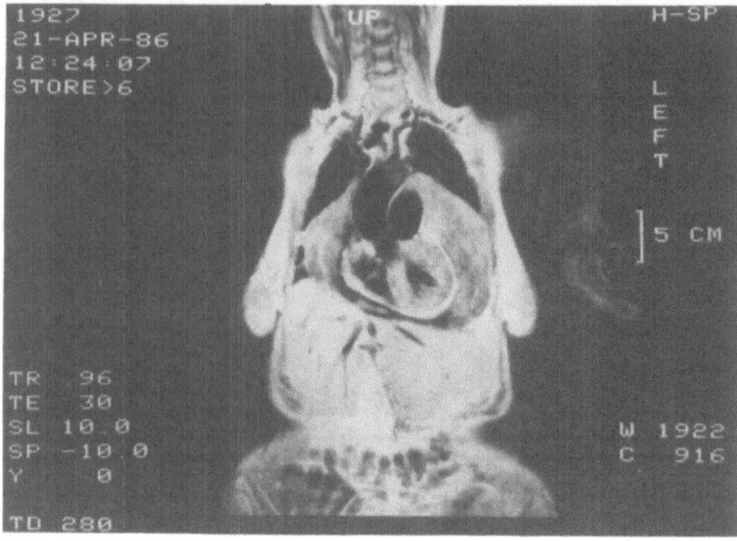

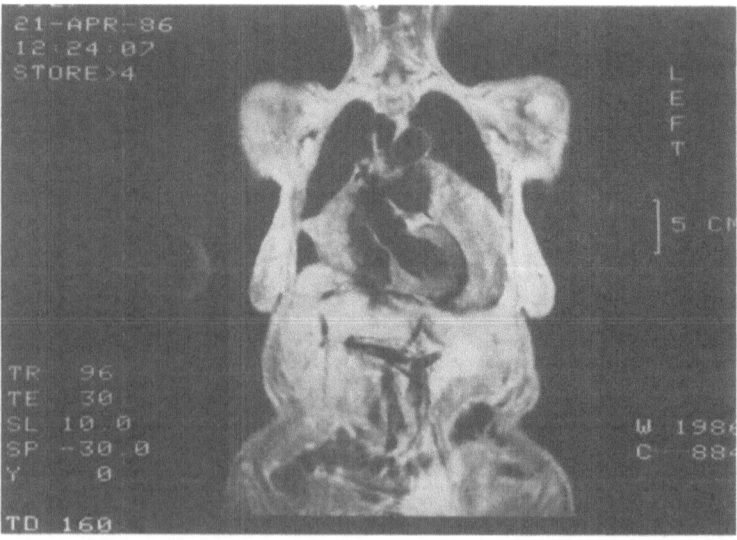

Fig. 5. MRI with ECG-gating in a 67-year-old woman after myocardial infarction with hemopericardium. Coronal scans demonstrating left and right ventricle in systole and diastole.

On the other hand, the second new digital technique, that is Magnetic Resonance Imaging, offers
– documentation of heart cavities,
– documentation of the myocardium,
– documentation of pericardial space;
and all of this without contrast medium, without puncture or catheterization, and without radiation.

If the appropriate software is available, MRI supplies noninvasively information about morphology and function of ventricles and myocardium. Myocardial metabolism can also be evaluated.

Thus, the first question can be answered as follows: DSA and MRI together with echocardiography can replace angiography in many patients:
– in most congenital heart diseases,
– in many acquired heart diseases,
– in pericardial and paracardial diseases,
– in pulmonary vascular diseases.

Second question: can digital angiography replace conventional techniques? Angiocardiography can be used in most cases with digital technique as well as with cineangiography. But selective coronary arteriography and aortocoronary bypass control are best done on a conventional basis.

Third question: can it offer more? And if so, how; and why does it not replace coronary arteriography?
1. Selective coronary catheterization is still necessary.
2. There is reduced spatial resolution compared to conventional coronary arteriography.
3. ECG-gating is only useful in patients without rhythm disorders.
4. When 4 DSA projections are used, there are more than 1000 frames that require postprocessing taking up to 60 minutes (Table 2).
5. Quantification of coronary arterial stenoses with DSA requires more time and does not yet offer more exact information in clinical practice. This can only be accomplished by the cardiologist and not by the technician.

Yet in contrast, there are important advantages to DSA in that other problems can be appreciated and in the case of an intravenous left ventriculogram it is less invasive [5] and can be used when radionuclide or cine-CT units are not available.

Other advantages to DSA include: in- and outflow of the heart can be demonstrated readily
– with or without ECG-gating,
– with less contrast medium and
– with more anatomic information obtained compared to conventional arteriography.

However, in the same way the more expensive MRI may provide important

advantages, e.g. in cases of hypersensitivity to contrast medium when a heart catheterization is rejected for whatever reason. Particular advantages include:
– MRI has high contrast resolution,
– fast imaging sequences are possible,
– neither catheter nor contrast media are necessary,
– real 3-dimensional analysis is possible.
The limitations of DSA in coronary studies include problems in the assessment of the peripheral outflow which may be of importance for surgical reconstruction, and the difficulty with quantitative evaluation of coronary stenoses. Is it a more or less exact visual interpretation?

Though processing programs generate a better morphologic assessment of coronary stenosis or sclerosis by means of X-ray cinematograms [6, 7], clinical practicability has not yet been achieved. A safe quantification with DSA units or arterial stenoses is feasible immediately after the investigation and there is no loss of time caused by the development of the film. Contour definition has to be made either manually or automatically, though false assessment due to motion artefacts or half-shadows cannot be excluded.

In the pelvic and carotid arteries, we determined the degree of stenosis geometrically and densitometrically and state the following:
1. the visual assessment of the degree of a stenosis varies considerably,
2. a 2-dimensional determination does not suffice,
3. a 3-dimensional definition of the stenosis still shows large scattering.
These observations demontrate the necessity
1. to train the radiologists and cardiologists by means of quantitative automatic measuring systems and to make them more critical,

Table 2. Cardangiography: biplane with DSA.

Advantages	Disadvantages
2 projections/scene	1. Spatial resolution (512 × 512)
↓	2. Required time for postprocess.
Decrease of CM used	10 sec × 25 fr./sec × 4 proj. =
↓	1000 frames (minimum)
Decrease of time/study and catheter placement	⇒ single hardcopies
	+ development 30'
↓	+ quantification 30'
Theoretical improvement as far as safety is	—————
concerned; but equalized more or less by	(minimum) 60'
using non-ionic CM	
	At least at the beginning: it is
	a cardiologist's job, not a technician's.

2. to add 3-dimensional evaluation if an automatic quantitative assessment of the arterial stenosis is required.

In the future, the flow imaging potential of Magnetic Resonance technology offers the possibility of applying digital subtraction technology. Only 3-dimensional *en bloc* data acquisition opens the possibility of documenting the coronary arteries noninvasively. However, this will not be possible for some time.

In the meantime software for angiographic programs of all arteries can be used and tested in vivo as to their quantitative safety. DSA may, in case Magnetic Resonance Imaging is not available, replace conventional angiography in the detection of congenital vitia or intra- and paracardiac masses as does computed tomography. Coronary angiography, however, will still have to be performed conventionally for the foreseeable future. The potentially outstanding quality of coronary DSA indicates, however, that it is reasonable to think that conventional cinematography will be discarded in favor or DSA in routine cardiac diagnostic units.

References

1. Heintzen PH, Brennecke R (eds): Digital imaging in cardiovascular radiology. Gg Thieme Verlag, Stuttgart/New York, 1983.
2. Felix R, Frommhold W, Lissner J, Meaney TF, Niendorf HP, Zeitler E (eds): Contrast media in digital radiography. Excerpta Medica, Amsterdam, 1983.
3. Thurn P, Felix R: Standortbestimmung der digitalen Subtraktions-angiographie (DSA). Schering AG, Berlin, 1984.
4. Guthaner DF, Wexler L, Bradley B: Digital subtraction angiography of coronary grafts: optimization of technique. AJR 1985; 145: 1185–1190.
5. Eichstädt H, Felix R: Kritischer Methodenvergleich zur Bestimmung ventrikulärer Funktionsparameter unter besonderer Berücksichtigung der DSA. In: Thurn P, Felix R (eds): Standortbestimmung der digitalen Subtraktions-angiographie (DSA); pp 111–122. Schering AG, Berlin, 1984.
6. Reiber JHC, Gerbrands JJ, Troost GJ, Kooijman CJ, Slump CH: 3-D reconstruction of coronary arterial segments from two projections. In: Heintzen PH, Brennecke R (eds): Digital imaging in cardiovascular radiology; pp 151–163. Gg Thieme Verlag, Stuttgart/New York, 1983.
7. Reiber JHC, Slager CJ, Schuurbiers JCH, Den Boer A, Gerbrands JJ, Troost GJ, Scholts R, Kooijman CJ, Serruys PW: Transfer functions of the X-ray-cine-video chain applied to digital processing of coronary cineangiograms. In: Heintzen PH, Brennecke R (eds): Digital imaging in cardiovascular radiology; pp 89–100. Gg Thieme Verlag, Stuttgart/New York, 1983.

2. Digital Angiography in Coronary Heart Disease

K. BACHMANN & R. GÄNSSER
University of Erlangen, Erlangen, FRG

Computerized digital imaging has gained considerable importance in the angiographic assessment of coronary heart disease. Today, computer acquisition and enhancement of radiographic images is feasible for 'road-mapping' during angioplasty, for the determination of coronary bypass graft patency by aortic root injection, for transvenous or low-dose direct left ventriculography, and for the computerized geometric and video-densitometric quantitation of focal coronary narrowing [1–16]. This steady advance in digital electronic imaging may eventually lead to replacement of filmbased selective coronary arteriography [16–18]. Though the 'filmless catheterization laboratory' is a promising new modality, it is nevertheless not yet available for routine diagnostic use. We are all willing to use real-time digital imaging instead of film as the primary storage medium for the angiographic examination in the catheterization laboratory. But the arguments for digital substraction angiography, which are well accepted in non-cardiac arteriography, are not so convincing in the visualization of coronary arteries. There are technical limitations introduced by the analog-digital conversion and the capacity of digital discs that are not yet overcome. As long as the architecture of the imaging chain does not change, digital information is not superior to analog information for coronary angiography.

Basically the conversion of analog to digital form involves information loss that cannot be restored by image processing modalities. This loss of information is mainly due to a reduction in spatial resolution, which has become the main limiting factor in the use of digital imaging techniques for the visualization of coronary arteries. In addition there may be misregistration of artefacts, oversaturation of the television camera, limited disc space for image storage, and slow data transfer during playback.

By using a high-resolution image intensifier of 7 inches, a focal spot of 1.2 mm, and a high dynamic video camera of 1249 lines the 512×512 matrix provides a spatial resolution of only 1.5 lp/mm as compared to 4 lp/mm in cine technique (Fig. 1). This limited spatial resolution can be increased up to a

P.H. Heintzen and J.H. Bürsch (eds), Progress in Digital Angiocardiography. ISBN 978-94-010-7093-5

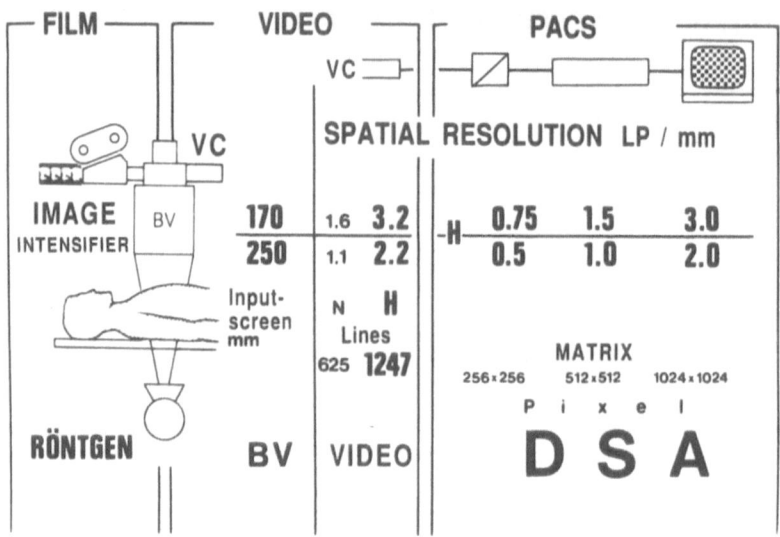

Fig. 1. Spatial resolution of digital imaging as a function of the image intensifier size, the video system and the matrix format.

maximum of 2.1 lp/mm at the object site by a magnification of 1.4. The 1024×1024 matrix provides improved spatial resolution but requires more and faster storage capabilities than offered by digital discs now routinely available.

Since the introduction of selective coronary angiography by Sones [19] it has been our primary aim to improve both the spatial and the temporal resolution. The progress in the imaging chain technology, especially in the image intensifier and in the high resolution video camera, has set today's standards in cine coronary angiography. These standards of imaging quality are defined by a spatial resolution of 4 lp/mm, a temporal resolution of 25 frames/sec, and an acquisition time of at least 10 seconds. So far, digital angiography is a trade-off between less spatial but higher density resolution. This compromise has produced substantial progress in peripheral angiography. For the evaluation of carotid, renal and femoral artery stenoses by non-selective contrast material injection a spatial resolution of 1.5 lp/mm and a temporal resolution of 6–8 frames/sec can be considered as diagnostically sufficient (Fig. 2). But the role of digital imaging in the angiographic diagnosis of coronary heart disease has still to be defined [2, 20, 21]. There is a tendency to accept reduced spatial resolution of digital coronary imaging by introducing the term 'significant coronary artery disease' in angiographic reports. Such a compromise could be accepted at routine if the enhanced density achieved by digitalization could be utilized for non-selective coronary angiography with contrast injection in the aortic root [22–24].

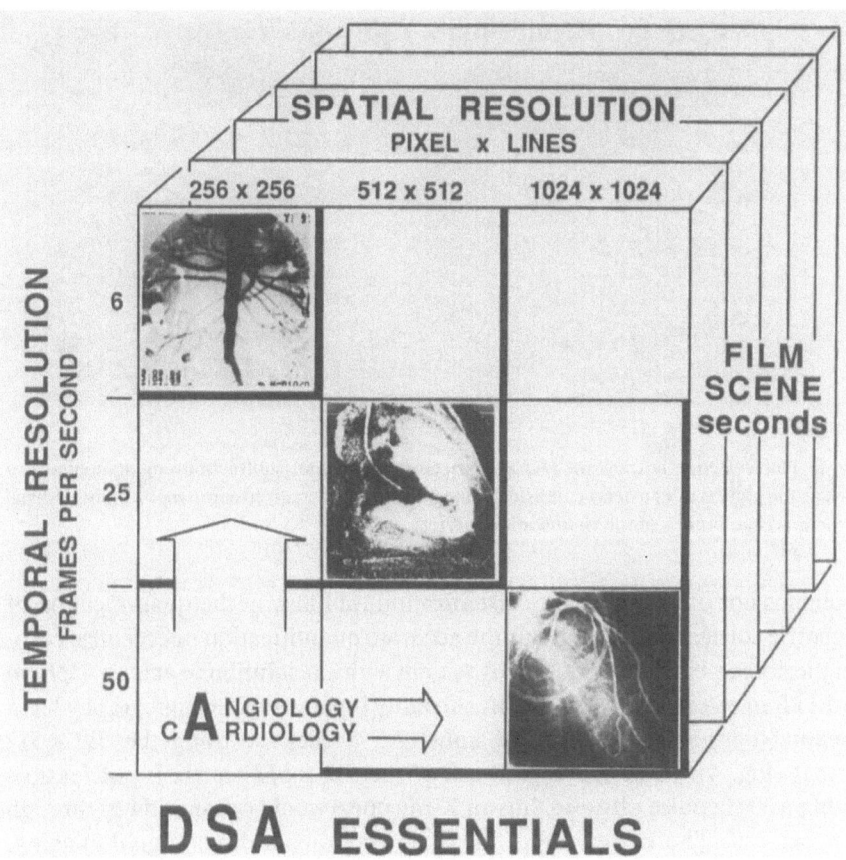

Fig. 2. Peripheral arteriography, left ventriculography and coronary angiography require different standards in spatial and temporal resolution. The requirement are highest for the visualization of the coronary arteries as a small and rapidly moving target.

This latter modality provides, however, a visualization of only the proximal segments of coronary arteries and coronary bypass grafts. Non-selective digital coronary angiograms of good quality can be obtained by chance only in patients with bradycardia, poor ventricular contraction, and coronary arteries with large diameters and without tortuosity or overlap (Fig. 3).

Nevertheless, digital aortic root coronary angiograms do not need to offer an equal image quality like selective coronary cine angiograms, if they provide the essential therapeutic information with more convenience for both the patient and the physician. Aortic root coronary angiography has to be considered as a prerequisite to accept degradation of image quality with the digital disc as the primary storage medium.

Today, limitations of digital imaging in coronary arteriography result in

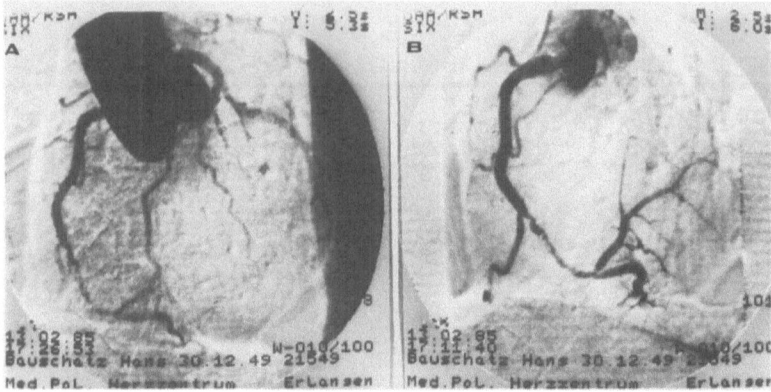

Fig. 3. Non-selective aortic root (A) and selective (B) digital subtraction angiographies in a 35-year-old patient after a heart contusion demonstrating a recanalized coronary thrombosis distal to the marginal branch of the right coronary artery.

problems not only in coronary visualization, but also in the quantification of eccentric coronary stenoses. For the accurate quantification of eccentric coronary lesions, a biplane angiography system with a resolution of at least 4 lp/mm and 25 frames/sec is necessary. But currently biplane digital angiography has a maximal temporal resolution of only 12.5 frames/sec using the 512×512 format (Fig. 4). Progressive read-out of the 512×512 matrix is not feasible within a 50 Hz pulse rate and thus an X-ray pulse would occur midway through the read-out. Therefore, one of the major options of direct digital imaging, namely the quantification of eccentric coronary stenoses, is still beyond the standard offered by computerized quantification or a video-digitized cineframe. Nevertheless, biplane digital coronary angiography and left ventriculography represent remarkable steps forward. When we compare selective digital coronary angiograms to conventional cine angiograms taken simultaneously, a very high correlation can be demonstrated in the measured coronary diameters with a regression coefficient of 0.96 (Fig. 5).

A high correlation was also found, when left ventricular ejection fraction and volume were measured in conventional and digital angiograms recorded simultaneously (Table 1).

Computer image processing makes direct ventriculography safer by reducing the amount of contrast material to 10–15 ml for a single injection. This low-dose direct digital ventriculography reduces the contrast-induced risk and thus permits serial studies without exceeding the upper limit of the contrast amount. Furthermore, radiation exposure per digital study is below that of film-based ventriculography. Thus quantitative digital coronary arteriography and left ventriculography offer promise in the objective evaluation of phar-

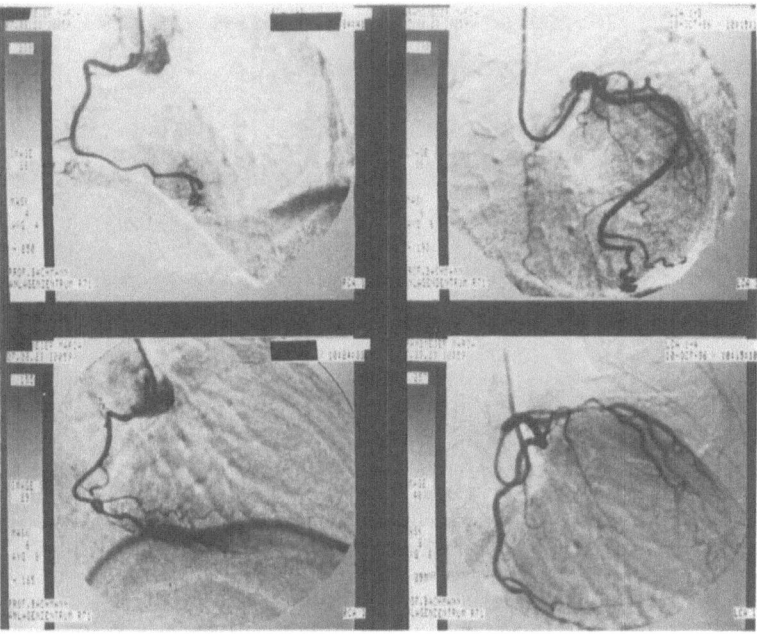

Fig. 4. Biplane selective digital subtraction coronary angiography in a 63-year-old woman with normal coronary anatomy. Digital imaging was carried out with the DIGITRON III (Siemens) using the 512 × 512 matrix and 12.5 frames/sec.

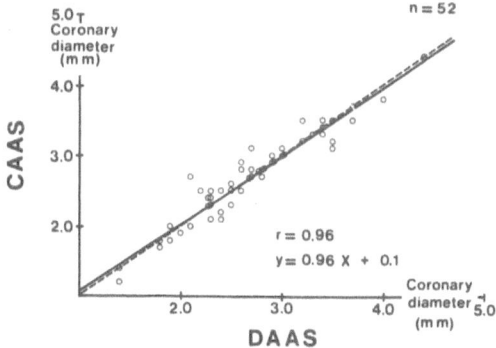

Fig. 5. Comparison of the coronary diameters measured by quantitative digital and cine coronary angiography. Quantitative studies were performed in 52 angiographically normal coronary segments from monoplane angiograms taken with 25 frames/sec simultaneously by digital and cine technique. Analyses were carried out with computer-based systems using full automated coronary contour detection in direct digital angiograms[1] and in optically magnified and video-digitized cineframes[2].

[1] Digital-Angiography-Analysis-System × DAAS using DIGITRON II with a 512 × 512 matrix (Siemens).

[2] Coronary-Angiography-Analysis-System × CAAS (Pie Data) [12, 32].

18

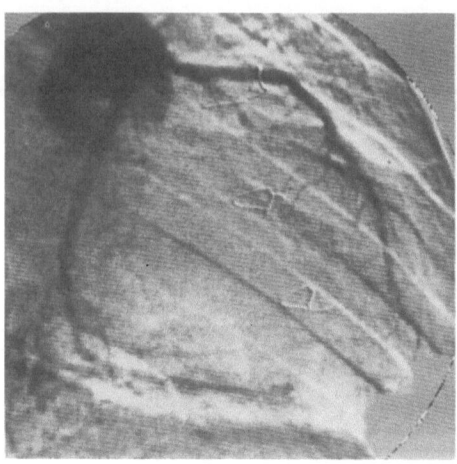

Fig. 6. Abnormal origin of the right coronary artery from the left anterior coronary sinus visualized by digital aortic root coronary angiography.

macological interventions (e.g. the assessment of coronary vasomotor tone) and left ventricular performance.

With the present state of technology non-selective digital coronary angiography can be recommended for diagnostic routine as an adjunct to conventional coronary angiography, and for identifying the origin of both abnormal coronary arteries and coronary bypass grafts (Fig. 6). Those who reduce the problem in symptomatic patients after coronary bypass surgery to the question of bypass patency may be satisfied with the digital contrast imaging in the proximal portion of a graft [2, 3, 6]. Non-selective digital angiography also facilitates the visualization of the internal mammary artery after implantation

Table 1. Comparison of quantitative digital and cine left ventriculography.[a]

	Digital	Cine	Correlation coefficient
EF (%)	78 ± 11	78 ± 11	0.99
EDV (ml)	141 ± 42	150 ± 42	0.94
ESV (ml)	33 ± 24	35 ± 24	0.98
SV (ml)	108 ± 29	116 ± 31	0.93

[a] Ejection fraction (EF), enddiastolic volume (EDV), endsystolic volume (ESV), stroke volume (SV).
Quantitative ventricular analyses were carried out with computer based calculating systems from user-defined ventricle contours. For the comparison temporal identical digital and cine monoplane ventriculograms were taken using the DIGITRON II (Siemens) with a 512 × 512 matrix and the AVD-system (Angiographic Ventricular Dynamics) (Siemens).

or transplantation for indirect or direct myocardial revascularization. Digital imaging techniques offer the option to perform transvenous left ventriculography as well as direct low-contrast ventriculography for the assessment of left ventricular pump function and mild mitral regurgitation due to papillary muscle insufficiency [25]. Moreover, selective digital coronary angiography has its place in daily routine in patients with marked overlap of the diaphragm or with obesity. In interventional cardiology selective digital coronary angiography offers a 'road-map' during percutaneous transluminal coronary angioplasty and has its place in coronary thrombolysis and recanalization [12, 14].

The combination of coronary cine and peripheral digital angiography allows the routine study of patients with multiple atherosclerotic disease [26–31]. Our own studies indicate an incidence of multiple atherosclerotic disease in 63.8% of patients who undergo coronary angiography [26, 28]. In this situation coronary cine angiography and digital ventriculography are followed by digital imaging of the extracranial arteries, the abdominal aorta, and the pelvic and femoral arteries in the same study [26–28]. In patients with arterial hypertension selective digital renal arteriography may be added easily. Thus 'total body angiography' [29] can be performed sequentially in a given patient without exceeding the upper limit of contrast material (Fig. 7). In the angiographic workup the radiologist may also take advantage of combined digital and cine angiography in patients with peripheral atherosclerotic lesions who may also have coronary heart disease. Furthermore, transbrachial angioplasty of peripheral or renal artery stenoses can be performed immediately after the diagnostic procedure using digital imaging as a 'road-map' and for assessing the results [27].

Summary

Digital imaging techniques have had a tremendous impact on clinical angiography and have converted conventional film-based non-cardiac angiography to digital arteriography. There is reason to believe that eventually digital electronic imaging will provide the same capabilities for cardiology.

Today, though, the coronary arteries still separate the analog from the digital world. When we overcome the technical limitations of spatial resolution and image storage, digital imaging will provide non-selective coronary arteriography by aortic root contrast injection.

Currently, we are using digital angiography primarily for the evaluation of bypass graft patency, for low-contrast direct ventriculography and for coronary 'road-mapping'. Furthermore, anomalies of the origin of coronary arteries are well documented by aortic root injection. In patients with multiple atherosclerotic disease, digital and conventional arteriography can be com-

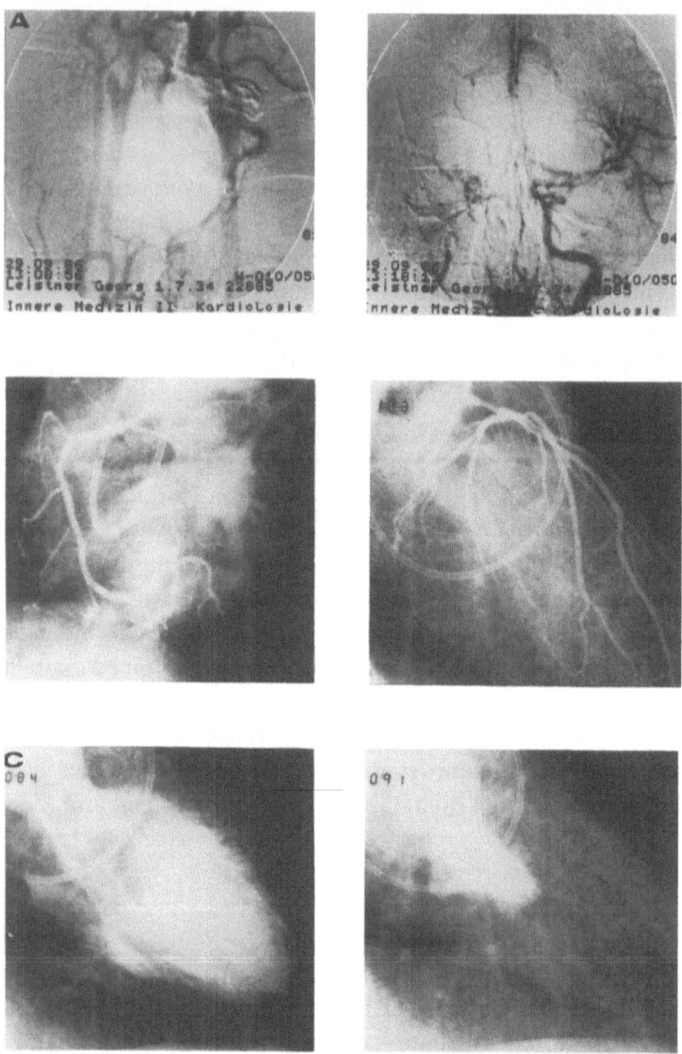

Fig. 7. 'Total body angiography' in a 52-year-old man with generalized atherosclerosis: angiographic workup was performed using conventional cardiac imaging (B, C) and digital imaging of the supra-aortic artery (A), abdominal aorta including proximal pelvic arteries and a femoro-femoral bypass (D), the femoral arteries and the trifurcation of the popliteal arteries (E, F). The angiographies demonstrate an occlusion of the right internal carotid artery with perfusion deficits of the right hemisphere (A), a moderate coronary main stem stenosis and wall irregularities of the right coronary artery (B), hypercontractility of the left ventricle (C), occlusion of the right common iliac artery with a femoro-femoral bypass (D) and a severe stenosis of the left superficial femoral artery (E). After the diagnostic procedure transbrachial dilatation of left femoral artery stenosis was performed and the primary success proven by a digital control angiography (E, F). (Total amount of contrast material 205 cc.)

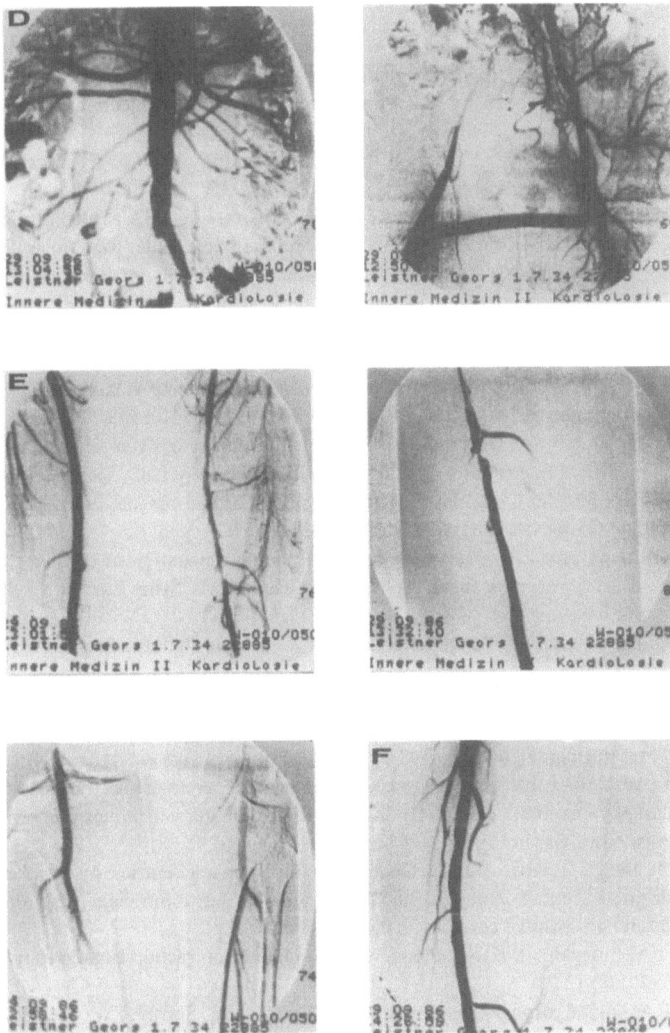

bined in a single study. It is likely that in the next decade, with the improvement in spatial resolution and storage capacity, non-selective digital subtraction angiography will gain widespread clinical use for the quantification of coronary anatomy, ventricular performance and myocardial perfusion. This progress in digital imaging will result in replacement of film-based angiography in cardiology.

References

1. Aldermann EL, Berte LE, Harrison DC et al.: Quantitation of coronary artery dimensions using digital image processing. Soc Photo-Optical Instrum Engineers-Digital Radiography 1981; 314: 273.
2. Hayward R, Hunter GJS: Digital subtraction angiography in coronary artery bypass graft assessment: clinical applicability. Br Heart J 1985; 54: 357.
3. Hauenstein HK, Schlosser V, Roeren T et al.: Intraarterielle DSA zur Kontrolle aortocoronarer Gefässbrücken – eine Alternative zur Coronarangiographie. Radiologe 1985; 25: 247.
4. Heintzen PH, Brennecke R, Bürsch HJ: Digital cardiovascular radiology. In: Hohne KH (ed.) Digital image processing in medicine; p 1. Springer, New York, 1981.
5. Heintzen PH, Brennecke R: Digital imaging in cardiovascular radiology. Georg Thieme, Stuttgart, 1983.
6. Heuser L, Krestin GP, Hannekum H, Wimmer G: Darstellung aortokoronarer Venenbrücken mit der digitalen Subtraktionsangiographie. DMW 1985; 110: 243.
7. Higgins CB, Norris SL, Gerber KH et al.: Quantitation of left ventricular dimensions and function by digital video subtraction angiography. Radiology 1982; 144: 461.
8. Mancini GBJ, Higgins ChB, Norris SL, Slutsky RA: Cardiac imaging with digital subtraction angiography. Cardiovasc Intervent Radiol 1983; 6: 252.
9. Rafflenbeul W, Heim R, Dzuiba B et al.: Morphometric analysis of coronary arteries. In: Lichten PR (ed.) Coronary angiography and angina pectoris. Symp Eur Soc Card; p 2. Georg Thieme, Stuttgart, 1976.
10. Ratib O, Rutishauser W: Recent developments of cardiac digital radiography. Int J Cardiac Imag 1985; 1: 29.
11. Selzer RH: Atherosclerosis quantification by computer image analysis. In: Bond (ed.) Conf on clinical diagnosis of atherosclerosis. Quantification methods of evaluation, p 43. Springer, Heidelberg/Stuttgart/New York, 1983.
12. Serruys PW, Reiber JHC, Wijns W et al.: Assessment of percutaneous transluminal coronary angioplasty by quantitative coronary angiography: Diameter versus densitometric area measurements. Am J Cardiol 1984; 54: 482.
13. Spiller P, Jehle J, Lauber A et al.: Digital imaging of the left ventricle by peripheral contrast injections-detection of impaired global and regional left ventricular function. Int symp advances in non-invasive cardiology, Aachen, 1982.
14. Turski PA, Stieghorst MF, Strother CM et al.: Digital subtraction angiography 'road map'. AJR 1982; 139: 1233.
15. Vogel RA: Digital coronary arteriography. In: Reiber JHC, Serruys PW (eds.) State of the art in quantitative coronary arteriography. Martin Nijhoff, Boston, 1986.
16. Whiting JS, Pfaff IM, Vas R et al.: Digital angiography in the assessment of coronary artery disease. In: Pohost GM, Higgins CB (eds.) New concepts in cardiac imaging; p 212. UCLA, Los Angeles, 1985.
17. Henry WL, Tobis J: The future of computerized cardiac angiography. Am J Cardiol 1984; 53: 1722.
18. Tobis J, Nacioglu O, Iseri L et al.: Detection and quantitation of coronary artery stenosis from digital subtraction angiograms compared with 35-millimeter film cineangiograms. Am J Cardiol 1984; 54: 489.
19. Sones FM, Shirey EK: Cine coronary arteriography. Mod Conc Cardiovasc Dis 1962; 31: 735.
20. Hessel SJ, Levy JM, Crowe JK et al.: Current experience with digital subtraction angiography in the community medical center. Cardiovasc Intervent Radiol 1983; 6: 280.
21. Mistretta CA, Crummy AB: Basic concepts of digital angiography. Progr Cardiovasc Dis 1986; 28: 245.

22. Bellmann S et al.: Coronary arteriography. I. Differential opacification of the aortic stream by catheters of special design. N Engl J Med 1960; 262: 325.

23. Nordenström B: Contrast examination of the cardiovascular system during increased intrabronchial pressure. Acta Radiol 1960; Suppl 200.

24. Paulin S: Non-selective coronary arteriography. Semin Roentgenol 1972; 7: 369.

25. Vas R, Diamond GA, Forrester JS et al.: Computer enhancement of direct and venous-injected left ventricular contrast angiography. Am Heart J 1981; 102: 119.

26. Bachmann K: Total cineangiography. In: Lichtlen PR (ed.) Coronary angiography and angina pectoris. Symp Eur Soc Card. Georg Thieme, Stuttgart, 1976.

27. Bachmann K, Raab G, Niederer W: Coronary angiography in combination with opacification of other arteries and simultaneous transbrachial dilatation of peripheral and abdominal arteries. In: Kaltenbach M et al. (eds.) Transluminal coronary angioplasty and intracoronary thrombolysis; p 144. Springer, Berlin/Heidelberg 1982.

28. Bachmann K, Bethge HD, Marhoff P: Combined cardiac cineangiography and peripheral digital subtraction angiography. In: Meyer J, Schweitzer P, Erbel R (eds.) Advances in non-invasive cardiology. Martinus Nijhoff, Boston, 1983.

29. Grinfeld LR, De la Fuente LM, Shinji K et al.: Total body angiography in patients with diffuse atherosclerosis (Abstract). Am J Cardiol 1974; 33: 141.

30. Kaufman STL, Chang R, Kadir S et al.: Intraarterial digial subtraction angiography: A comparative view. Cardiovasc Intervent Radiol 1983; 6: 271.

31. Myerowitz PD, Turnipseed WD, Swanson K et al.: Digital subtraction angiography as a method of screening for coronary artery disease during peripheral vascular angiography. Surgery 1982; 69: 1042.

32. Reiber JHC, Booman F, Tan HS et al.: Computer processing of coronary occlusions from X-ray arteriograms. INSERM 1979; 88: 79.

3. Digital Coronary Arteriography in the Outpatient Clinic

HIROYUKI ABE & KAZUHISA HIMI
Division of Cardiovascular Diagnostic and Interventional Medicine, Faculty of Medicine, Nihon University, Tokyo, Japan

Introduction

Left heart catheterization and coronary arteriography are generally performed on patients who have been admitted in the hospital because the procedure is thought to be accompanied with some risk and to necessitate rest of more than several hours.

Recently, we have employed the percutaneous left brachial approach for selective coronary arteriography using 5F sheath and 5F high-flow preformed catheters. As a recording system of the coronary arteriograms, we proposed to use a digital system and compared the diagnostic quality with the conventional cine film recording. This method permits us to study the coronary patients in an outpatient clinic and allows us to give reports to the patients shortly after the study.

Materials and methods

Patient selection for outpatient coronary arteriography is of prime importance to have a successful study and to avoid serious complications. The following criteria are applied in the selection of the patients:
1. patients with stable angina,
2. asymptomatic patients with ECG abnormalities, and
3. follow-up studies after coronary artery bypass graft (CABG) or percutaneous transluminal coronary angioplasty (PTCA).
These three best fit the outpatient clinic study.

At present, an age limitation is set at 60 years. The patients with unstable angina and suspected main left coronary artery disease are recommended to have the procedure as an in-hospital study.

Following is the proposed selective coronary arteriographic technique. Currently, the left brachial approach using a 5F sheath and 5F preformed catheters

P.H. Heintzen and J.H. Bürsch (eds), Progress in Digital Angiocardiography. ISBN 978-94-010-7093-5

is most often employed, although in some patients such as small-sized women the femoral approach is occasionally required.

In Table 1, the seven steps for the outpatient coronary arteriography technique are shown. After left arm preparation, the brachial artery is punctured with a 22 gauge needle in a routine fashion in order to insert a 5F sheath. The sheath should be fixed by a sterilized patch to prevent untoward movements during catheter manipulation. Then, 2500 units of heparin are given through the side arm of the sheath. Preformed catheters are now introduced through the hemostat valve using a guide wire. A 5F pigtail catheter is first introduced to measure aortic and ventricular pressures as well as to obtain left ventriculograms. Then, preformed (Judkins or Amplatz type) catheters are introduced for selective coronary arteriography. Non-ionic contrast media are recommended to visualize the coronary arterial tree. The contrast material is not diluted and arteriograms are recorded on a digital system. After the procedure, hemostasis is accomplished by applying digital compression for about fifteen minutes. Protamin is not required to reverse the effect of heparin. The patient is then instructed to keep his arm straight for the next four hours, and is allowed to return home (Fig. 1).

The DSA system and digital recording techniques are summarized in Fig. 2. Digiformer DFP-50A (Toshiba) is the system used in this study. For ECG gated or non-gated coronary arteriography, a 10 msec width cine pulse is applied and images are processed at a maximum rate of 7.5 f/s on progressive mode in 1024×1024 matrix. On the other hand, ECG gated or non-gated left ventriculography is performed on cine pulse exposure or TID mode at a maximum rate of 30 f/s on progressive or interlace mode, and processed on 512×512 matrix. On a practical point, coronary arteriograms are also obtained in the same manner as left ventriculograms with or without ECG gating. These images are displayed on a high resolution CRT with 1024×1024 matrix. Then, the final images selected by physicians are filmed by a high resolution multi-imager.

Table 1. Seven steps of outpatient clinic coronary arteriography technique.

---

1. Skin prep. in the left or right antecubital area or groin.
2. Puncture of the brachial or femoral arteries.
3. Insertion of the 5F sheath with hemostat valve.
4. Intra-arterial heparin 2500 U.
5. Insertion of the 5F catheter using guidewire.
6. Coronary arteriography using non-ionic contrast media.
7. Hemostasis.

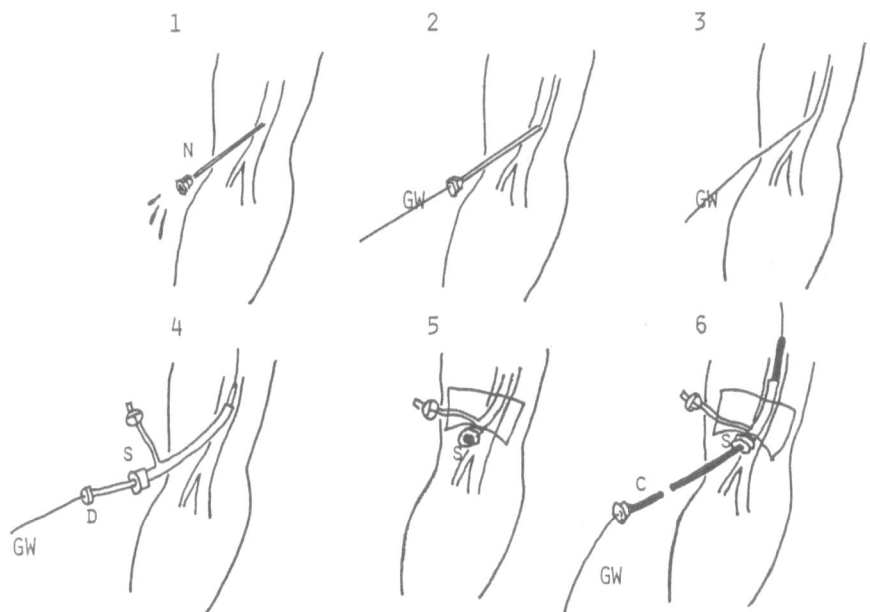

Fig. 1. Technique for brachial artery puncture and catheter insertion. N, puncture needle; GW, guidewire; S, sheath (5F); D, dilator; C, angiographic catheter (5F).

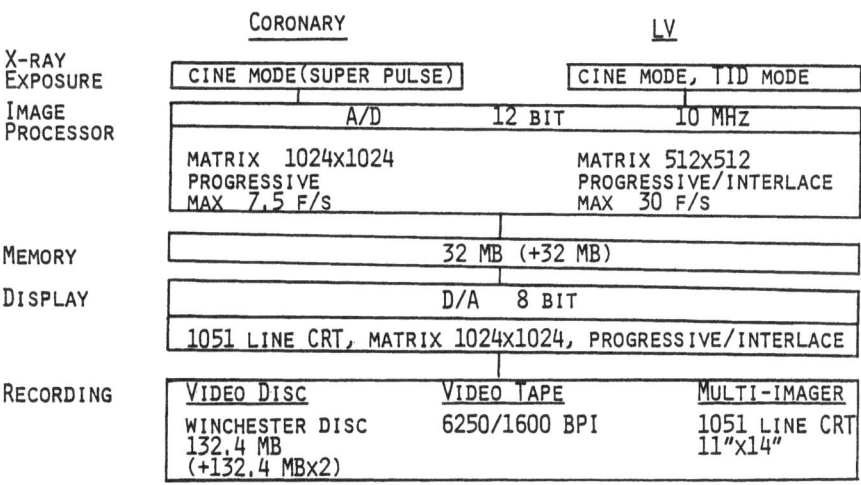

	CORONARY		LV
X-RAY EXPOSURE	CINE MODE(SUPER PULSE)		CINE MODE, TID MODE
IMAGE PROCESSOR	A/D	12 BIT	10 MHZ
	MATRIX 1024x1024 PROGRESSIVE MAX 7.5 F/S		MATRIX 512x512 PROGRESSIVE/INTERLACE MAX 30 F/S
MEMORY	32 MB (+32 MB)		
DISPLAY	D/A 8 BIT		
	1051 LINE CRT, MATRIX 1024x1024, PROGRESSIVE/INTERLACE		
RECORDING	VIDEO DISC	VIDEO TAPE	MULTI-IMAGER
	WINCHESTER DISC 132.4 MB (+132.4 MBx2)	6250/1600 BPI	1051 LINE CRT 11"x14"

Fig. 2. Digital fluorography system and recording technique. 'Super pulse' indicates a high-frequency exposure of X-ray pulse of 10 msec width.

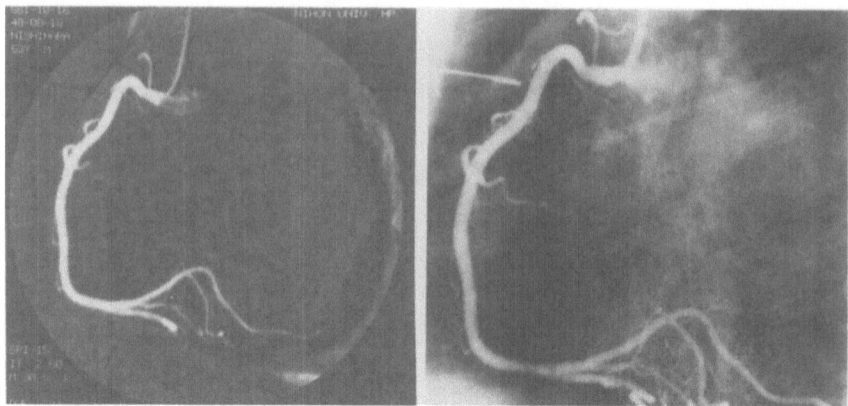

Fig. 3. Right coronary arteriograms obtained in LAO projection. Left: a non-ECG gated digital image on 512 × 512 matrix. Right: a conventional cine film image.

Results

For the first series of fifty cases of outpatient clinic coronary arteriography, all had diagnostic studies without major complications. Subcutaneous hematoma of moderate degree was experienced in only two cases. The coronary images obtained on 512 × 512 matrix without ECG gating are found to be as good quality as conventional cine arteriograms. Figure 3 is a good example of the comparison in the right coronary artery between digital and cine film recording. The digital left coronary arteriogram shown in Fig. 4 demonstrates an equivalent finding for clinical judgement (subtotal occlusion of the left ante-

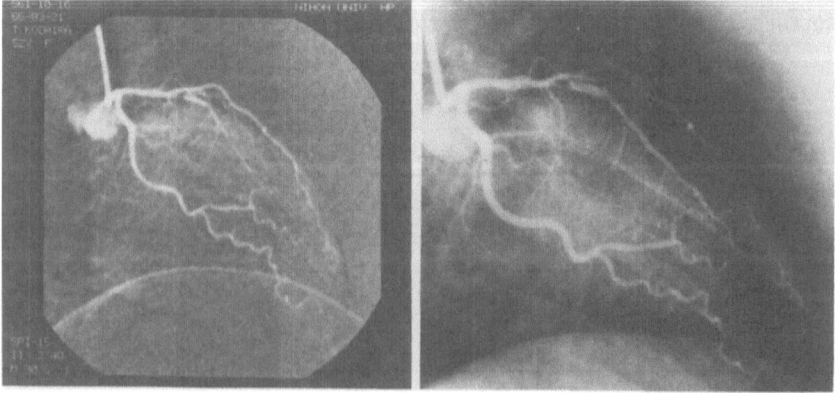

Fig. 4. Left coronary arteriograms obtained in RAO projection. Left: a digital image. Right: a conventional cine film image.

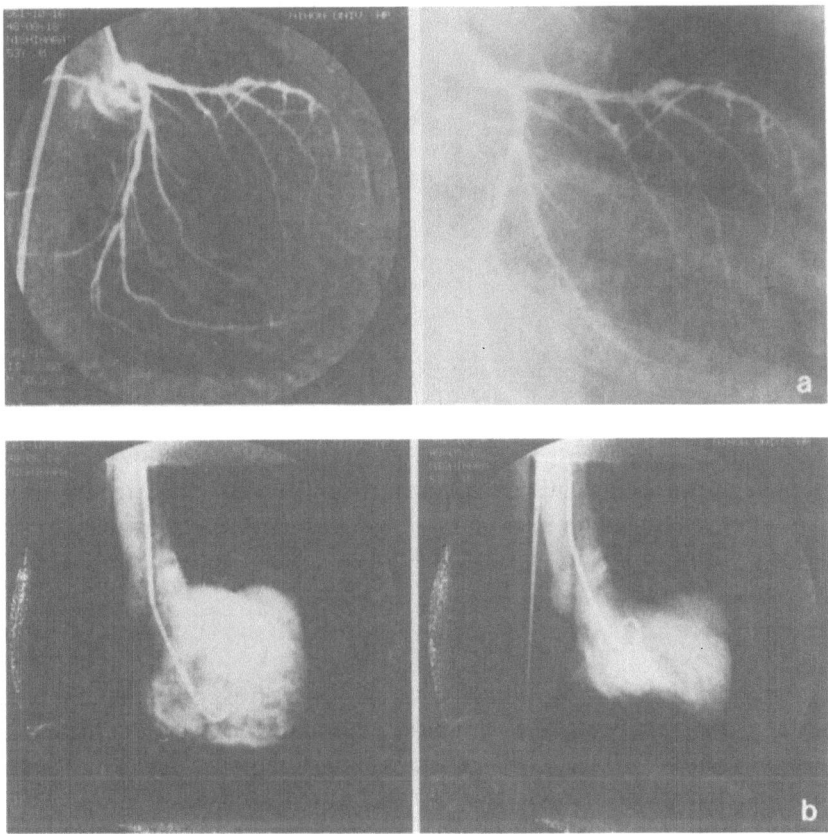

Fig. 5. A: left coronary arteriograms obtained in RAO and hepato-clavicular angled view (femoral approach). Left: a digital image. Right: a conventional cine film image. Note, better deliniation of the LAD and the circumflex system in the digital image. B: digital left ventriculograms in RAO projection (15 f/s). Left: end-diastole. Right: end-systole.

rior descending; LAD), compared to the cine film image. In the digital image, the superimposed hemi-diaphragm does not interfere with the image of the coronary artery. Fig. 5A is another example demonstrating the efficacy of digital coronary arteriography. This is a hepato-clavicular angled view of the patient who underwent left ventricular aneurysmectomy. His digital arteriogram shows a narrowed proximal LAD and surgically amputated distal LAD. The circumflex artery is better deliniated than in the conventional cine arteriogram. His left ventriculograms in end-diastole and end-systole show deformity of the cavity and a non-contractile segment as well. This is 15 f/s and 512×512 matrix image (Fig. 5B).

These examples suggest that 512×512 matrix coronary arteriograms offer

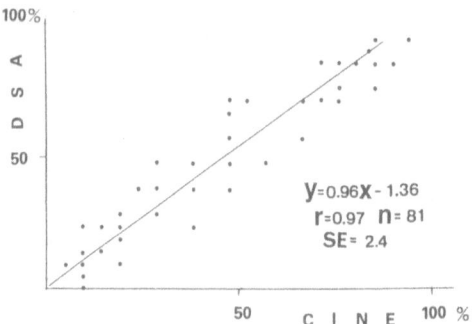

100%

y=0.96X - 1.36
r=0.97 n= 81
SE= 2.4

50   C I N E   100 %

Fig. 6. Comarison of per cent diameter stenosis in the coronary arteries between digital images (DSA) and conventional cine film images (CINE).

pertinent information useful in clinical practice. In eighty-one coronary artery lesions, per cent diameter stenosis on digital images (DSA) was compared to that on conventional cine films (CINE). An excellent correlation was found between the two (Fig. 6):

$$Y = 0.96X - 1.36 \; (r = 0.97).$$

If coronary arteriograms are obtained with ECG gated exposure and displayed on 1024×1024 matrix, it seems to improve the anatomical detail by increasing spatial resolution. However, it is known that images on 512×512 matrix provide sufficient information to make a clinical judgement.

Discussion

Performing coronary arteriography as an outpatient procedure provides the patients benefits and also improves the cost-effectiveness of the cardiac catheterization laboratory. We have realistically approached this goal with a combination of the percutaneous technique using smaller catheters and the digital recording system.

The method described here is one of the practical ways of improving coronary arteriography. Recent progress in catheter technology permits us to use smaller catheters which provide high flow rates. Because of this, the puncture at the catheter insertion site is smaller and no blood flow obstruction occurs in the punctured artery during the study. And hemostasis is easier after catheter and sheath removal. We are using 5F sheat for catheter entry rather than 5.5F sheath [1]. The incidence of complications of this technique is quite low. Especially, the left brachial approach is anatomically feasible for smaller catheter manipulation. 5F high flow catheters have a large enough lumen for contrast delivery into the coronary artery or the left ventricle. Supposing that digital coronary arteriograms on a 512 × 512 matrix provide sufficient clinical information, the conventional cine film may be eliminated as a recording media.

As far as frame rate is concerned, it is known that 16 f/s is highly reproducible with 96% accuracy in the left ventricular volume curve. This is based on the study of sampling theory. Therefore, we believe that frame rates of 15 f/s for left ventriculogram and 7.5 f/s for coronary arteriogram are feasible in clinical use [2]. By digital image, the bones and a diaphragm which superimpose with the coronary artery may be subtracted and improve diagnostic accuracy. Furthermore, quantitation of coronary stenosis may become easy and reproducible by the videodensitometric technique [3, 4]. Assessment of myocardial perfusion [5] is one of the advantages of selective coronary arteriography.

In conclusion, outpatient digital coronary arteriography using 5F catheters would provide a new method of visualizing and assessing coronary artery pathology.

Summary

Digital coronary arteriography approached through the left brachial artery in the outpatient clinic may be performed effectively and safely. Stenoses in coronary arteries are well recognized and in excellent accordance with the findings in conventional cine coronary arteriography. And, it provides more accurate assessment of coronary lesions or myocardial perfusion by applying a videodensitometric technique. Finally, the technique described above offers a less invasive and more economical alternative to the conventional Sones or Judkin's methods.

References

1. Eugster GS et al.: Percutaneous left brachial catheterization using 5-French preformed (Judkin's) catheters. Catheterization Cardiovasc Diagnosis 1986; 12: 274–276.
2. Abe H: Image diagnosis in ischemic heart disease: cine angiography vs digital radiography. Eizo-joho (medical) 1985; 17 (1): 28–35.
3. Abe H et al.: Coronary flow analysis by digital technique. Gazo-shindan 1986; 6 (8): 803–808.
4. Brown BG et al.: Quantitative coronary arteriography: Estimation of dimensions, hemodynamic resistance, and atheroma mass of coronary artery lesions using the arteriogram and digital computation. Circulation 1977; 55: 329–337.
5. Vogel RA et al.: Visualization of myocardial perfusion using application of digital radiographic technique to selective coronary arteriography. Am J Cardiol 1982; 49: 935.

4. Digital Subtraction Angiography, the New Standard in Pediatric Cardiology?

HARVEY L. CHERNOFF
Pediatric Cardiac Catheterization Laboratory, Boston Floating Hospital for Infants and Children, New England Medical Center, Boston, and Department of Pediatrics, Tufts University School of Medicine, Boston, MA, USA

Radiographic cardiac imaging with contrast medium is one of the oldest and most accurate methods for diagnosing cardiac anatomic malformations. The techniques used have been governed by the level of X-ray exposure and the dose of contrast medium required. This for many years limited the use of this modality in infants and small children. As surgeons became more expert in correcting defects the requirement for accurate preoperative diagnosis became increasingly important. For this reason imaging has been a modality that is directed primarily to surgical intervention. This is understandable since the detailed delineation of anatomy is essential to the surgery.

In the 1950s the use of image intensification systems came increasingly into use allowing imaging of the heart in motion. This was a great advance over the then standard angiographic techniques which at best were limited to 12 frames per second.

The next major step occurred with the availability of biplane units which allowed cineangiographic imaging in two planes 'simultaneously'. This reduced both the amount of contrast medium used and reduced the duration of a catheterization. This remained the state of the art until the late 1970s when equipment allowing compound angulated views in two planes was developed. The next major advance was the ability to perform compound angulated images isocentrically or non-isocentrically. In the 1980s motion digital subtraction angiography (DSA) became available.

The clarity of the images in cineangiography and DSA is determined by a number of factors. The imaging chain must be in good working order. The X-ray exposure must be adequate to excite the input phosphor of the image intensifying tube; the camera and lens system must collect the data without undue interference from scatter radiation. The duration of the X-ray exposure is important since a prolonged exposure does not 'stop motion' and may cause blurring of the image. This need has resulted in the use of pulsed exposures rather than continuous fluoroscopic exposure. In cineangiography film with optimal grain-to-contrast is used to ensure adequate detail of the stored

P.H. Heintzen and J.H. Bürsch (eds), Progress in Digital Angiocardiography. ISBN 978-94-010-7093-5

images. With DSA the recording medium is the computer. It must have a matrix sufficient to store the very large amount of digital data needed to produce detailed images.

DSA imaging is presently in the same relation to cineangiography as was cineangiography to cut-film angiography in the 1950s. Now, as ocurred in the 1950s, many angiographers fear that with the new technique it may not be possible to obtain the details necessary to surgeons to confidently embark on surgery. Now, as with the change from cut film to cineangiograms, I find that surgeons confidently embark on surgery in patients who have undergone studies in the new modality, DSA. Their concern now, as it was then, is delineation of the anatomy, not the imaging technique.

Many angiographers complain that the medium is cumbersome to process. Both angiographers and surgeons complain that viewing requires special equipment which makes reviewing difficult, and also makes it dificult to send studies to colleagues since facilities for viewing these studie are not standardized.

Some of the complaints are valid. The lack of standardized post-study reviewing techniques can limit the locations even within the same institution. When portable viewing equipment is available it is not as compact and easily moved as the currently available 35 mm film projectors. This complaint is reminiscent of the difficulties in the early days of cineangiography before 35 mm film had been adopted as the standard and studies were being done using 16, 35 and 70 mm film.

The complaint about processing is one based for the most part on lack of experience with DSA and should be easily surmountable. The majority of DSA studies for diagnosis of congenital defects can be prepared for viewing during the catheterization by technicians who have been trained in processing digital subtraction angiograms. Those situations in which DSA processing requires physician time to delineate not easily discernible anatomic details is well worth that effort. It will often eliminate the need inherent in standard angiography for making further injections to clarify the anatomy, and does not add, overall, to the time of a study.

In our catheterization laboratory we employ a biplane unit which allows use of compound angulated views in both planes either isocentrically or non-isocentrically (Coronix III using Philips electronics and image intensifiers). The DSA unit is an add-on and uses a dedicated television camera (Fischer Digital Imaging System, DA 100).

DSA is used in the same role as standard cineangiography. Injections are made selectively. We early abandoned fluorographic imaging in favor of pulsed half-msec exposures. At the same time the matrix size was increased from 256×256 to 512×512. There was concern initially that the limitation of 30 frames per second acquisition with DSA would impose a problem since with

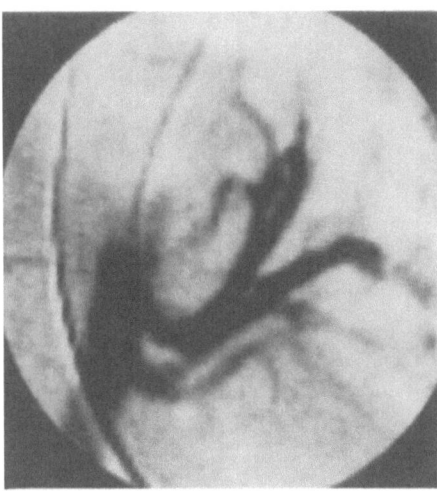

Fig. 1. Single frame from a postero-anterior DSA study acquired at 30 frames per second showing the catheter tip at the orifices of opacified arteries supplying a pulmonary sequestration in a 1.5 kg infant. Contrast medium injected 0.75 ml Renografin 60.

standard pediatric cineangiography about 60 frames per second has been found necessary to ensure capture of the needed information. We found, however, that with DSA image processing, 30 frames per second does not result in loss of information.

Unmasked images are collected in digital mode. This allows tailoring of masks to enhance different segments of a run. In addition, availability of the unmasked images aids in locating the areas of interest in relation to other anatomic landmarks which at times may be helpful, especially in interventional procedures.

Radiation exposure can be reduced significantly using DSA. By slowing the frame rate from 60 to 30 frames per second, there is an immediate 50% savings in the radiation dose. Furthermore, with DSA, good images can be obtained using 60% of the radiation dose required for filming. This represents, overall, about a four-fold reduction in the exposure dose when compared with cineangiography.

The volume of contrast medium for most selective cineangiographic studies is 1.0 ml/kg/injection. Using DSA the volume of contrast medium can usually be reduced by 50%. It is still necessary to increase the volume and injection pressure for the same situations in which increases are needed when performing standard cineangiography.

In our laboratory even those who prefer to use cineangiography recognize the advantages of being able to process images. We now routinely simultaneously record television images when cineangiograms are done. These video

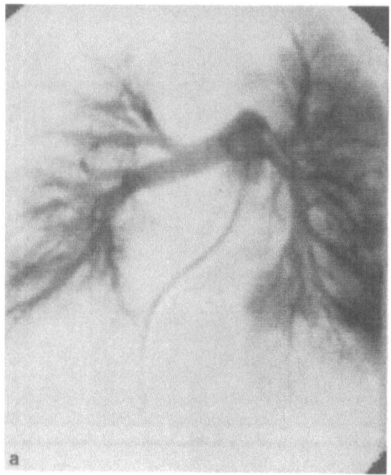 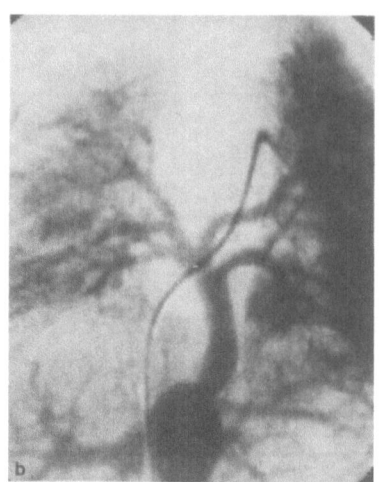

Fig. 2. Two single frames from a DSA postero-anterior view acquired at 30 frames per second showing the catheter tip in the left pulmonary artery of a 2.9 kg infant. Contrast medium injected 5.0 ml Renografin 60. A: selective injection into the pulmonary artery. B: levophase showing infradiaphragmatic anomalous pulmonary venous return.

images can be acquired on the digital unit for processing. The images are not as clear as those acquired using the digital system as the primary recording modality. Nevertheless, they can be processed on the DSA unit with delineation of information that may not be evident in the cineangiograms. This additional information may preclude the need for further cineangiographic views.

Certainly, for anatomic delineation of congenital heart defects DSA is at least as good and usually superior to standard cineangiography. As of the time of these deliberations biplane motion DSA is becoming available. With this and the reduction in radiation and contrast medium doses DSA will have reached the stage of becoming the angiographic procedure of choice for imaging congenital heart defects.

Summary

Radiographic cardiac imaging with contrast medium and film, one of the oldest and most accurate methods for diagnosing cardiac anatomic malformations has progressed from cut-film imaging to biplane cineangiography. With the advent of digital subtraction angiography with units capable of high quality 30 frames per second motion imaging, this modality has reached the stage at which it can replace standard cineangiography.

Part II: Digital Ventriculography

i. Quantitation of Valvular Insufficiency
ii. Assessment of Cardiac Dynamics

5. Quantitation of Valvular Regurgitation by Digital Ventricular Angiocardiography

J.H. BÜRSCH, J. ZERBST & P.H. HEINTZEN

Department of Pediatric Cardiology and Biomedical Engineering, University of Kiel, Kiel, FRG

The development of digital angiocardiography has provided new diagnostic approaches to quantitatively assess hemodynamic parameters by radio-opaque contrast absorption measurements. Aside from the advent of new image processing capabilities, the technical characteristics of X-ray systems have been substantially improved with the generation of stabilized roentgen pulses and the linear transfer of roentgen absorption intensities by the image intensifier-television chain. Thus, it appears that digital angiography equipment now facilitates high quality densitometric measurements. On the other hand, roentgen densitometry has more than a 20-year history and numerous concepts have been developed and experimentally tested with analog densitometric equipment [1–7]. Among these, the assessment of valvular regurgitation proved to be of particular diagnostic value. The preferred method was to quantitate phasic variations (ejection and regurgitation) of the total amount of contrast medium in the ventricle by integral density measurements over the entire projection area of that chamber. Even though the feasibility and diagnostic significance were clearly demonstrated for aortic, pulmonic and mitral valve insufficiency [8–11], this technique was not generally accepted due to the inconvenience of handling the analog densitometer as well as technical variables difficult to control.

But currently available improvements have led to an increasing interest in applying these techniques. Consequently, approved principles have been reappraised and in addition, specific advantages of the digital imaging mode have been considered for densitometric analysis [12, 13].

This paper describes our preliminary experience with digital densitometry primarily for valvular regurgitant fraction measurements. Basically, the severity of valvular insufficiency was estimated by measuring the regurgitant amount of contrast medium as a fraction of the amount of ventricular ejection after selective contrast injections into either the left or the right ventricle.

P.H. Heintzen and J.H. Bürsch (eds), Progress in Digital Angiocardiography. ISBN 978-94-010-7093-5
© 1988, Kluwer Academic Publishers, Dordrecht

Densitometric principle

Roentgen densitometry has been developed to obtain objective measurements of the transport of roentgen contrast media in the circulatory system. This technique measures the brightness at selected sites in angiographic images. Regional brightness levels are approximately proportional to roentgen intensities of the image intensifier input screen. A more complex relationship exists between the radiation intensities and the mass of material transradiated and assuming monochromatic radiation, roentgen attenuation relates exponentially to the absorbent mass. If two measurements are performed, namely, without and with contrast medium, the ratio of intensities (I_1/I_2) is related exponentially to the amount of contrast medium (M):

$$I_1/I_2 \sim e^M.$$

This relationship is theoretically valid for a single roentgen beam and practically applies to each individual picture element. Experimental data conformed to the theory even under non-ideal conditions using a narrowed roentgen spectrum for angiocardiography (filtering of radiation).

Densitometric analysis using an anatomically defined region of interest (ROI) requires two basic processes, namely, the logarithmic conversion of picture element data and the subsequent integration of the converted data of an ROI. Thus, a relative value for the total amount of medium is obtained from the difference of two measurements:

$$M \sim \Sigma(\log I_1 - \log I_2)\triangle a.$$

The indices indicate the two measured intensities (I) before and during contrast opacification. $\triangle a$ corresponds to the minute area of each picture element.

This principle has been applied to estimate the severity of valvular insufficiency by quantitating the change in amount of ventricular contrast medium during the systolic and diastolic phases. If a complete dilution curve is recorded, several cycles can be analyzed to compare regurgitant measurements.

An example is illustrated in Fig. 1 depicting two density curves as examples for competent and incompetent valve closure. Regurgitant fraction is calculated from the phasic variations of curve amplitudes in one or more cardiac cycles. Each diastolic deflection in relation to the preceding systolic deflection gives a direct measure of regurgitant fraction amount. Assuming homogeneous indicator mixing in the ejected blood volume this ratio reflects regurgitant fraction volume. In addition, the end-diastolic and end-systolic amplitudes may be used to determine the ratio of left ventricular volumes. Consequently, a single densogram facilitates both regurgitant fraction and ventricular ejection fraction measurements.

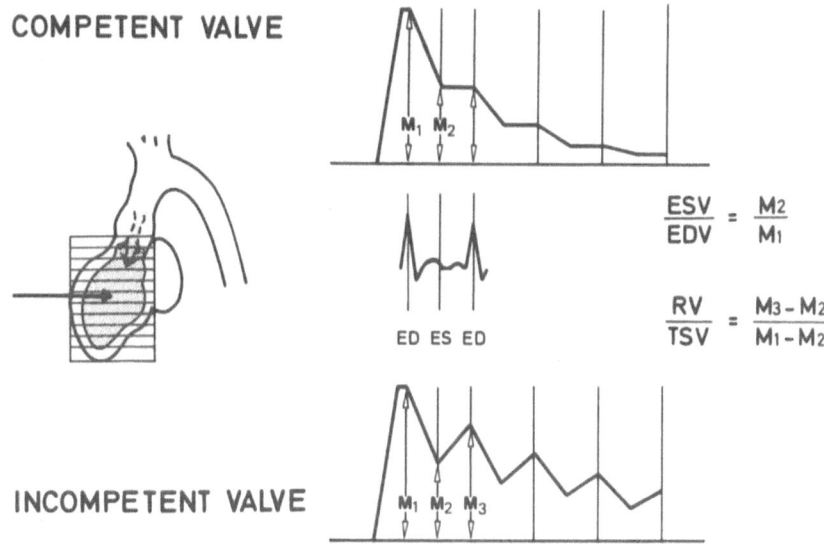

COMPETENT VALVE

$$\frac{ESV}{EDV} = \frac{M_2}{M_1}$$

$$\frac{RV}{TSV} = \frac{M_3 - M_2}{M_1 - M_2}$$

ED ES ED

INCOMPETENT VALVE

Fig. 1. Schematic drawing of ventricular radio-opaque dilution curves for illustration of the determination of residual fraction (ESV/EDV) and regurgitant fraction (RV/TSV). In the upper curve competent valve closure is assumed indicated by diastolic plateaus. The lower curve shows diastolic increases in ventricular contrast amounts due to aortic (pulmonic) valve insufficiency. ESV = end-systolic volume; EDV = end-diastolic volume; RV = regurgitant volume; TSV = total stroke volume; M = amplitudes of densogram proportional to the amount of contrast medium in the ventricle.

Image processing

Only recently DSA systems have become commercially available to obtain densitometric recordings from manually outlined regions of interest. The particular system used in our studies was specifically designed for the quantitative analysis of image series. The basic components are depicted in Fig. 2. Basically, video images were digitally acquired at a rate of 25/sec and stored on semiconductor memory with a capacity of up to 256 digitized images (256 × 256 picture elements per image, 8 bit resolution per picture element). Selection of single images for instant display on the video monitor was facilitated by positioning a potentiometer on the processor console. Likewise, a second image could be selected for real time subtraction providing DSA images for further densitometric analysis. Subtraction images were transferred to a separate contour processing device connected to a resistor foil for manual outlining of ROIs. Summated data of logarithmically converted densities were obtained and used as relative measures of the contrast amount within each ROI. The system was operated for DSA densitometry studies taking into account corresponding cardiac and respiratory phases. Our approach in those

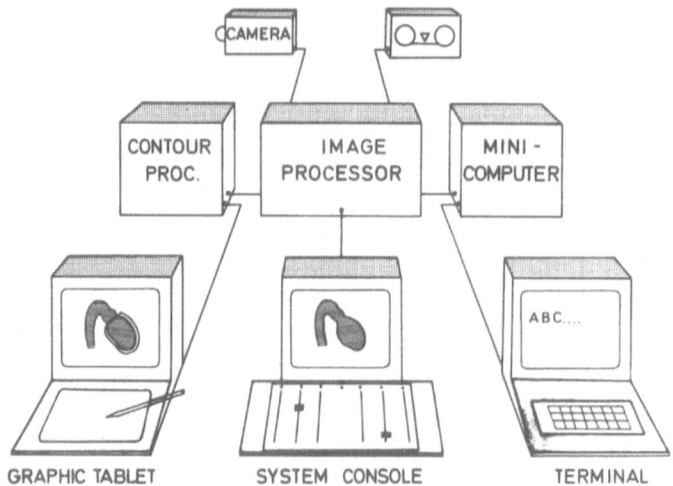

Fig. 2. Block diagram of the digital processing system for serial image sequence acquisition and processing. The central image processor is connected to a contouring device for outlining of regions of interest and summated density measurements. Another option is to feed selected images into a minicomputer for complex arithmetic calculations.

patients who were not cooperative was to accomplish regular respiration by sedation and to acquire images over the period of two respiratory cycles prior to the injection of contrast medium. Further analysis involved:

1. the selection of a specific contrast image followed by
2. the selection of an appropriate pre-injection image that produced minimal subtraction artefacts.

This technique proved to be most practical and reliable achieving correspondence of images from identical respiratory and cardiac phases for mask mode subtraction.

Densitometric methods

Aortic and pulmonary insufficiency

The following example is used to illustrate differences between densitometric analysis of the conventional non-subtracted angiogram and DSA images for comparison. Figure 3 depicts a left ventricular angiogram in the non-subtracted and in the mask subtraction mode. The ROI is outlined according to the end-diastolic cardiac phase. In each of the two images the contour defines the ventricular ROI for summated densitometric measurements. Figure 4

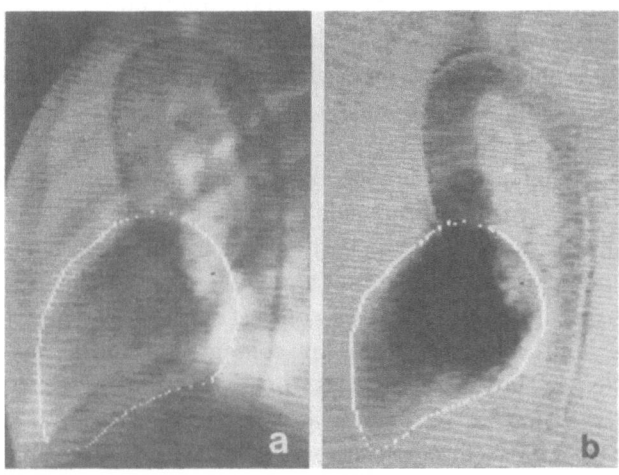

Fig. 3. Video monitor pictures from a patient study with left ventricular contrast injection (lateral projection) in the original (a) and the subtraction mode (b) for comparison. The brightened line encompasses the end-diastolic contour of the ventricle and defines the region of interest for integrated density measurements.

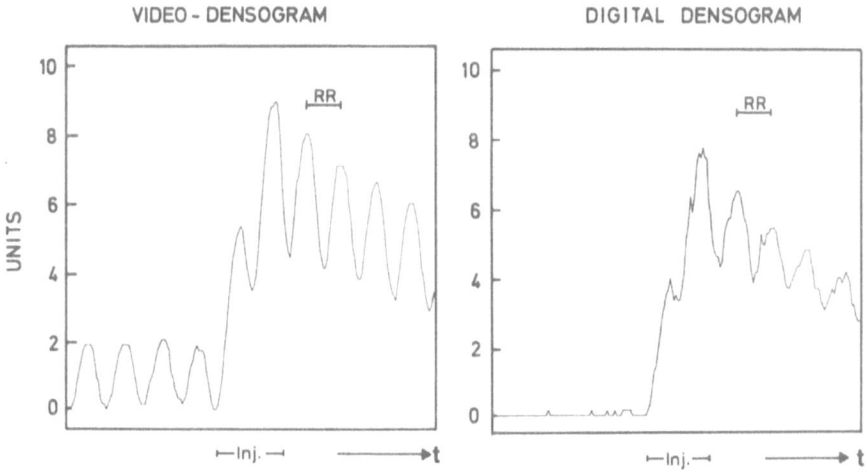

Fig. 4. Ventricular densograms from the patient study depicted in Fig. 3. The left densogram results from subsequent measurements of the original, non-subtracted video images. This record is affected by cyclic density variations superimposing with the specific signal of contrast absorption. The curve on the right was derived from density measurements in the subtraction images. Density variations relate to the pure contrast material. These amplitudes are proportional to ventricular contrast amounts. The washout part of the curve indicates significant diastolic regurgitation of contrast medium.

illustrates ventricular densograms by a frame-by-frame analysis using the end-diastolic ROI without any change in size and position of the densitometric sampling area. The resulting two ventricular densograms differ in shape with respect to phasic variations in non-contrast induced roentgen densities. Curve processing in the 'non-subtraction mode' yields cyclic variations, clearly visible in the pre-injection phase. On the contrary, densitometry of subtraction images reveals a zero line without density fluctuations. The latter curve is suitable to directly measure the regurgitant fraction of contrast medium from the washout phase of the densogram. Otherwise, in the non-subtraction mode these signals are superimposed by non-contrast density variations. The further processing of ventricular densograms that contain pure contrast information is depicted in Fig. 5. Three cardiac cycles from the washout of contrast medium are designated. These curve sections are analyzed by setting the maximum amplitude of each of the three cycles to a 100% value. Subsequently, the data from each of the individual cycles are plotted in relation to the end-diastolic peak amplitude. Superimposition of the normalized data indicates good consistency of the measurements (Fig. 6). It is apparent that not only valvular regurgitation but also ventricular ejection fraction may be estimated.

For simplicity the processing of only seven subtraction images was applied in our studies using four end-diastolic and three end-systolic contrast images. Thus, three values of regurgitant fraction as well as the ratio of end-systolic to end-diastolic volumes from a single angiographic study were obtained. These data were used to estimate the reliability of both the regurgitant fraction measurements and fractional volume determinations namely ESV/EDV.

Mitral insufficiency

A characteristic feature of image subtraction is the elimination of non-specific background densities. The resulting zero background ideally meets the requirements of integral density measurements, irrespective of the size and position of the ROI. Thus, variations in the shape of opacified cardiac structures can readily be accomplished by using adequately shaped ROIs of different size. This feature allows quantitation of mitral regurgitation in a fast and highly practical manner. Principally, the reflux of contrast medium is quantitated from an atrial ROI outlined to the end-diastolic and end-systolic silhouette of this chamber (Fig. 7). The difference in densitometric values from the onset to the end of systole is a relative measure of regurgitant blood volume. In order to calculate regurgitant fraction, a second measurement is performed using a differently shaped left ventricular ROI. The systolic ejection of ventricular contrast amount relates to the total stroke volume. In order to keep to the basic assumption of identical concentrations in both the ventricular total stroke volume and the regurgitant volume, measurements must be compared

DIGITAL DENSOGRAM

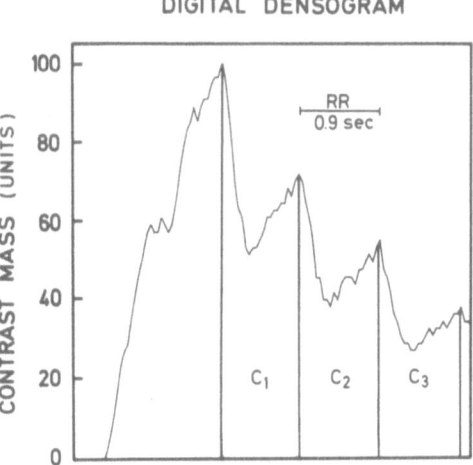

Fig. 5. DSA-densogram (Fig. 4, right) displayed for detailed ejection and regurgitation measurements. C_1, C_2 and C_3 indicate three consecutive cardic cycles to be analyzed.

SUPERPOSITION

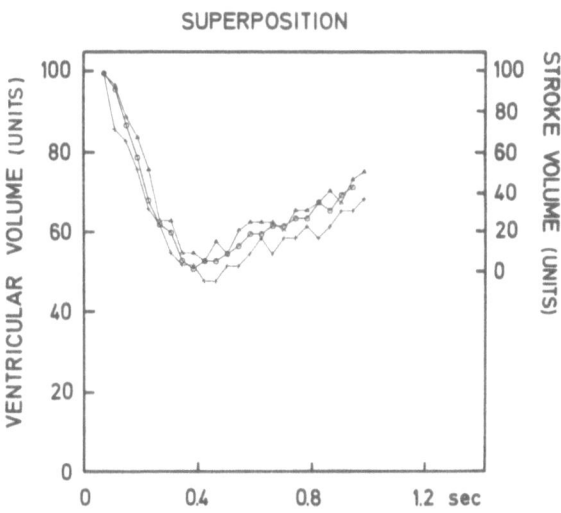

Fig. 6. Variations of densities (Fig. 5) of three cardiac cycles that are superimposed by setting the maximum deflections (end-diastolic amplitudes) of curve sections to a 100% value. The temporal course shows good agreement of normalized data from the three cycles. The scaling on the left axis indicates fractional ventricular volumes. The scale on the right indicates per cent stroke volume. The latter scaling is based on the minimum deflection of each curve to be set to zero.

46

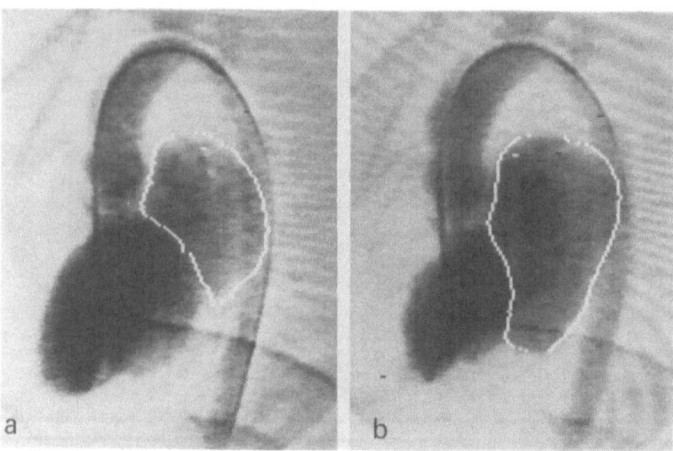

Fig. 7. Video monitor pictures in a patient with mitral regurgitation. The brightened contour indicates left atrial borders according to the ventricular end-diastolic (a) and end-systolic (b) phases.

from the one particular cardiac phase. It is important that the shape of the ROI can be modified easily to accurately outline the atrium, particularly in respect to the plane of the mitral valve (lateral or oblique roentgen projection). Nevertheless, inaccuracies may result from the inability to completely separate the left atrial chamber from the descending aorta if the atrium is signif-

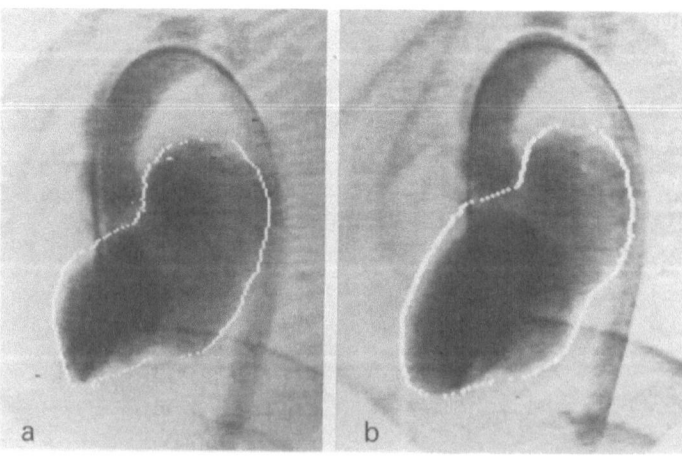

Fig. 8. Levogram in a patient with combined aortic and mitral valve insufficiency. Both left cardiac chambers, the ventricle and the atrium, are outlined to define a common region of interest in the end-systolic (a) and end-diastolic (b) phase. Thus, aortic regurgitation can be detected in spite of mitral valve incompetence.

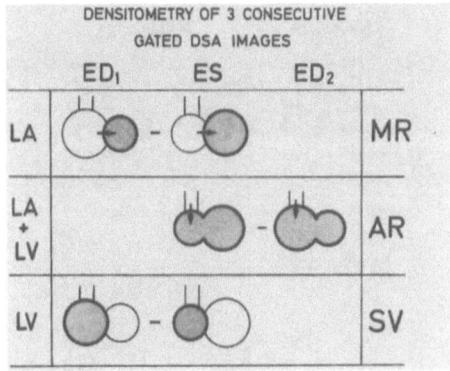

Fig. 9. Diagrammatic presentation of the regions of interest (gray shaded) for distinct analysis of mitral regurgitation (MR) and aortic regurgitation (AR) in combined valvular insufficiency. The phasic change in contrast amounts in each of the indicated chambers is related to the fractional change of ventricular amount and stroke volume (SV), respectively. LA = left atrium; LV = left ventricle; ED = end-diastole; ES = end-systole.

DENSITOMETRY DATA FROM

A SINGLE DSA STUDY

(MITRAL AND AORTIC INSUFFICIENCY)

| | CARDIAC CYCLES | | | |
	I	II	III	MEAN
MI RGF	60	50	55	55 %
AO RGF	8	9	16	11 %
LV EF	52	59	56	56 %

Fig. 10. Example of individual measurements in the patient with combined valvular insufficiency (Fig. 8).

icantly enlarged (Fig. 7). In cases with combined mitral and aortic regurgitation the latter can be separately measured using an ROI that encompasses both the left ventricle and the left atrium (Fig. 8). The increase of contrast amount from end-systole to the following end-diastole is a relative measure of aortic regurgitation. This value can be related to the amount ejected from the left ventricle in the preceding cardiac cycle in order to estimate aortic regurgitant fraction separately from mitral regurgitation. Figure 9 displays schematically the different ROIs according to the three different phases of one cardiac cycle for detailed analysis of combined mitral and aortic regurgitation. A numerical

48

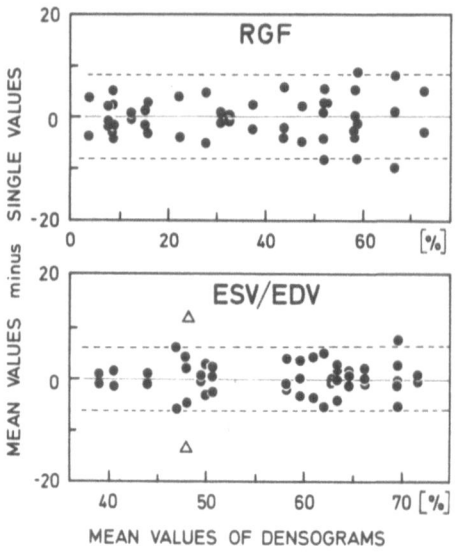

Fig. 11. Graphic representation of patient data for illustration of the reproducibility of individual densitometric measurements. The differences between single values and the mean in each angiographic study are plotted against the respective mean values of regurgitant fraction (RGF) and ventricular residual volume (ESV/EDV). The scatter range of 2 SD is delineated. The triangles (lower panel) have not been considered in this statistical analysis.

example from such a case is given in Fig. 10. It illustrates the reproducibility of regurgitant fraction data as well as ejection fraction values from three consecutive cardiac cycles.

Patient studies

Twenty children (1 month–16 years) with suspected aortic (n = 10) or pulmonary (n = 10) insufficiency were studied by DSA. Selective contrast injections of about 0.5 ml/kg body weight were made into either the left or the right ventricle. Ventriculograms were recorded in the lateral projection with a rate of 25 images/sec. Eight of the children were not able to willingly suspend respiration. In these children contrast injection was delayed for two respiratory cycles in order to select pre-injection images of any desired phase.

In the other patients (with suspended respiration) the contrast injection was delayed for only 2 seconds after onset of radiation. Subtraction images were processed according to the largest and the smallest size of the opacified chamber immediately following the termination of contrast injection. Thus, 2 or 3 consecutive cardiac cycles were analyzed for replicate determination of valvular regurgitation (RGF) and fractional volume changes of the ventricle (ESV/EDV). A representative value of fractional volumes was calculated as the mean of 3 values in each of the studies. Valvular regurgitation varied between 4 and 73% RGF. In order to estimate the reproducibility of the individual measurements the difference between single values and their respective mean RGF in each study was determined. Statistical analysis revealed adequate reproducibility of data with a standard deviation of ± 4.2% of RGF. Similarly, the fractional volume data resulted in a standard deviation of ± 3.1% of ESV/EDV (Fig. 11).

Based on these preliminary clinical data, it has become our routine to use the 2-standard deviation values, namely, ± 8.4% RGF and ± 6.2% ESV/EDV as confidence limits indicating a sufficiently accurate study. We presently aim to calculate data during the course of angiocardiography in order to repeat the study if necessary and to potentially improve unsatisfactory conditions, such as patient motion, irregular respiration, poor contrast mixing or unsuitable roentgen projections.

Comment

Ventricular densitometry offers a direct assessment of the severity of valvular insufficiency by measuring the regurgitant amount of contrast medium as a fraction of the amount of ventricular ejection. Previous studies using 'analog videodensitometry' were affected by uncontrollable roentgen density variations, such as cardiac, respiratory and spontaneous motion. DSA as a preprocessing mode of densitometric analysis allows visual control of such inappropriate conditions and potentially eliminates the contribution of background structures to the absorption by contrast medium. This study demonstrates that DSA provides reproducible values of regurgitant fraction and ventricular ejection fraction even in children with spontaneous respiration, providing a considerable advantage over conventional videodensitometry. The accuracy of clinical data has not yet been clinically established. However, the reproducibility in the order of ± 8% RGF forms the basis to derive diagnostic conclusions from these densitometric parameters. Furthermore, previous experimental comparisons of electromagnetic flow measurements with analog videodensitometry using the same principle revealed no systematic deviation of values and a scatter range similar to that of DSA densitometry [2, 10, 14, 15].

Another important aspect of DSA relates to the ability to vary the size and position of densitometric sampling areas for the optimal outlining of cardiac chambers. This feature has been found to be essential for assessing mitral regurgitation by delineating the mitral valve plane in different cardiac phases.

From this limited experience, we believe that DSA combined with densito-metric analysis is a proven, valuable, and practical technique in the assessment of valve function.

References

1. Bürsch JH, Simon R: Methodisch einfache Quantifizierung von Herzklappeninsuffizienzen durch videodensitometrische Kontrastmittel-Mengenmessungen. Verh.-Berichte der Deutschen Gesellschaft für Kreislaufforschung 1972; 38: 317–320.
2. Bürsch JH, Heintzen PH, Simon R: Videodensitometric studies by a new method of quantitating the amount of contrast medium. Eur J Cardiol 1974; 1: 437–446.
3. Heintzen PH (ed): Roentgen-, cine- and videodensitometry. Fundamentals and applications for blood flow and heart volume determination. Thieme, Stuttgart, 1971.
4. Heintzen PH, Bürsch JH: Methods for angiocardiodensitography. Circulation 1965; 32 (Suppl II): 110.
5. Rutishauser W, Stucky J, Schad N, Wirz P: Kreislaufmessungen mittels Röntgen-Cine-densitometrie. Verh Dtsch Ges Kreislaufforschg 1966; 32: 252–256.
6. Trenholm BG, Winter DA, Mymin D, Landsdown EL: Computer determination of left ventricular volume using videodensitometry. Med Biol Eng 1972; 10: 163.
7. Wood EH, Sturm RE, Sanders JJ: Data processing in cardiovascular physiology with particular reference to roentgen videodensitometry. Mayo Clin Proc 1964; 39: 849–865.
8. Bürsch JH, Ritman EL, Wood EH, Sturm RE: Roentgen videodensitometry. In: Bloomfield DA (ed) Dye curves; pp 313–333. University Park Press, Baltimore, 1974.
9. Heintzen PH, Bürsch JH (eds): Roentgen video techniques for dynamic studies of structure and function of the heart and circulation. Thieme, Stuttgart, 1978.
10. Heintzen PH, Brennecke R, Bürsch JH, Hahne HJ, Lange PE, Moldenhauer K, Onnasch D, Radtke W: Quantitative analysis of structure and function of the cardiovascular system by roentgen-video-computer techniques. Mayo Clin Proc 1982; 5: I–78–91.
11. Lange PE, Hüttig G, Bürsch JH, Bernhard A, Heintzen PH: Videodensitometrische, angio-kardiographische und hämodynamische Untersuchungen bei korrigierten Fallotschen Tetralogien. Z Kardiologie 1975; 64: 120–137.
12. Bürsch JH: Densitometric studies in digital subtraction angiography: Assessment of pulmonary and myocardial perfusion. Herz 1985; 10: 208–214.
13. Gaux JC, Curuvija S, Angel CY, Brenot PH, Parola JL, Pernes JM, Raynaud A: Calculation of left ventricle ejection fraction (LVEF) by digital videodensitometric analysis. Annales de Radiologie 1984; 28, II: 189–192.
14. Falliner A, Bürsch JH, Wessel A, Faltz HC, Heintzen PH: Zuverlässigkeit der Röntgen-Videodensitometrie für Klappeninsuffizienzmessungen und für die Bestimmung der ventrikulären Auswurffraktion. Z Kardiol 1981; 70: 754–760.
15. Simon R, Callesen C, Heintzen PH: Bestimmung der Regurgitationsfraktion von Pulmonalinsuffizienzen durch videodensitometrische Indikator-Mengenmessung. Basic Res Cardiol 1973; 68: 509–520.

6. Quantification of Aortic Regurgitation

P.-A. DORIOT, J. DIVERNOIS, P. CHATELAIN & W. RUTISHAUSER
Cardiology Center, University Hospital, Geneva, Switzerland

Introduction

The aortic regurgitation fraction RGF is defined as 'volume regurgitating from the aorta during diastole' divided by 'volume expelled into the aorta in the previous systole'. Assuming a competent mitral valve yields:

$$\text{RGF (\%)} = [(\text{SV-FSV})/\text{SV}] \times 100, \tag{1}$$

where SV is the left ventricular stroke volume and FSV the 'forward' stroke volume. Conventional assessment of RGF requires determination of SV and FSV. SV is obtained from a contrast ventriculogram by volumetry (area-length or Simpson's method). FSV is calculated from heart rate and cardiac output (CO), obtained usually by help of an indicator dilution technique. Since SV and FSV measurements are several minutes apart, RGF is affected by temporal variations of these two parameters. Moreover, all steps involved in the calculation of enddiastolic and endsystolic volumes of the left ventricle (LV) can produce together a considerable error of SV. The accuracy of FSV is no better than the accuracy of routine CO measurements. RGF can thus be very inaccurate.

Videodensitometric methods requiring neither volumetry nor CO measurement allow to overcome these limitations [1–3]. The method presented in this contribution is similar to a method validated by Falliner and co-workers [3]. While they used a videotape recorder and an analog videodensitometer to establish the 'densogram' of a contrast medium amount injected into the LV, we used to this purpose our equipment for digital subtraction angiography (DIGITRON 2, Siemens) which allows to compute densograms for defined regions of interest (ROIs) directly from the digitally recorded angiographic sequence. This simplifies greatly apparative and operative aspects. The major difference between our approach and Falliner's one consists, however, in the proposed solution to the problem of drifting baselines of the densogram.

P.H. Heintzen and J.H. Bürsch (eds), Progress in Digital Angiocardiography. ISBN 978-94-010-7093-5
© 1988, Kluwer Academic Publishers, Dordrecht

Theoretical basis

The densitometric approach requires basically:

a) A model describing the left ventricular washout M(t) of a contrast medium amount injected into the LV. M(t) shall be proportional to the mass m(t) of contrast medium in the LV at time t, but have the physical dimension and unit of a densogram.

b) A link between M(t) and RGF.

c) A means to measure M(t).

In order to obtain a simple but reasonable model, we require the following assumptions to be fulfilled in the washout time interval selected for determination of RGF:

a) The mitral valve is competent.

b) The concentration of contrast medium in the LV is homogeneous during each systole.

c) The concentration of contrast medium in the regurgitating volume is equal to the concentration in the LV during the just terminated systole.

d) T (cardiac period), T_s (systole duration), EDV (enddiastolic volume), ESV (endsystolic volume), and RGF are constant.

Under these assumptions, enddiastolic and endsystolic amounts of contrast medium represented by $M(t_i)$ and $M(t_i+T_s)$ decrease exponentially in the selected time interval, as shown in the simplified diagram of Fig. 1 (right ordinate scale):

$$M(t_i) = B_d \exp[Ct_i], \tag{2}$$
$$M(t_i + T_s) = B_s \exp[C(t_i + T_s)]; \tag{3}$$

i is the order number of the considered cardiac cycle, C is common to both equations. The 2 exponentials $M_d(t)$ and $M_s(t)$ carrying the points $M(t_i)$ and $M(t_i + T_s)$ of the washout phase are thus:

$$M_d(t) = B_d \exp[Ct], \tag{4}$$
$$M_s(t) = B_s \exp[Ct]. \tag{5}$$

If T, T_s, B_d, B_s and C can be determined, the ejection fraction EF, the 'forward ejection fraction' FEF and RGF can be calculated from the equations:

$$EF(\%) = [1 - (B_s/B_d) \exp(CT_s)] \times 100, \tag{6}$$
$$FEF(\%) = [1 - \exp(CT)] \times 100, \tag{7}$$
$$RGF(\%) = [1 - FEF/EF] \times 100. \tag{8}$$

Densograms will be called 'time-dilution-curves' or 'TDCs', according to the terminology of the DIGITRON. We assume next that M(t) is reflected, up to an additive constant A, in the TDC obtained by summing in each image of the sequence the gray values of all pixels included in a ROI drawn around an

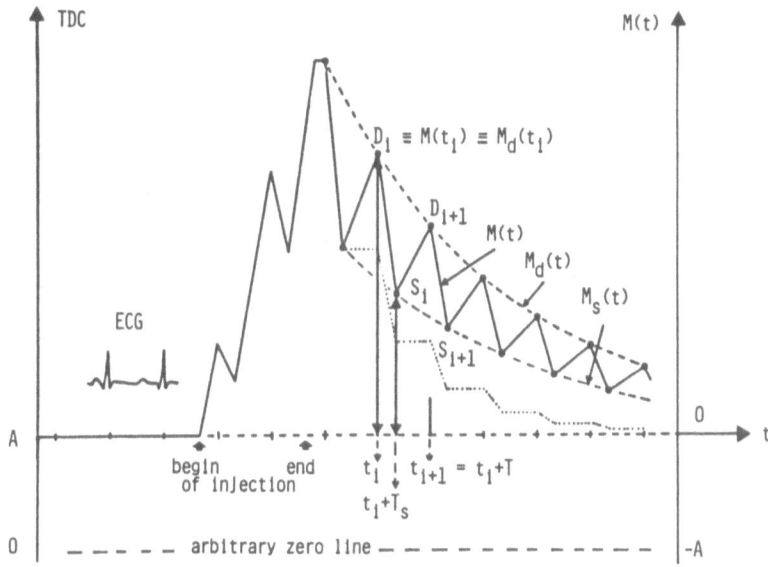

Fig. 1. Simplified left ventricular time-course M(t) of a contrast medium amount injected into the LV. M(t) can also be viewed as a simplified enddiastolic TDC, since it is also dimensionless and has the same arbitrary unit. Enddiastolic and endsystolic points of the hypothetical TDC (pointed curve) one would obtain if regurgitation disappeared at the end of the injection lie also on 2 exponentials since the model is also valid for RGF = 0.

enddiastolic silhouette: 'TDC value at time t' = A + M(t). (The gray value of a pixel (x, y) is equal to the logarithmic videosignal log S (x, y).) The constant A depends on the reference zero line of the TDC, which can be arbitrarily chosen. Although only enddiastoles and endsystoles are needed for determination of $M_d(t)$ and $M_s(t)$, the TDC is computed over all images of the sequence for correct identification of the former. M(t) in Fig. 1 is thus equivalent to a simplified 'enddiastolic' TDC (left scale). Increasing ordinate corresponds to increasing opacification of the ROI. The enddiastolic and endsystolic points D_i and S_i of this TDC, identical to the points $M(t_i) = M_d(t_i)$ and $M(t_i+T_s) = M_s(t_i+T_s)$, are related to these latter ones according to:

$$D_i = A + M_d(t_i) = A + B_d \exp[Ct_i], \qquad (9)$$
$$S_i = A + M_s(t_i+T_s) = A + B_s \exp[C(t_i+T_s)]. \qquad (10)$$

However, experience shows that the non-enddiastolic points of a real enddiastolic TDC do not reflect accurately the actual amounts of contrast medium in the LV, mainly because of the periodic incursion of the aortic valvular tract into the enddiastolic ROI [4]. In order to obtain more accurate endsystolic values $M_s(t_i+T_s)$, an 'endsystolic' TDC must also be computed, using a ROI drawn around an endsystolic silhouette. The points S_i are then measured on this TDC. Simplified enddiastolic and endsystolic TDCs having the same scale and the same offset A relatively to the zero line (up to here), equations (9) and (10) remain temporarily valid.

Figure 2 shows a pair of real enddiastolic/endsystolic TDCs. The zero line is arbitrary as already stated. Both TDCs are 'normalized' to one pixel (the DIGITRON divides the sum of gray levels in each image by the number of pixels of the ROI). Consequently, the respective scales of these TDCs are different. This explains why the endsystolic TDC lies above the enddiastolic one in a great part of the washout phase (the average gray level of the endsystolic TDC is momentarily darker than the average gray level of the enddiastolic TDC). For simplicity, we will, however, assume in this section that these TDCs have the same scale as $M(t)$. The periodic oscillation of each TDC before onset of the injection is due to variations in X-ray attenuation of the various tissues and blood thicknesses contributing to the sum of gray levels inside the respective ROI. If these 2 periodic 'background' oscillations could be validly extended into the washout phase, the necessitated points of $M_d(t)$ and $M_s(t)$ could be measured relatively to the enddiastolic and endsystolic horizontal baselines A_d = const and A_s = const depicted in dashed lines. Unfortunately, 'background' oscillations and thus enddiastolic/endsystolic baselines begin to drift after onset of the injection (cf. [3]), because of rapid opacification of myocardium and thoracal tissues, recirculation and maybe other reasons. Thus, equations (9) and (10) must be modified to:

$$D_i = A_d(t_i) + M_d(t_i) = A_d(t_i) + B_d \exp [Ct_i], \qquad (11)$$
$$S_i = A_s(t_i+T_s) + M_s(t_i+T_s) = A_s(t_i+T_s) + B_s \exp[C(t_i+T_s)], \qquad (12)$$

where most probably $A_s(t) \neq A_d(t)$ − constant. Obviously, $A_d(t)$ ad $A_s(t)$ should also be known in order to determine the EF, FEF and RGF using equations (6), (7) and (8).

One could assume that $A_d(t)$ and $A_s(t)$, although unknown, are sufficiently constant (that means horizontal) during the first 2 consecutive cardiac cycles i and i+1 of the washout phase ('method of differences', cf. [3]). This is equivalent to assume that the points D_i and S_i of these 2 cycles decrease exponentially, which allows to use the simple formulas below:

$$EF_i(\%) = [1 - (S_i - S_{i+1})/(D_i - D_{i+1})] \times 100, \qquad (13)$$
$$FEF_i(\%) = [1 - (D_{i+1} - D_{i+2})/(D_i - D_{i+1})] \times 100, \qquad (14)$$
$$RGF_i(\%) = [1 - FEF_i/EF_i] \times 100. \qquad (15)$$

Thus, 2 consecutive cardiac cycles would yield one set of values EF_i, FEF_i and RGF_i, and 3 consecutive cycles would allow for some averaging of EF, FEF and RGF. Unsatisfying points of this approach are, however, that all involved differences must accurately reflect the actual changes in left ventricular contrast medium amount (for simple mathematical reasons), and that these

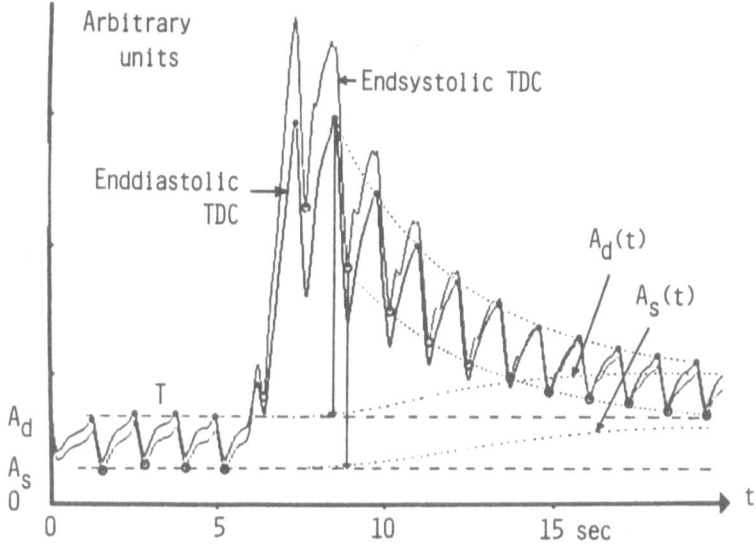

Fig. 2. Pair of 'normalized' enddiastolic/endsystolic TDCs. Problematic is that the real enddiastolic and endsystolic baselines $A_d(t)$ and $A_s(t)$ are unknown in the washout phase.

changes should themselves accurately correspond in each considered cardiac cycle to the theoretical representation of the washout process resulting from assumptions a to d. This is not the case, and the fiability of EF_i, FEF_i and RGF_i decreases rapidly with increasing order number i (cf. [3]). One could try to eliminate (partially) these difficulties by injecting a greater amount of contrast medium, but this could worsen the potential problem of assumed linearity between true amount of contrast medium in the LV at time t and corresponding TDC value.

Therefore, an algorithm was designed to 'reconstruct' the 2 unknown baselines in the washout phase. Its principle is to find 2 artificial baselines such that the points D_i and S_i of the TDCs lie best on exponential curves when measured with respect to these artificial baselines, according to equations (4) and (5) or, equivalently, (11)and (12). Each baseline is composed of a sinusoidal segment beginning at the end of the known baseline segment (begin of the injection), and of a horizontal segment (Fig.3; the 2 TDCs are 'normalized' but this will still be ignored for simplicity). The exact location of the left ends of the 2 sinusoidal segments is not critical and is set by the operator at the approximate onset time of injection. The right end of the 2 horizontal segments can be chosen by the operator or set by the computer program at the lowest point of the washout part of the endsystolic TDC. The best amplitude and best half-period of each sinusoid, as well as the best coefficients B_d, B_s and C are found automatically and simultaneously by the optimizing algorithm according to the

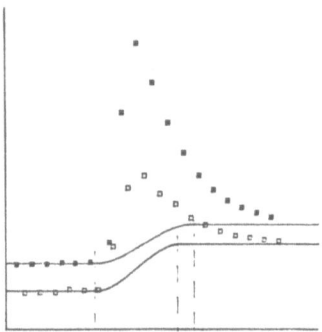

Fig. 3. Principle of 'reconstruction' of the 2 unknown baseline portions. Enddiastolic (filled squares) and endsystolic points are the initial points obtained from the 2 'normalized' native TDCs. Accordingly, both baselines found by the algorithm have been 'normalized', which explains that the offset between both is smaller after the injection than before ('normalization' of the baselines consists in multiplying the amplitude of the endsystolic baseline by the ratio 'number of pixels of the enddiastolic ROI' over 'number of pixels of the endsystolic ROI', the initial horizontal baseline segment being equal to zero).

criterion above. Each baseline is thus determined independently of the other, excepted the constraint of common coefficient C. EF, FEF and RGF are then calculated using equations (6), (7) and (8).

The algorithm was tested on many exact or noisy simulated TDCs. The obtained EF, FEF and RGF were regularly within a few percents of the expected ones. Variations of the results induced by simulated moderate irregularities such as extrasystoles, unstable cardiac period, etc. were observed but were within acceptable limits.

Patient study

Patients with clinical aortic regurgitation (and believed free of mitral regurgitation) were examined, as well as patients without suspected aortic or mitral regurgitation (called 'normal' in the following). The first few patients received a 40 ml selective injection of Iohexol (Omnipaque-350, 15 ml/sec). The dose was then lowered to 20 ml in order to reduce eventual nonlinear effects. The sequence was recorded in 'CONTINUOUS MODE' (DIGITRON), which provides constant radiographic parameters throughout the sequence (kV, mA, iris setting, videoamplification). Imaging rate was 25 i./sec and resolution $256 \times 256 \times 10$ bits. The injection was delayed by 5 sec in order to secure the needed initial baselines (the DIGITRON regulates the exposure parameters in 2 sec). Sequence duration was 15 to 20 sec. Using the available DIGITRON software, 2 ROIs were drawn around the enddiastolic and endsystolic silhouettes of the LV on adequate mask subtracted images. The corresponding 2 TDCs were computed from the original (unsubtracted) image sequence, rescaled (using same additive and multiplicative factors) but not 'denormalized' (see previous section), and recorded on a film document (MULTISPOT device of the DIGITRON).

The 2 TDCs yield as explained previously 'normalized' points $D_{i,norm}$ and $S_{i,norm}$ instead of the points D_i and S_i of our equations. The points $D_{i,norm}$ of the enddiastolic TDC and the points $S_{i,norm}$ of the endsystolic TDC were entered from the film document by means of a graphic tablet into a VAX-11/750 computer. Enddiastolic, respectively endsystolic points of the respective initial baselines were also entered. All entered points were 'denormalized' by multiplying all endsystolic points by the ratio 'number of pixels of the endsystolic ROI' over 'number of pixels of the enddiastolic ROI'. The algorithm determined then the best artificial baselines $A_d(t)$ and $A_s(t)$, and the best coefficients B_d, B_s and C, in the sense explained in the previous section. EF, FEF and RGF were calculated according to equations (6), (7) and (8).

Each patient had also biplane LV cine angiography before or after the DIGITRON sequence. The enddiastolic volume EDV_v, the endsystolic volume ESV_v and the ejection fraction EF_v were obtained by the area-length method (v stands for volumetry. In some patients calculations were performed for the RAO 30° view only because of poor LAO 60° view). Cardiac output of patients with regurgitation was measured from 2 Cardiogreen injections into the aortic root with sampling in the femoral artery using the 3 points method. RGF_v was calculated according to the formula:

$$RGF_v \ (\%) = [(EDV_v - ESV_v - FSV)/(EDV_v - ESV_v)] \times 100. \qquad (16)$$

Elimination of some patients in both groups for reasons given in the next section left 10 patients with regurgitation and 11 normal subjects.

Results and discussion

Table 1 summarizes the correlations between our EF, FEF, RGF and the reference values EF_v, FEF_v and RGF_v. Table 2 shows similarly the results obtained by the 'method of differences' (3 cycles). The correlations are clearly lower than in Table 1.

The EF are slightly lower than the EF_v, in both patients groups (Table 1). An immediate explanation would be that TDCs and contrast medium amounts in the LV are not linearly related because of too elevated contrast medium concentrations (non-applicability of Lambert-Beer's absorption law). However, inflating a balloon in a water bath (20 cm depth) with different contrast medium solutions, from 0 to 200 or 300 ml, under the same radiographic conditions (CONTINUOUS MODE, etc.) yielded regularly an almost perfect straight line (it could be shown that the expected non-linearity is compensated by a decrease of the scattered radiation amount). So, there is no evidence for non-linearity. Some authors have suggested that blood is preferentially ejected during systole becaue of its lower density compared to the density of contrast medium. However, maximum acceleration occurring during systole is approximately 1 g, which is not sufficient to achieve fast separation of a mixture blood/contrast medium (because of viscosity). Experiments in a centrifuge at higher accelerations also do not support this view.

Thus, the following hypothetical explanations must still be investigated:

A) Some contrast medium remains trapped in the LV cavity (violation of assumption b).

B) Apnoe lowers progressively the ejection fraction (the 'method of differences' yielded statistically higher EF_d).

C) The EF are accurate and the EF_v overestimate the true ejection fractions. The results of Falliner and co-workers [3] were similar to ours in this respect. However, their underestimation of their reference EF may be due to the fact that only an enddiastolic ROI was used. In our study, EF obtained from an enddiastolic ROI were regularly lower than the corresponding '2 ROIs' EF.

Table 1. Correlations between the EF, FEF, RGF and the reference values EF_v, FEF_v, RGF_v.

	Range	n	r
EF (%) = 0.90 EF_v + 0[a]	39 to 78[b]	21	0.77
FEF (%) = 0.86 FEF_v + 0[a]	13 to 47[b]	10[c]	0.91
RGF (%) = 1.04 RGF_v + 0[a]	34 to 69[b]	10[c]	0.90

[a] All y-offsets were forced to 0 because none was significantly different from 0.
[b] Ranges of reference values.
[c] 'Normal' patients have been excluded from the regression analysis.

Table 2. Correlations between the EF_d, FEF_d, and RGF_d obtained by the 'method of differences', and the reference values EF_v, FEF_v, RGF_v.

	Range	n	r
EF_d (%) = 1.02 EF_v + 0[a]	39 to 78[b]	21	0.71
FEF_d (%) = 0.96 FEF_v + 0[a]	13 to 47[b]	10[c]	0.71
RGF_d (%) = 1.10 RGF_v + 0[a]	34 to 69[b]	10[c]	0.60

[a] All y-offsets were forced to 0 because none was significantly different from 0.
[b] Ranges of reference values.
[c] 'Normal' patients have been excluded from the regression analysis.

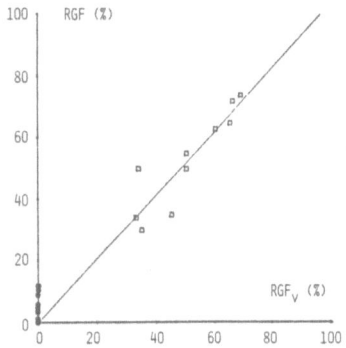 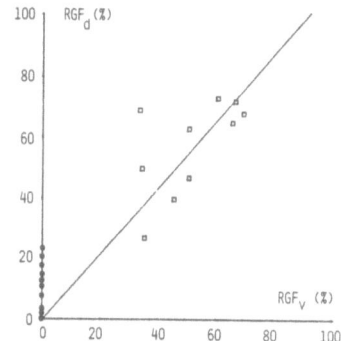

Fig. 4. a: correlation between the RGF and the RGF$_v$. Cardiac output of normal patients was not measured; their RGF$_v$ are therefore zero and have been excluded from the regression analysis (see Table 1). b: correlation between the RGF$_d$ obtained by the 'method of differences' and the RGF$_v$ (see Table 2).

The FEF of patients with aortic regurgitation are clearly lower than the corresponding FEF$_v$ (Table 1; since cardiac output of the 'normal' patients was not measured, their FEF$_v$ were taken equal to the EF$_v$ and excluded from the regression analysis). The FEF of 'normal' patients were often lower than the corresponding EF. This may be due to a regurgitation induced by the catheter which was not always pulled back into the aorta immediately after the injection. If the EF really underestimate the true EF while the RGF are accurate, the FEF will also underestimate the true FEF because of the interdependence of EF, FEF and RGF explicited in equations (6), (7) and (8). Underestimation of the true EF is also possible if assumption c) is not well fulfilled, for instance if the concentration of contrast medium in the regurgitating volume is higher than in the just previously ejected volume. This would imply, however, that the RGF overestimate the true RGF (which is of course possible despite the high correlation between RGF and RGF$_v$). Fig. 4a shows the surprisingly high correlation between RGF and RGF$_v$ of regurgitating patients (the RGF$_v$ of 'normal' patients having not been measured, they were taken equal to zero and excluded from the regression analysis. The corresponding RGF were zero or positive, with one exception: RGF= −1%. The clearly positive RGF of some of these 'normal' patients may reflect the regurgitation induced by the catheter remaining in the LV after the injection). Fig. 4b shows that calculating the RGF$_d$ by the 'method of differences' yields a lower correlation.

In the introduction, some unsatisfying aspects of the conventional measurement of RGF were pointed out. However, an advantage of the conventional method is its greater tolerance for irregularities of the cardiac cycle. Marked irregularities in the TDCs produced EF, FEF and RGF values clearly different from the expected ones (EF$_v$, FEF$_v$ and RGF$_v$). Patients presenting such irregularities were excluded from the study, as were patients who could not hold respiration.

Conclusion

Densitometric and conventional regurgitation fractions are well correlated. This is due to the use of enddiastolic and endsystolic ROIs, and to the performed 'reconstruction' of enddiastolic and endsystolic baselines. If the manufacturers of DSA equipment would develop hardwired ROI integrators for TDCs computation in video-times, videodensitometric methods could become very attractive. One could for instance compute the time-course of the left ventricular volume over one cardiac cycle much faster than presently feasible.

Summary

Assessment of the aortic regurgitation fraction RGF by videodensitometry avoids several drawbacks of the conventional method based on left ventricular volumetry and cardiac output measurement. Early techniques required video-tape recording of a left ventricular injection of contrast medium, and an analog videodensitometer to establish the left ventricular time-course (densogram) of the injected contrast medium amount. We used to this purpose our equipment for digital subtraction angiography (DIGITRON 2, Siemens). In order to improve the accuracy of RGF, a published method was modified in two points:
a) Two densograms were computed, an enddiastolic one, obtained from a ROI (Region Of Interest) drawn around the enddiastolic silhouette of the left ventricle (LV), and an endsystolic one obtained from an endsystolic ROI.
b) The baseline of each densogram, unknown in the washout phase, was reconstructed by means of a multiparametric fitting algorithm running on a VAX-11/750 computer. The left ventricular ejection fraction (EF) and the forward ejection fraction (FEF) were obtained from the washout parts of the baseline corrected densograms. RGF was calculated from the equation RGF(%) = (1-FEF/EF)×100.
The method has been applied to 10 patients presenting aortic regurgitation and to 11 patients with intact aortic valves. All patients had also conventional ventriculography. In the first group of patients, the RGF was also measured conventionally (Biplane cineangiography and Cardiogreen dilution). Following correlations were obtained: EF = 0.90 EF$_v$ + 0 (n=21), FEF = 0.86

$FEF_v + 0$ (n=10), $RGF = 1.04\ RGF_v + 0 =$ (n=10) (v denotes the conventional method requiring volumetry of the LV).

References

1. Bürsch JH, Heintzen PH, Simon R: Roentgenvideodensitometric determination of the residual fraction of the normal left ventricle and regurgitation fraction in experimental aortic regurgitation. Physiologist 1972; 15: 3.
2. Simon R, Steiger U, Wirz P, Krayenbühl HP, Schönbeck M, Rutishauser W: Quantifizierung von Aortenklappeninsuffizienzen durch videodensitometrische Kontrastmittelmessungen. Schweiz Med Wschr 1974 104: 1562.
3. Falliner A, Bürsch JH, Wessel A, Faltz H-C, Heintzen PH: Zuverlässigkeit der Roentgen-Videodensitometrie für Klappeninsuffizienzmessungen und für die Bestimmung der ventrikulären Auswurffraktion (Accuracy and performance of Roentgen-Videodensitometry for valvular regurgitation and ventricular ejection measurements). Z Kardiol 1981; 70: 754–760.
4. Divernois J: Mesure de la régurgitation aortique par vidéodensitométrie numérisée. Thèse no 7034. Faculté de Médecine de l'Université de Genève. Edition du Grillon, Genève, 1986.

7. Quantitative Assessment of Aortic Regurgitation by Digital Subtraction Angiography

PAUL A. GRAYBURN & STEVEN E. NISSEN
Division of Cardiology, Department of Medicine, University of Kentucky College of Medicine, Lexington, KY, USA

The severity of aortic regurgitation has been traditionally assessed by visual interpretation of cineaortograms utilizing a 1 to 4+ scale [1]. This method is subjective and may be influenced by variations in left ventricular volume, radiographic technique, contrast dose, and interobserver agreement [2]. Despite these limitations, this semiquantitative technique continues to be the most widely accepted clinical measurement of the magnitude of aortic regurgitation.

Aortograms acquired in digital format can also be analyzed by semi-quantitative visual grading. Booth et al. [3] studied 12 patients with aortic regurgitation in whom both cineaortography and digital subtraction aortography had been performed. All studies were analyzed in blinded fashion by two observers using conventional visual grading. Although interobserver agreement was excellent for both studies, visual interpretation digital aortography systemically overestimated the degree of aortic regurgitation as assessed by cineaortography. This was attributed to enhancement of myocardial contrast by digital subtraction.

Klein et al. [4] utilized a computer-based method to evaluate the degree of aortic regurgitation in 17 patients in whom digital subtraction aortograms had been performed. R-wave gated images were acquired in digital format using a $512 \times 512 \times 8$ bit pixel matrix. After subtraction, a 30×30 pixel region of interest was positioned over both the aortic root and the left ventricle. Time intensity curves were generated by computer for each region of interest. The ratio of left ventricular to aortic contrast density (LV_d/Ao_d) at end-injection was taken as an index of the severity of aortic regurgitation and compared to visual grading of cineaortography. The correlation between the two methods was quite good. In addition, reproducibility as well as inter-and intra-observer agreement were excellent. Despite these encouraging results, this index provides only semi-quantitative data in that it can distinguish between mild, moderate, and severe aortic regurgitation as determined by visual inspection of cineaortograms.

P.H. Heintzen and J.H. Bürsch (eds), Progress in Digital Angiocardiography. ISBN 978-94-010-7093-5

Regurgitant fraction

Regurgitant fraction is the only clinically available measurement providing truly quantitative information regarding the severity of aortic regurgitation. Unfortunately, calculation of regurgitant fraction at catheterization by the Sandler Dodge method is limited in accuracy and has been shown to correlate poorly with electromagnetic flow measurements in patients undergoing open heart surgery [5]. Dye dilution techniques have long been used to quantitate regurgitant fraction in aortic insufficiency and have been shown to correlate closely with electromagnetic flow measurements [6, 7]. Von Bernuth et al. [8] adapted dye dilution principles to analog videodensitometry to accurately quantify aortic regurgitant fraction in dogs. In similar fashion, dye dilution methods can be applied to digital subtraction aortography to calculate regurgitant fraction using radiographic contrast as the indicator [9].

Theoretical considerations

To determine regurgitant fraction by dye dilution methods, an indicator such as indocyanine green is injected into the aortic root. Following injection, timed blood samples are collected via cuvette from both the left ventricle and the aorta distal to injection. Time-concentration curves are then constructed for both sampling sites. Regurgitant fraction is equal to the area under the left ventricular time-concentration curve divided by the area under the aortic time-concentration curve. Time-intensity curves can be easily generated by computer analysis of digitally acquired aortograms following injection of radiographic contrast into the aortic root. The area under time-intensity curves generated from aortic and left ventricular regions of interest represents mass of contrast rather than concentration. However, because mass equals concentration times volume, concentration can be obtained by dividing the area under the time-intensity curve by the volume of its corresponding region of interest. Accordingly, aortic regurgitant fraction can be determined from analysis of digital subtraction aortograms using the following formula:

$$RF = \frac{A_{LV}/V_{LV}}{A_{Ao}/V_{Ao}} = \frac{A_{LV}V_{Ao}}{A_{Ao}V_{LV}},$$

where RF is regurgitant fraction, A_{LV} and A_{Ao} are the areas under left ventricular and aortic time-intensity curves, and V_{LV} and V_{Ao} are the volumes of the left ventricular and aortic regions of interest.

Experimental model

To test the hypothesis that aortic regurgitant fraction could be accurately quantified by digital subtraction aortography, we studied six open-chest dogs in whom aortic regurgitation of varying severity was produced by an expandable basket catheter. All dogs were instrumented with a tightly fitted electromagnetic flow probe as a means of determining regurgitant fraction. The flow probe was calibrated in vivo using thermodilution cardiac outputs and the zero line was re-established following each grade of aortic insufficiency by withdrawing the basket catheter above the aortic valve plane. For each animal, several degrees of aortic regurgitation were produced by incremental expansion of the basket catheter. Simultaneous electromagnetic flow, ECG, and aortic pressure were recorded and a digital aortogram performed. Aortograms were obtained by R-wave triggered injection of 18 ml of radiographic contrast over 2 seconds via a 6F NIH catheter positioned just above the aortic leaflets. Images were obtained by continuous fluoroscopy at 30 frames/sec and underwent real-time analog-to-digital conversion into a $256 \times 256 \times 8$ bit pixel matrix. The digital images were then stored on 10 megabyte high-density floppy disks for subsequent analysis.

Image processing

All aortograms were analyzed using a dedicated medical image processing computer (MIPRON I, Kontron Electronics). Logarithmic transformation was performed in order to account for the non-linear relationship between contrast concentration and optical brightness (Beer-Lambert Law). Gated digital subtraction was then performed such that each mask frame was subtracted from the contrast-containing frames corresponding to its portion of the cardiac cycle. Rectangular regions of interest were then positioned over the left ventricle and aorta. Size and angulation of the regions of interest were adjusted so that they were perpendicular to the long-axis of the aorta and left ventricle and completely encompassed the largest diameter of the corresponding cardiac chamber. Time-intensity curves were then generated for each region of interest as summated pixel intensity versus time. Figure 1 illustrates the positioning of the regions of interest and their respective time-intensity curves. The area under each time-intensity curve was determined and divided by the volume of its corresponding region of interest. This volume was calculated assuming a circular cross-section of both the aorta and left ventricle such that volume equals $\pi(D/2)^2h$ where D is the diameter and h the thickness of the region of interest in pixels. Regurgitant fraction was then calculated by the previously derived formula:

$$RF = \frac{A_{LV}/V_{Ao}}{A_{Ao}/V_{LV}}.$$

66

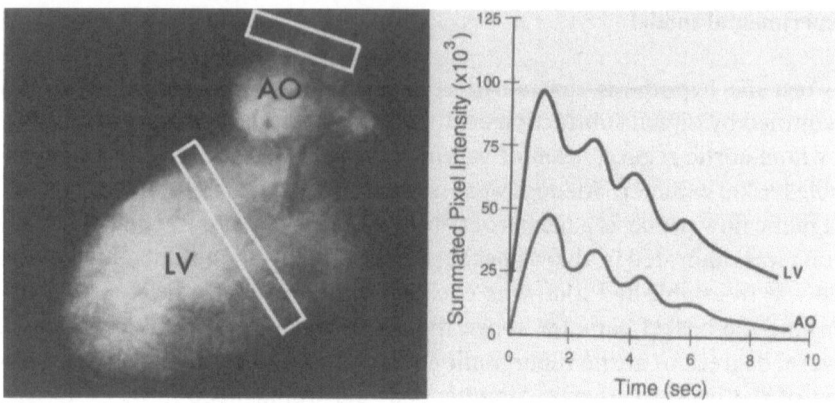

Fig. 1. Left panel: digital subtraction angiogram demonstrating the positioning of the aortic and left ventricular regions of interest. Right panel: time-intensity curves derived from the regions of interest shown in the left panel. The image has been scaled for reproduction purposes. Ao = aorta, LV = left ventricle.

Results

Regurgitant fractions ranged from 5.3 to 72.8 per cent by electromagnetic flow and from 2.4 to 78.2 per cent by digital subtraction angiography. A close correlation (r = 0.94) was observed between regurgitant fractions by the two methods (Fig. 2). The regression approximated unity (y = 0.98× + 0.46) and the standard error of the estimate was minimal (7.4 per cent). Regurgitant fraction by electromagnetic flow was also compared to visual grading of the

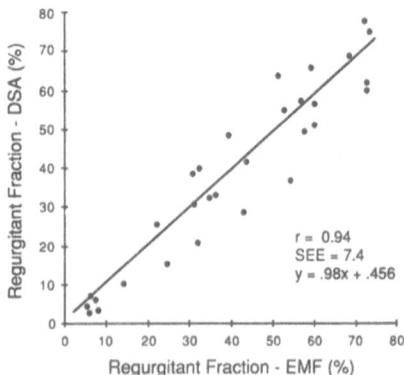

Fig. 2. Regression plot depicting the relationship between regurgitant fractions measured by digital subtraction angiography and electromagnetic flow. A close correlation is observed (r = 0.94) with a small standard error of the estimate (7.4%).

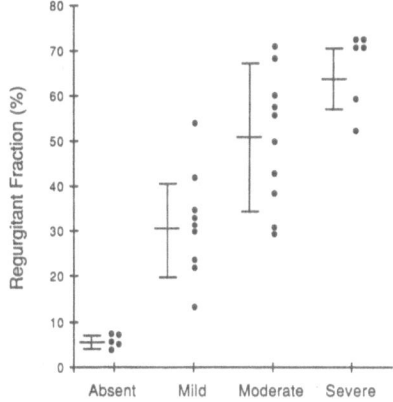

Fig. 3. Graph showing the regurgitant fractions obtained by electromagnetic flow according to the angiographic grade of aortic regurgitation. Although higher regurgitant fractions are present with increasing severity by visual grading, considerable overlap is observed.

angiograms. The angiograms were graded on a 1 to 4+ scale by consensus of two observers who were unaware of the calculated regurgitant fraction. The results of this comparison are shown in Fig. 3. Considerable overlap was present among the various grades of aortic regurgitation confirming that visual grading is limited in its ability to quantitate the magnitude of this lesion.

Discussion

Digital subtraction aortography offers several advantages over conventional angiographic assessment of aortic regurgitation. Because it offers the ability to determine regurgitation fraction, digital angiography is quantitative and thus superior to subjective visual grading. Further, digital formatting facilitates image analysis, is reproducible, and avoids difficulties associated with non-linearity of film.

Several limitations to the above technique deserve emphasis. The appearance of contrast in the myocardium overlying the left ventricular region of interest contributes to the time-intensity curve and may tend to cause a slight overestimation of regurgitant fraction. In addition, streaming or inadequate mixing of blood and contrast could affect the time-intensity curves. Finally, we studied acute aortic regurgitation in dogs and the results could differ in humans with chronic aortic regurgitation. In particular, the geometric assumptions used in this model may not be accurate in the presence of chronic aortic regurgitation with a dilated left ventricle.

Despite these limitations, we believe that the determination of regurgitant fraction by digital aortography may provide a better gold standard than visual grading of cineaortograms. Accordingly, this method may be useful in evaluating non-invasive methods of quantitating aortic regurgitation such as Doppler or radionuclide imaging. It may also provide a method of assessing changes in regurgitant fraction with afterload manipulation as a means of evaluating left ventricular function in patients with aortic regurgitation.

Future directions

Digital subtraction angiography offers the potential to calculate aortic regurgitant fraction by a variety of algorithms. For example, information contained in the washout phase of time-intensity curves may provide quantitative data [10]. The possibility exists to perform separate injections in the pulmonary artery and left ventricle using a single region of interest positioned over the proximal aorta. The difference between time-intensity curves from the two injections should reflect regurgitant flow and volume considerations should cancel out if the region of interest is constant. This technique could also be utilized to measure mitral regurgitation or shunt flow.

Conclusions

Regurgitant fraction in aortic insufficiency can be determined by analysis of aortic and left ventricular time-intensity curves generated from digital subtraction aortograms. This method has been validated in an animal model of acute aortic regurgitation and is superior to semi-quantitative visual grading of cineangiograms. Prospective evaluation of this method in patients with aortic regurgitation may provide an accurate method for quantifying the severity of this lesion.

References

1. Sellers RD, Levy MJ, Amplatz K, Lillehei CW: Left retrograde cardioangiography in acquired cardiac disease. Technic, indications, and interpretations in 700 cases. Am J Cardiol 1964; 14: 437–451.
2. Croft CH, Lipscomb K, Mathi K, Firth BG, Nicod P, Tilton G, Winniford MD, Hillis LD: Limitations of qualitative angiographic grading in aortic or mitral regurgitation. Am J Cardiol 1984; 53: 1593–1598.
3. Booth DC, Nissen SE, DeMaria AN: Assessment of the severity of valvular regurgitation by digital subtraction angiography compared to cinaortography. Am Heart J 1985; 110: 409–416.
4. Klein LW, Agarwal JB, Stets G, Rubinstein RI, Weintraub WS, Helfant RH: Video-

densitometric quantitation of aortic regurgitation by digital subtraction aortography using a computer-based method of analyzing time-density curves. Am J Cardiol 1986; 58: 753–756.

5. Mennel RG, JoynerCR Jr, Thompson PD, Pyle RR, MacVaugh H III: The preoperative and operative assessment of aortic regurgitation. Am J Cardiol 1972; 29: 360–366.

6. Malooly DA, Donald DE, Marshall HW, Wood EH: Assessment of an indicator-dilution technic for quantitating aortic regurgitation by electromagnetic flowmeter. Circ Res 1963; 12: 487–507.

7. Armelin E, Michaels L, Marshall HW, Donald DE, Cheesman RJ, Wood EH: Detection and measurement of experimentally produced aortic regurgitation by means of indicator-dilution curves recorded from the left ventricle. Circ Res 1963; 12: 269–290.

8. Von Bernuth G, Sakiris NG, Wood EH: Quantitation of experimental aortic regurgitation by roentgen videodensitometry. Am J Cardiol 1973; 31: 265–272.

9. Grayburn PA, Nissen SE, Elion JE, Evans J, DeMaria AN: Quantitation of aortic regurgitation by computer analysis of digital subtraction aortography (Abstract). J Am Coll Cardiol 1986; 7: 154A.

10. Bursch JH, Heintzen PH, Simon R: Videodensitometric studies by a new method of quantitating the amount of contrast medium. Eur J Cardiol 1974; 1: 437–446.

8. Quantitation of Ventricular Dynamic Geometry by Digital Angiocardiography

P.E. LANGE, W. BUDACH, B. EWERT, D.G.W. ONNASCH &
P.H. HEINTZEN
Department of Pediatric Cardiology and Bioengineering, University of Kiel, Kiel, FRG

Introduction

Conventional angiocardiography requires a large amount of contrast medium, which is especially detrimental in infants and children. In addition, a ventricular injection is often associated with catheter-induced ventricular ectopic rhythm [1–5], precluding optimal analysis of ventricular function, necessary in the pre- and postoperative assessment. To avoid these difficulties and to reduce the amount of contrast medium required, computer-enhancement techniques, based on digitization of the photon density of video images, have been used to provide high-resolution images of right [5] and left [1–4, 6–10] ventriculograms after intravenous and selective ventricular injection of contrast medium. Studies systematically analyzing spatial orientation, size, shape, and function of the right and left ventricle do not exist. We therefore used image enhancement techniques [6] to determine the extent to which digital subtraction angiocardiography after left and right ventricular injection of small amounts of contrast medium with reduced flow can provide information previously available only after large intraventricular contrast administration.

Methods

Patients

All patients were undergoing routine diagnostic cardiac catheterization for clinically indicated reasons.

RV study: 25 patients were studied including 3 infants under 1 year of age, 9 children between 1 and 6 years, and 13 between 13 and 20 years. They were 18 days to 20 years old (mean 8.7), they were 50 to 193 cm tall (mean 124), weighed 3 to 71 kg (mean 30.6), and their body surface area was 0.203 to 1.99 m^2 (mean 1.004). Diagnoses included pre- and postoperative tetralogy of

P.H. Heintzen and J.H. Bürsch (eds), Progress in Digital Angiocardiography. ISBN 978-94-010-7093-5
© 1988, Kluwer Academic Publishers, Dordrecht

Fallot (5 patients), ventricular septal defect (3 patients), pulmonary stenosis (3 patients), aortic stenosis (2 patients), patent ductus arteriosus (2 patients), congestive cardiomyopathy (1 patient) and combined lesions (9 patients).

LV study: 29 patients were studied including 4 infants under 1 year of age, 4 children between 1 and 6 years, and 21 between 6 and 60 years. They were 18 days to 60 years old (mean 14.4), they were 50 to 180 cm tall (mean 134.4), weighed 3 to 81 kg (mean 31.3), and their body surface area was 0.203 to 1.991 m² (mean 1.165). Diagnoses included combined valvular aortic stenosis and insufficiency (6 patients), valvular aortic stenosis (3 patients), aortic insufficiency (2 patients), atrial septal defect (5 patients), coarctation of the aorta (4 patients), tetralogy of Fallot (3 patients), ventricular septal defect (1 patient), mitral insufficiency (1 patient), complete transposition of the great arteries (1 patient), vascular abnormalities without ventricular overloading (3 patients).

Cardiac catheterization was performed with local lidocaine anesthesia and sedation (infants younger than 6 months: no medication, infants between 6 and 12 months 10 mg/kg acidum phenylbarbituricum; older children: pethidone, 1 to 1.5 mg/kg, atropine 0.01 to 0.015 mg/kg, acidum phenylbarbituricum 10 mg/kg (up to 200 mg).

In the RV study 16 patients (LV study: 18 patients) underwent conventional angiocardiography before digital angiocardiography, 9 patients (LV study: 11 patients) underwent digital angiocardiography first.

Data acquisition

Conventional and digital angiocardiography were performed with a 6F or 7F Berman catheter inserted into the femoral artery or femoral vein, using the percutaneus Seldinger technique.

RV study: diatrizoate meglumine (Urografin^R, Schering)0.97 ml/kg body weight (0.63 to 1.55) was injected at a rate of 13.70 ml/s (4 to 25 ml/s) into the right ventricle for conventional angiocardiography and 0.29 ml/kg (0.17 to 0.39 m/kg) at a rate of 7.40 ml/s (4 to 14 ml/s) for digital angiocardiography.

LV study: diatrizoate meglumine 0.78 ml/kg body weight (0.45 to 1.22) was injected at a rate 15.60 ml/s (4 to 25 ml/s) into the left ventricle for conventional angiocardiography and 0.28 ml/kg (0.15 to 0.47 ml/kg) at a rate 8.1 ml/s (range 4 to 18 ml/s) for digital angiocardiography.

The injection was always initiated at the rapid filling phase of diastole by the ECG-triggered injection delay control to achieve complete mixing of the contrast material with blood. Anterior-posterior and lateral projections of the right and left ventricle were obtained using both techniques (X-ray generator Siemens Pandoros) with the patient in the supine position and recorded side by side at a rate of 50 frames/s on videotape. For calibration purposes a steel

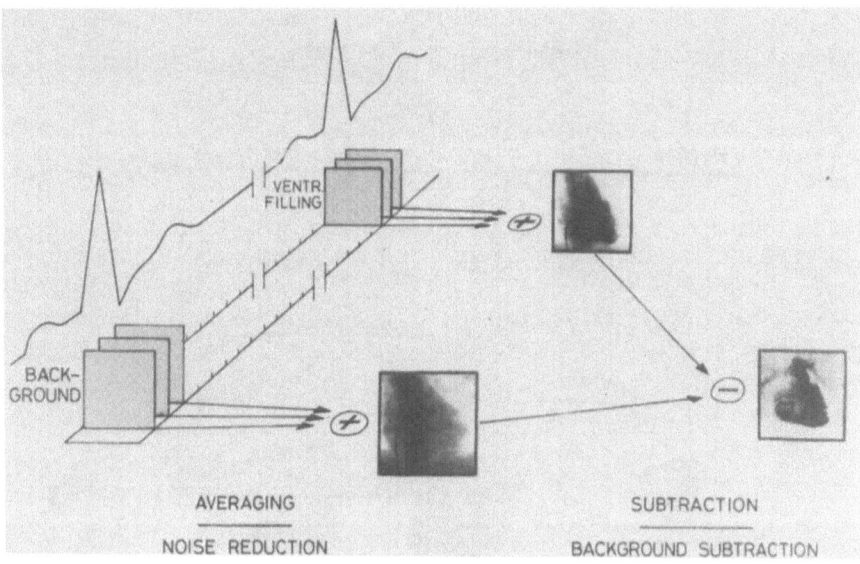

AVERAGING   SUBTRACTION

NOISE REDUCTION   BACKGROUND SUBTRACTION

Fig. 1. For off-line background subtraction a cardiac cycle was selected by the operator at a dia-phragmatic level similar to the best opacified cycle (or second postextrasystolic beat) of the ventricular filling phase. End-diastolic and end-systolic frames as well as the preceding and the following frames of the selected background and opacified cycles were digitized (1 television field = 256 × 256 pixels at 256 gray levels) and stored on digital disc. For noise reduction the gray level of each pixel was averaged for the 3 background and the 3 opacified frames. After the logarithmic subtraction of the background picture from the opacified picture linear rescaling was performed to match the 256 gray levels of the output device.

sphere of known diameter was recorded at the location occupied by the ventricle [11]. Suspended respiration, used to minimize diaphragmatic motion, was achieved only in older children.

For conventional angiocardiograms the image intensifier output screen was imaged through a partly transparent mirror to both the cine and the television camera, whereas for digital processing the entire information was imaged to the television camera (Plumbicon). The X-ray equipment was pulsed with 50 frames/s and 2 ms pulse length alternatively in the two planes. Blanking the anterior-posterior image intensifier during lateral radiation and vice versa prevented X-ray scattering from the orthogonal plane. For a preselected X-ray current (depending on the patients' size: 250 to 400 mA) in a test mode before each injection the voltage was automatically tuned to achieve a distinct level at the image intensifier output screen. This level corresponded to 10 μR per image at the input screen (25 cm diameter) for normal cine angiocardiograms and was reduced to 4 μR for digital angiocardiography. For the 17 cm input screen the dose was twice as high. On the average, the resulting voltages were

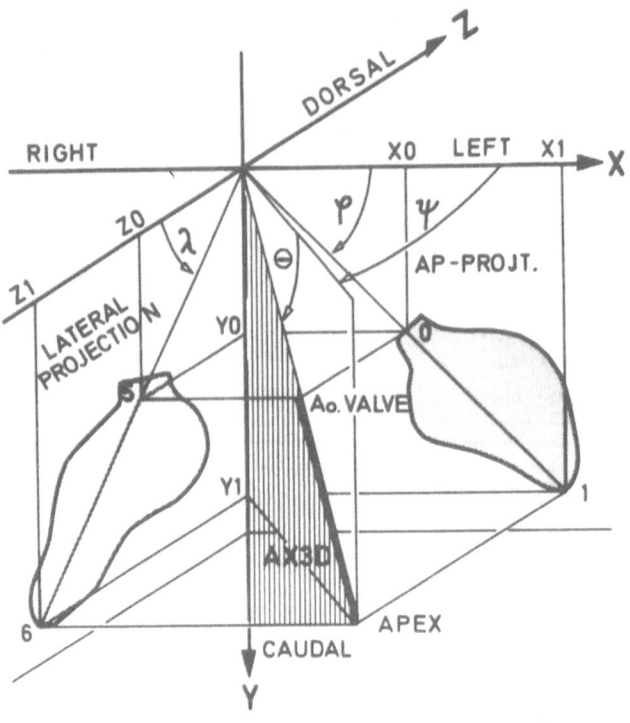

Fig. 2. The spatial orientation of the long ventricular axis (AX3D) of the left ventricle is determined on the basis of the anatomic landmarks center of semilunar valve / apex marked on the anterior-posterior and lateral ventricular projections and characterized by the spatial angles psi (φ) and theta (θ).

77 and 70 kV, respectively. The mean currents were 370 and 320 mA and the recording times were 9.2 and 7.9 seconds, respectively.

The largest ventricular projections were assumed to represent end-diastole and the smallest end-systole. The system used to obtain off-line digital angiocardiography has been described in detail [6]. For background subtraction a cardiac cycle was selected by the operator at a diaphragmatic level similar to the best opacified cycle (or the second postextrasystolic beat) of the ventricular filling phase. End-diastolic and end-systolic frames as well as the preceding and the following frames of the selected background and opacified cycles were digitized (1 television field = 256 × 256 pixels at 256 gray levels) and stored on digital disc (80 Mbyte = 1.225 images) (Fig. 1). The gray level of each pixel was logarithmically converted and averaged for the 3 background and the 3 opacified frames. After subtraction of the background picture from the opacified picture linear rescaling was performed to match the 256 gray levels of the output device.

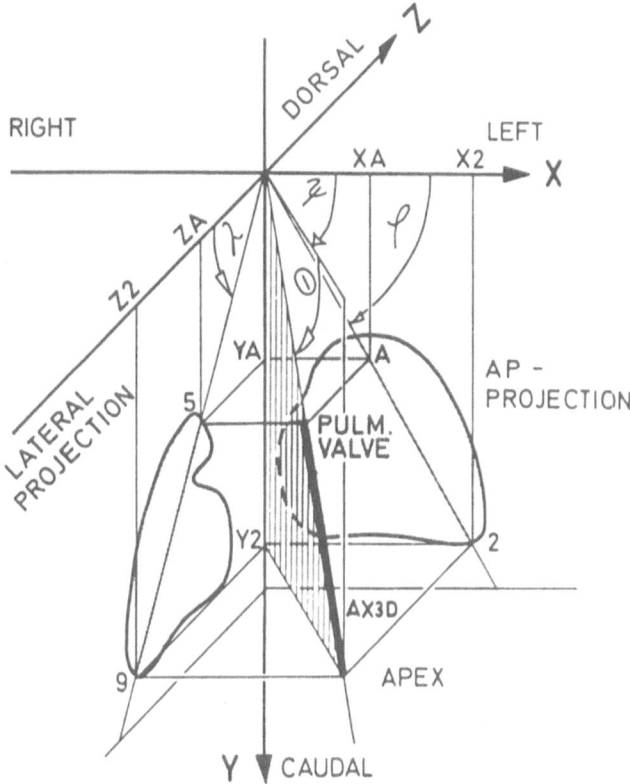

Fig. 3. The spatial orientation of the long ventricular axis (AX3D) of the right ventricle is determined on the basis of the anatomic landmarks center of semilunar valve / apex marked on the anterior-posterior and lateral ventricular projections and characterized by the spatial angles psi (φ) and theta (θ).

Measurements

Biplane ventricular projections obtained by both techniques were assessed in an identical manner. Displayed on a television monitor side by side the biplane silhouettes (steel sphere and ventricles in sinus beats) were traced by 2 independent observers (A and B) using a resistance foil and stored in a digital computer (PDP 11/60). In addition to biplane outlines up to 10 anatomically defined landmarks were marked allowing, for example, the determination of the long ventricular axis between the center of the semilunar valve ring and the apex (Figs. 2, 3) [11]. To minimize memory bias 2 days to 3 months (mean 34 and 36 days for RV and LV, respectively) elapsed between the interpretations of the angiocardiograms of a single patient. RV volumes at end-diastole and end-systole calculated with the multiple slices methods as well as LV volumes

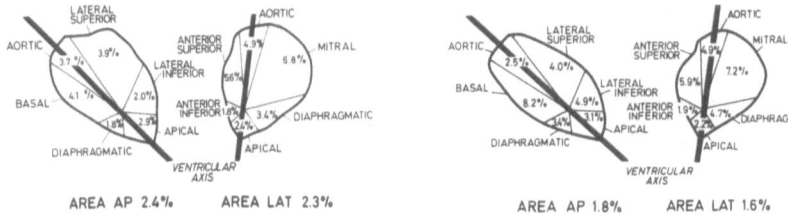

Fig. 4. Accuracy of regional border recognition of left ventricular anterior-posterior (AP) and lateral (LAT) projections in end-diastole (left) an end-systole (right) was assessed on the basis of a fixed radial reference system the center being at 69% of the long ventricular axis between the center of the semilunar valve and the apex (see also Fig. 2). The difference between digital and conventional angiocardiography is expressed in per cent of the respective projection area.

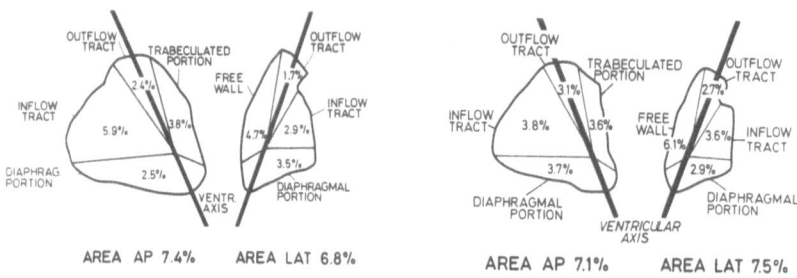

Fig. 5. Accuracy of regional border recognition of the right ventricular anterior-posterior (AP) and lateral (LAT) projections in end-diastole (left) and end-systole (right) was assessed on the basis of a fixed radial reference system the center being at 69% of the long ventricular axis beween the center of the semilunar valve and the apex (see also Fig. 3). The difference between digital and conventional angiocadiography is expressed in per cent of the respective projection area.

calculated with the area-length method [11] were corrected with factors appropriate for position and cardiac phase [12, 13]. For the regional assessment a fixed radial reference system (Figs. 4, 5) was used.

A least-squares correlation was used to compare volume parameters obtained by both techniques. Significances of differences were calculated using the paired t-test.

Results

RV study: 25 of 47 patients in whom conventional (CA) and digital (DA) angiocardiography were performed were included in this study. The reasons for exclusion were two or more premature ventricular contractions (PVC) during CA in 17 patients, precluding adequate opacification of the second postextrasystolic beat; a single PVC during DA in 1 patient, preventing opacification of the trabeculated portion; poor quality of CA and DA in 1 patient, poor position of the injection catheter during CA and DA in 3 patients, preventing opacification of the total RV chamber. No PVCs were observed in 30 DAs and 18 CAs. Two PVCs were noted in 4 DAs and in 5 CAs, and 3 or more noted in 24. The second postextrasystolic beat could be included in 15 (9 CAs and 6 DAs).

Parameters of ventricular geometry are summarized in Table 1. Intra- and interobserver variability for end-diastolic (EDV) and end-systolic (ESV) volumes was excellent, correlation coefficients being slightly higher for EDV. There was no significant difference between DA and CA. For parameters of spatial orientation and shape correlation coefficients were lower but not different for DA and CA. Comparing DA and CA the highest correlation coefficients were observed for EDV and ESV with r = 0.996 and r = 0.990, respectively (Fig. 6), being lower for parameters of spatial orientation and shape. For the ejection fraction there was no significant difference between DA and CA.

LV study: 29 of 54 patients in whom CA and DA were performed were included in this study. The reasons for exclusion were 1 PVC in 9 patients, 2 PVCs in 2 patients and more than 2 PVCs in 14 patients during CA, precluding adequate opacification of the second postextrasystolic beat. DA of 12 of these patients could not be assessed because of 1 PVC in 9 patients, of 2 PVCs in 1 patient and more than 2 PVCs in 2 patients. Poor quality of CA and DA was noted in 5 of these children. No PVC was observed in 16 CAs and 43 DAs. The second postextrasystolic beat could be included in 13 CAs and no DAs. In all DAs including the 20 of 28 children, in whom breathing was not suspended, quantitative assessment was possible.

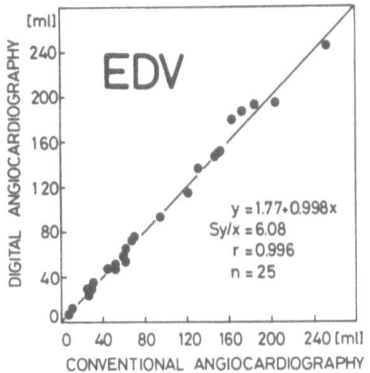 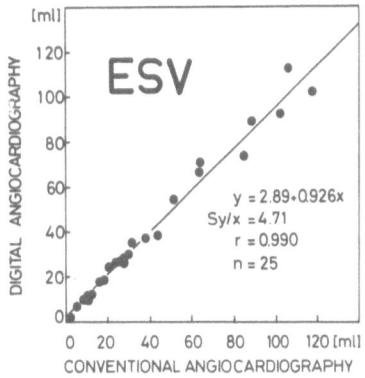

Fig. 6. Relationships of the right ventricular end-diastolic (EDV) and end-systolic (ESV) volume determined with digital and conventional angiocardiography.

Table 1. Right ventricular geometry.

	n	a	b	sy/x	r
Observer A: CA versus DA					
Psi d	25	6.485	0.858	7.674	0.925
Theta d	25	1.962	0.954	2.568	0.904
AX/MD d	25	0.145	0.901	0.051	0.902
EDV	25	− 1.201	1.049	11.030	0.988
Psi s	25	9.308*	0.839*	5.213	0.943
Theta s	25	9.282	0.855	2.471	0.912
AX/MD s	25	0.324	0.794	0.061	0.890
ESV	25	2.594	0.916	7.073	0.977
EF	25	0.141	0.767	0.061	0.781
Observer B: CA versus DA					
Psi d	25	2.300	0.982	7.381	0.911
Theta d	25	7.152	0.892	2.820	0.907
AX/MD d	25	0.169	0.862	0.049	0.907
EDV	25	1.712	0.999	6.114	0.996
Psi s	25	3.199	0.899	6.209	0.975
Theta s	25	4.219	0.936	2.938	0.895
AX/MD s	25	0.329	0.766	0.061	0.863
ESV	25	2.890	0.926	4.711	0.990
EF	25	0.091	0.833	0.042	0.871
Interobserver variability CA: A versus B					
Psi d	25	2.485	0.852	8.493	0.909
Theta d	25	− 3.569	1.029	1.707	0.960
AX/MD d	25	0.204*	0.846*	0.030	0.957
EDV	25	0.380	1.001	5.166	0.997
Psi s	25	3.276	0.860	7.912	0.946
Theta s	25	5.146	0.894	3.545	0.851
AX/MD s	25	0.273	0.798	0.051	0.920
ESV	25	0.516	1.001	3.229	0.996
EF	25	0.060	0.884	0.026	0.959
Interobserver variability DA: A versus B					
Psi d	25	− 3.844	1.055	7.846	0.938
Theta d	25	2.805	0.946	2.634	0.907
AX/MD d	25	0.154	0.867	0.050	0.898
EDV	25	2.132	0.971	5.719	0.997
Psi s	25	− 7.085	1.090	8.070	0.953
Theta s	25	6.893	0.873	3.309	0.847
AX/MD s	25	0.247	0.800	0.053	0.896
ESV	25	1.091	1.014	5.510	0.987
EF	25	0.075	0.843	0.041	0.894

Table 1. Continued.

	n	a	b	sy/x	r
Intraobserver variability CA: B1 versus B2					
Psi d	25	− 8.112	1.164	7.485	0.933
Theta d	25	8.514*	0.868*	1.736	0.959
AX/MD d	25	0.186	0.847	0.047	0.911
EDV	25	1.002	0.980	2.097	0.997
Psi s	25	7.338*	0.763*	7.788	0.948
Theta s	25	− 0.174	0.996	2.506	0.929
AX/MD s	25	0.308	0.767	0.082	0.786
ESV	25	0.239	1.004	2.435	0.998
EF	25	0.002	0.970	0.022	0.971
Intraobserver variability DA: B1 versus B2					
Psi d	25	− 7.009	1.188	7.796	0.939
Theta d	25	7.066	0.884	1.859	0.954
AX/MD d	25	0.142	0.886	0.057	0.874
EDV	25	− 0.782	1.007	2.854	0.999
Psi s	25	4.082	0.910	7.326	0.961
Theta s	25	6.438	0.894	2.051	0.944
AX/MD s	25	0.388	0.718	0.080	0.732
ESV	25	− 0.357	1.027	3.050	0.996
EF	25	− 0.008	1.006	0.031	0.941

Abbreviations: CA: conventional angiocardiography; DA: digital angiocardiography; *significant deviation from the line of identity ($p < 0.01$); d: end-diastole; s: end-systole; psi and theta: angles characterizing the spatial orientation of the long ventricular axis (see also Fig. 2); AX/MD: shape parameter spatial long ventricular axis/mean diameter of a sphere with the ventricular volume; EDV: end-diastolic volume; ESV: end-systolic volume; EF: ejection fraction.

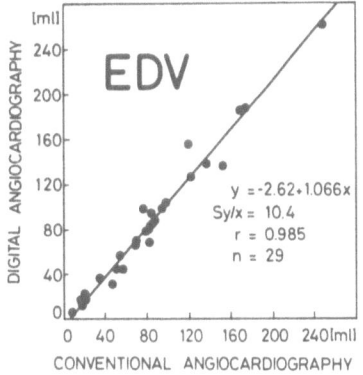
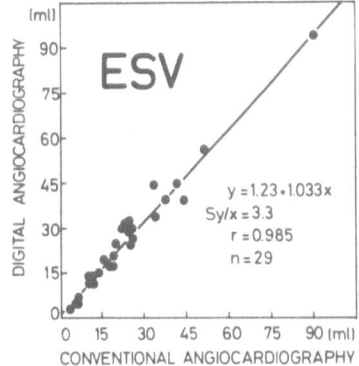

Fig. 7. Relationships of the left ventricular end-diastolic (EDV) and end-systolic (ESV) volume determined with digital and conventional angiocardiography.

Table 2. Left ventricular geometry.

	n	a	b	sy/x	r
Observer A: CA versus DA					
Psi d	29	4.790	0.857	4.479	0.950
Theta d	29	6.596	0.853	3.551	0.960
AX/MD d	29	0.374	0.751	0.094	0.694
EDV	29	− 1.097	1.048	9.197	0.983
Psi s	29	0.660	0.962	5.761	0.992
Theta s	29	4.294	0.912	3.810	0.941
AX/MD s	29	0.122	0.929	0.086	0.909
ESV	29	0.224	1.114	2.710	0.983
EF	29	0.066	0.885	0.044	0.840
Observer B: CA versus DA					
Psi d	29	8.009*	0.739*	5.011	0.925
Theta d	29	7.982	0.826	3.299	0.948
AX/MD d	29	0.601	0.602	0.100	0.593
EDV	29	0.554	1.008	10.340	0.979
Psi s	29	1.025	0.943	5.092	0.929
Theta s	29	4.505	0.908	3.681	0.936
AX/MD s	29	0.132	0.898	0.101	0.876
ESV	29	0.764	1.058	3.351	0.972
EF	29	0.112	0.821	0.036	0.880
Interobserver variability CA: A versus B					
Psi d	29	− 0.524	0.992	3.526	0.975
Theta d	29	2.885	0.971	2.161	0.985
AX/MD d	29	0.354	0.765	0.069	0.798
EDV	29	2.627	0.953	4.441	0.995
Psi s	29	5.375	0.791	6.881	0.853
Teta s	29	4.108	0.939	3.912	0.941
AX/MD s	29	0.001	1.000	0.122	0.857
ESV	29	3.273	0.901	3.735	0.952
EF	29	0.111	0.822	0.035	0.878
Interobserver variability DA: A versus B					
Psi d	29	− 2.124	1.046	5.674	0.934
Theta d	29	4.193	0.949	2.682	0.971
AX/MD d	29	0.316	0.788	0.066	0.839
EDV	29	1.404	0.984	5.550	0.998
Psi s	29	2.606	0.929	3.374	0.971
Theta s	29	7.442	0.847	3.356	0.943
AX/MD s	29	− 0.025	0.978	0.112	0.875
ESV	29	2.476	0.930	3.676	0.965
EF	29	0.157*	0.766*	0.030	0.884

Table 2. Continued.

	n	a	b	sy/x	r
Intraobserver variability CA: B1 versus B2					
Psi d	29	2.812	0.929	3.096	0.980
Theta d	29	− 1.948	1.044	2.267	0.984
AX/MD d	29	0.256	0.835	0.055	0.880
EDV	29	5.079	0.914	5.612	0.992
Psi s	29	0.867	0.930	4.067	0.951
Theta s	29	− 1.642	1.042	2.956	0.967
AX/MD s	29	− 0.119	1.066	0.106	0.900
ESV	29	1.003	0.963	3.102	0.971
EF	29	0.105	0.848	0.027	0.931
Intraobserver variability DA: B1 versus B2					
Psi d	29	− 3.617	1.129	5.325	0.942
Theta d	29	− 2.965	1.075	1.870	0.986
AX/MDd	29	0.189	0.869	0.057	0.884
EDV	29	0.807	0.990	6.076	0.993
Psi s	29	0.067	1.015	2.921	0.979
Theta s	29	1.689	0.949	1.895	0.982
AX/MD s	29	0.029	0.967	0.106	0.888
ESV	29	− 0.394	1.030	2.963	0.980
EF	29	0.083	0.881	0.025	0.934

Abbreviations: See Table 1.

Parameters of ventricular geometry are summarized in Table 2. Intra- and interobserver variability for EDV and ESV was excellent, correlation coefficient being slightly higher for EDV. There was no significant difference between DA and CA. For parameters of spatial orientation and shape correlation coefficients were higher but not different for DA and CA. Comparing DA and CA the highest correlation coefficients were observed for EDV and ESV with $r = 0.979$ and $r = 0.972$, respectively (Fig. 7), being lower for parameters of spatial orientaton and shape. For the ejection fraction there were no significant difference between DA and CA.

Discussion

For the quantitative evaluation of left and right ventricular size and function by digital angiocardiography contrast medium has been injected into peripheral [1] and central [2–4, 8–10, 14] veins as well as into the left [7, 15–17] and right [5] ventricle, preferably utilizing a power injector [1–10, 14–17]. This means that digital angiocardiography for quantitation of ventricular geometry, as it is used today, is not a noninvasive technique.

In most instances an ECG-gated mask mode direct video subtraction technique was used [1–6, 9, 10, 15–17], rarely the time-interval difference mode [8, 14] and seldom a combination of film and video [7, 8, 14]. Studies in adults were performed during held inspiration to prevent motion artefacts [1–3, 7–10, 14–16] while in most children a normal respiration had to be accepted [5, 17]. To minimize such motion artefacts we selected for background subtraction a cardiac cycle at a diaphragmatic level similar to the best opacified cycle of the ventricular filling phase, utilizing the end-diastolic and end-systolic frame as well as the preceding and the following frames (Fig. 1).

For the assessment of the accuracy with which ventricular geometry can be quantitated by digital angiocardiography in a clinical setting conventional angiocardiography remains the gold standard. One has to be aware, however, that it does not provide true reference values for comparison; it is a biological method with its own limitations [12, 13].

For digital as well as conventional angiocardiography the input information available for analysis are manually [1–6, 8–10, 14–19] and rarely automatically [7] traced mono- [1–4, 7–10, 14–16] and biplane [5, 6, 17] ventricular projections. In addition, we mark manually anatomic landmarks [11, 19] which allow the determination of the spatial orientation of ventricular axes as well as certain shape and muscle volume parameters [18].

Reproducibility of left ventricular border recognition is excellent for digital angiocardiography. Intra- and interobserver variability do not differ from that of conventional angiocardiography (Table 2), being in accordance with the reported interobserver variability in adult patients [3, 4, 14]. Surprisingly, the results are similar for the geometrically complex right ventricle (Table 1).

The low statistical as well as systematic error, comparing end-diastolic and end-systolic volumes gained by digital and conventional angiocardiography (Fig. 7; Table 2), indicate accurate tracing of left ventricular borders. In contrast to other authors who found a somewhat lower accuracy for the basilar regions in adults [2, 10] the error was not significantly different for the selected regions in infants and children (Fig. 4). Surprising is again the high accuracy with which the borders of the right ventricle with the morphologically quite different compartments inflow and outflow tract as well as trabeculated portion can be recognized globally and also regionally (Figs. 5, 6; Table 1). The somewhat lower correlation coefficients for the left and right ventricular ejection fraction in infants and children (Tables 1, 2) as compared to the left ventricular one in adult patients [1–3, 9, 14, 15] is probably related to the larger range of values in adult patients with impaired myocardial function in some.

Anatomic landmarks are more difficult to define with digital angiocardiography. Landmark dependent parameters like angles characterizing ventricular spatial orientation [19] and shape parameters [18] of the left and right ventricle do not correlate as well with those determined on the basis of conventional angiocardiography (Table 1, 2). It is probably due to the lack of morphologic detail in a single digitized frame. Superimposition of an original frame – as the new equipment allows – should improve results.

Digital angiocardiography has several advantages. First, the amount of contrast medium can be reduced considerably. Thirty per cent for right and 35% for left ventricular injection of the amount used for conventional angiocardiography was required to obtain adequate visualization of posterior-anterior and lateral projections. Confirming the results for the left ventricle in adult patients [7, 15] it is especially important for small babies with complex heart defects, since hemodynamic and toxic side effects of the contrast medium will be diminished [20]. For the visualization of the left ventricle after peripheral and central vein injection, however, the amount of contrast medium could not be decreased [1–4, 8–10, 14].

A second advantage of the technique is that only about 50% of the flow rate used for conventional angiocardiography was necessary for right and left ventricular injection. Both the reduction of the amount of contrast medium and flow rate decrease recoil of the injection catheter, which is probably why digital angiocardiography results in a considerably lower incidence of ventricular ectopic activity. No premature ventricular contractions were observed in 64% of the digital and 38% of conventional angiocardiography after right ventricular injection as well as 80% and 20%, respectively after left ventricular injection. Also, more than 2 premature ventricular contractions were rare in digital and common in conventional angiocardiography.

The X-ray energy necessary for digital angiocardiography has rarely been addressed explicitly in the literature [21]. It seems, however, that it is at least as high for conventional angiocardiography, especially after peripheral injection for the visualization of the left ventricle with its rather long X-ray series. The X-ray energy level to which our infants and children were exposed is somewhat lower than that used for conventional angiocardiography. The exact amount of reduction, however, is difficult to assess, because both kilovoltage and milliamperage were altered. Because the dose at the intensifier input screen was reduced to 40% and since th X-ray series were 1.3 seconds shorter for digital angiocardiography, it appears justified to assume a considerable dose reduction. It could be reduced further, because for the utilized off-line digitization the signal-to-noise ratio is mainly determined by the video cameras and the tape recorder.

Thus, after ventricular injection digital angiocardiography for the quantitative assessment of left and right ventricular geometry enables the utilization of multiple injections during he monitoring of physiological and potential therapeutic interventions.

84

Summary

To analyze the value of digital angiocardiogaphy (DA) for the quantitative assessment of dynamic ventricular geometry after the injection of a small amount of contrast medium parameters of left (LV) and right ventricular (RV) spatial orientation, size, shape, and function were determined on the basis of manually marked biplane ventricular projections and anatomic landmarks after the injection of 0.28 ml/kg body weight at a rate of 8.10 ml/s into LV (n = 29) and 0.29 ml/kg at 7.40 ml/s into RV (n = 25) and compared to those gained on the basis of conventional angiocardiography (CA) after the injection of 0.78 ml/kg at 15.62 ml/s into LV and 0.97 ml/kg at 13.70 ml/s in infants and children with various congenital heart diseases undergoing routine diagnostic cardiac catheterization. No premature ventricular contractions (PVC) were observed in 64% of DA and 38% of CA after RV injection as well as 80% and 29% respectively after LV injection. More than 2 PVCs were rare in DA and common in CA. The X-ray energy for DA was considerably reduced compared to CA. Intra- and interobserver variability of LV as well as RV border and anatomic landmark recognition in DA and CA did not differ. The highest correlation without systematic error between DA and CA was observed for end-diastolic and end-systolic volumes with correlation coefficients of $r = 0.985$ and 0.985 for LV as well as 0.996 and 0.990 for RV, respectively. Ventricular spatial orientation and shape, that is parameters dependent on the accuracy of locating anatomic landmarks, correlated less well for LV and RV with correlation coefficients between 0.593 and 0.975. Comparing the accuracy of regional border recognition there was no significant difference between the selected regions, neither for LV nor RV.

Digital angiocardiography after ventricular injection allows the accurate determination of left and right ventricular dynamic geometry, especially that of volume parameters. Advantages are the reduction of contrast medium, injection flow, X-ray energy, and ventricular ectopy, thus permitting the utilization of multiple injections during the monitoring of physiological and potential therapeutic interventions. It is, however, an invasive method.

Acknowledgement

The authors thank Isa Schulze Brexel, Ines Fey, and Traudel Hansen for continuous invaluable assistance.

References

1. Tobis J, Nacioglu O, Johnston WD, Seibert A, Iseri LT, Roeck W, Elkayam U, Henry WL: Left ventricular imaging with digital subtraction angiography using intravenous contrast injection and fluoroscopic exposure levels. Am Heart J 1982; 104: 20–27.
2. Kronenberg MW, Price RR, Smith CW, Robertson RM, Perry JM, Pickens DR, Domanski MJ, Partain CL, Friesinger GC: Evaluation of left ventricular performance using digital subtraction angiography. Am J Cardiol 1983; 51: 837–842.
3. Nissen SE, Booth D, Waters J, Fassas T, DeMaria AN: Evaluation of left ventricular contractile pattern by intravenous digital subtraction ventriculography: Comparison with cineangiography and assessment of interobserver variability. Am J Cardiol 1983; 52: 1293–1298.
4. Norris SL Slutsky RA, Mancini GBJ, Ashburn WL, Gregoratos G, Peterson KL, Higgins CB, Einsidler E, Dillon W: Comparison of digital intravenous ventriculography with direct left ventriculography for quantitation of left ventricular volumes and ejection fractions. Am J Cardiol 1983; 51:1399–1403.
5. Lange PE, Budach W, Radtke W, Onnasch DGW, Heintzen PH: Right ventricular imaging with digital subtraction using intraventricular contrast injection. Am J Cardiol 1984; 54: 839–842.
6. Brennecke R, Brown TK, Bürsch JH, Heintzen PH: Computerized video-image preprocessing with applications to cardio-angiographic roentgen-image series. In: Nagel HH (ed) Digital image processing; pp 244–262. Springer, Berlin/Heidelberg/New York, 1977.
7. Sasayama S, Nonogi H, Kawai C, Fujita M, Eiho S, Kuwahara M: Automated method for left ventricular volume measurement by cineventriculography with minimal doses of contrast medium. Am J Cardiol 1981; 48: 746–753.
8. Lauber A, Fischbach T, Jehle J, Pölitz B, Schmiel FK, Spiller P, Loogen F: Digitale Subtraktionsangiokardiographie: Genauigkeit der linksventrikulären Volumenbestimmung bei intravenöser Kontrastmittelinjektion. Z Kardiol 1983; 72: 262–267.
9. Goldberg HL, Borer JS, Moses JW, Fisher J, Cohen B, Skelly NT: Digital subtraction intravenous left ventricular angiography: comparison with conventional intraventricular angiography. J Am Coll Cardiol 1983; 1: 858–862.
10. Mancini GBJ, Norris SL, Peterson KL, Gregoratos G, Widmann TF, Ashurn Wl, Higgins CB: Quantitative assessment of segmental wall motion abnormalities at rest and after atrial pacing using digital intravenous ventriculography. JACC 1983; 2: 70–76.
11. Onnasch DGW, Malerczyk V, Pilarczyk J, Lange PE, Heintzen PH: A system for acquisition, documentation, and analysis of manually outlined ventricular angiograms. In: Heintzen PH, Bürsch JH (eds) Roentgen-video-techniques; pp 139–145. Thieme Verlag, Stuttgart, 1978.
12. Lange PE, Onnasch DGW, Farr F, Heintzen PH: Angiocardiographic left ventricular volume determination. Accuracy, as determined from human casts, and clinical application. Eur J Cardiol 1978; 8: 449–476.
13. Lange PE, Onnasch DGW, Farr F, Heintzen PH: Angiocardiographic right ventricular volume determination. Accuracy, as determined from human casts, and clinical application. Eur J Cardiol 1978; 8: 477–501.
14. Birchler B, Hess OM, Murakami T, Niederer MP, Anliker M, Krayenbühl HP: Comparison of intravenous digital subtraction cineangiocardiography with conventional contrast ventriculography for the determination of the left ventricular volume at rest and during exercise. Eur Heart J 1985; 6: 497–509.
15. Nichols AB, Martin EC, Fles TP, Stugensky KM, Balancio LA, Casarella WJ, Weiss MB: Validation of the angiographic accuracy of digital left ventriculography. Am J Cardiol 1983; 51: 224–230.

16. Tobis J, Iseri LT, Johnston WD, Nalcioglu O, De Boer C, Shah A, Paynter J, Henry WL: Determination of the optimal timing for performing digital ventriculography during atrial pacing stress test in coronary heart disease. Am J Cardiol 1985; 56: 426–433.

17. Lange PE, Ewert B, Radtke W, Hahne HJ, Onnasch DGW, Heintzen PH: Angiocardiographic volume determination of the left ventricle in children. Value of digital subtraction techniques after selective injection. In: Doyle EF, Engle MA, Gersony WM, Rashkind WJ, Talner NS (eds) Pediatric cardiology; pp 312–315. Springer Verlag, New York, 1986.

18. Lange PE: Clinical relevance of video-angiocardiometry in the pediatric age group. Herz 1985; 4: 238–247.

19. Lange PE, Onnasch DGW, Schaupp GH, Zill C, Heintzen PH: Roentgenanatomic determination of left and right ventricular spatial orientation in congenital heart disease. In: Just HJ, Heintzen PH (eds) Angiocardiography – current status and future developments; pp 120–128. Springer Verlag, Berlin/Heidelberg, 1986.

20. Lange PE, Neubert D, Onnasch DGW, Sievers HH, Heintzen PH: Effects of angiocardiographic contrast media on the pulmonary circulation in pigs. Am J Cardiol 1984; 54: 1125–1130.

21. Vas R, Diamond GA, Forrester JS, Whiting S, Swan HJC: Computer enhancement of direct and venous-injected left ventricular contrast angiography. Am Heart J 1981; 102: 719–728.

9. Accuracy of Digital Subtraction Angiocardiography for the Assessment of Global and Regional Left Ventricular Function at Rest and during Exercise*

OTTO M. HESS, DANIEL GROB, JÖRG GRIMM, BERNHARD
BIRCHLER, PETER NIEDERER & HANS P. KRAYENBÜHL
*Medical Policlinic, Cardiology, University Hospital, and Institute of Biomedical Engineering,
University and Federal Institute of Technology, Zürich, Switzerland*

Introduction

Left ventricular function is an important determinant for prognosis and post-operative outcome of patients with severe coronary or valvular heart disease. Digital subtraction angiocardiography is a semi-invasive technique with a high temporal and spatial resolution which allows the assessment of left ventricular function from the measurements of volumetric parameters at rest and also during supine exercise [1–4]. Due to the fact that contrast dye is injected into a peripheral vein, this technique is less invasive and more convenient for the patient than conventional left ventricular angiocardiography. Most authors [1, 2, 4] have used on-line video recordings for data acquisition; since temporal and spatial resolution of the video system can be a limiting factor especially under exercise conditions at high heart rates, digital subtraction angiocardiography based on cinefilm as data carrier was evaluated for assessing global and regional left ventricular function in 30 patients.

Patients and methods

Thirty patients with a mean age of 52 years were included in the present study. Twenty-six of the 30 patients had coronary artery disease and 4 had normal coronary arteries. Twenty of the 30 patients were studied at rest and 10 patients during supine bicycle exercise.

Study protocol

First conventional left ventricular angiocardiography (LVA) was performed in the right anterior oblique projection (RAO) with injection of 45 ml Urogra-

* This study was supported by a grant of the EMDO foundation, Zürich.

P.H. Heintzen and J.H. Bürsch (eds), Progress in Digital Angiocardiography. ISBN 978-94-010-7093-5

phin 76% at a flow rate of 12 ml/s. The angiocardiogram was recorded on cinefilm at a rate of 50 frames/s. After the conventional angiocardiogram was carried out, an interval of 15 minutes was allowed for dissipation of the hemodynamic effects of the contrast medium. Then, a second injection of 45 ml Urographin 76% at a flow rate of 15 ml/s was performed into the superior vena cava. The entire sequence starting one or two heart cycles before the injection and ending after the contrast medium had passed through the left ventricle was recorded on cinefilm at a rate of 50 frames/s. During the passage of the contrast medium the patients were asked to stop breathing to avoid misregistration.

Ten patients were studied during supine bicycle exercise at a mean workload of 64 watts for 2 minutes. The exercise test was carried out at a low workload because it had to be performed twice. Conventional angiocardiography was carried out at the end of the exercise test with injection of 60 ml Urographin 76% at a flow rate of 16 to 18 ml/s. After an interval of 15 minutes the exercise test was repeated at the same workload and duration; then, 60 ml Urographin 76% were injected at a flow rate of 16 to 18 ml/s into the superior vena cava.

Digital image processing

The cinefilm was scanned on a computer-assisted (VAX 750) image processing system with a modified film projector Vanguard XR-35 and a high resolution photodiode camera (Eikonix 78/99). The observer entered the frame numbers of the cinefilm at the computer terminal. The cinefilm was then automatically positioned on the projector at the desired cineframe. The image was digitized, stored on disk, averaged and subtracted on the DeAnza image processor (IP 8500). After subtraction, the image was linearly amplified to extend the brightness over the whole dynamic range of the image processing system [3].

Three different subtraction modes were tested: *mask mode subtraction* (MMS): two to four images were averaged and a mask from the beginning or the end of the film sequence was subtracted. *Time interval difference subtraction* (TID): one cineframe during the passage of the contrast medium through the left ventricle was digitized and a mask 60 to 100 ms before or after the digitized cineframe was subtracted (Fig. 1). *MMS and TID subtraction* (MMS + TID): as a new technique a combined subtraction mode with sequential superposition of MMS and TID subtracted images was used. The combination of both subtraction modes allowed to take advantage of the relative imaging strengths of each method, i.e. the MMS image detects slowly moving parts of the left ventricle, whereas the TID image detects rapidly moving parts of the left ventricular wall (Fig. 1).

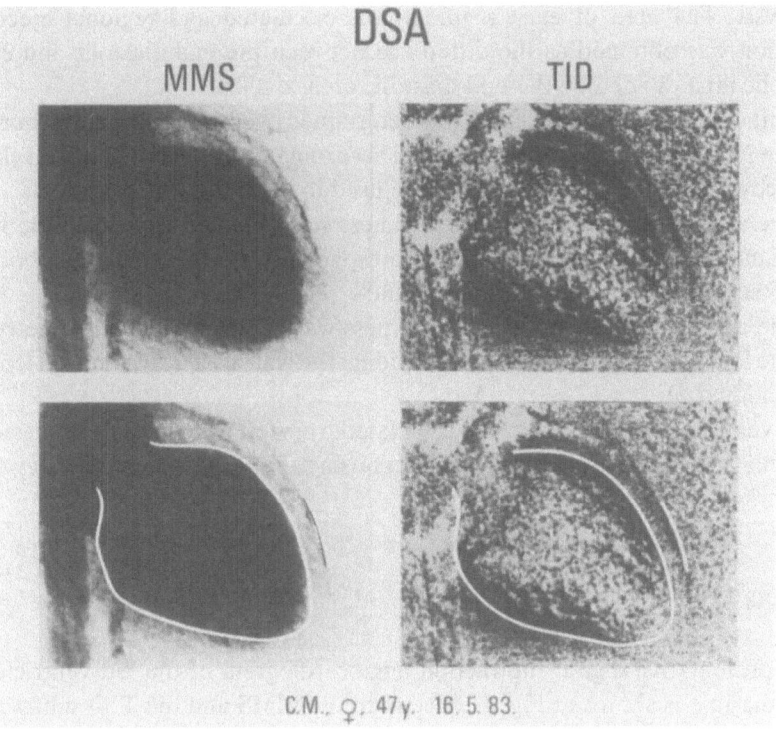

Fig. 1. Digital subtraction angiocardiogram in a patient with normal left ventricular function. The left ventricular angiogram at end-diastole is shown after mask mode (MMS; left hand panel) and time interval difference (TID; right hand panel) subtraction. The upper panels show the subtracted images as they are displayed on the video monitor and the lower panels after completion of contour detection. Left ventricular wall thickness can be delineated easily in both MMS and TID subtracted images over the anterolateral border of the left ventricle.

Contour detection and quantitative analysis

The left ventricular silhouette was outlined by a semi-automatic system which allowed to select boundary points either in the MMS or the TID mode using a 'mouse' controlled cursor. Individual points were connected by a spline function [3]. Usually a set of 10 to 15 points resulted in an acceptable definition of the left ventricular contour. Then left ventricular volume and ejection fraction were calculated using the 'area-length' method [5] for volume calculation.

Regional ejection fraction was determined using a radial axis system with a reference point in the center of the left ventricular long axis from the aorto-mitral junction to the apex [3]. There superior and 3 inferior regions were defined using this reference point and dividing the superior and inferior part of the left ventricle in 3 equal segments excluding the aortic valve area from the analysis. The area of each segment was calculated and regional ejection fraction was obtained as the difference between the end-diastolic and end-systolic area divided by the end-diastolic area $\times$ 100.

Left ventricular wall thickness was determined over the anterolateral border of the left ventricle in RAO projection according to the technique of Rackley and coworkers [6]. Two methods were used to calculate wall thickness:

1. the average end-diastolic wall thickness was obtained from multiple wall diameters which were inscribed orthogonally to the epicardial border (Rackley's technique; method 1), and

2. the average end-diastolic wall thickness was determined by planimetry of the left ventricular wall segment dividing the wall area by its midwall length (method 2).

Left ventricular muscle mass was calculated from left ventricular end-diastolic volume and end-diastolic wall thickness using the technique of Rackley and coworkers [6].

Results

A representative digital subtraction angiocardiogram of the left ventricle at end-diastole is shown in Fig. 1. Given are the MMS and the TID subtracted images in the RAO projection. Left ventricular wall thickness can be identified over the anterolateral border of the left ventricle. The left ventricular contour and wall thickness are inscribed in the lower two panels for the MMS and TID subtracted image. Best results were obtained with the combined subtraction mode (MMS + TID); only these results are reported in the present analysis.

Global left ventricular function parameters (Table 1 and Fig. 2)

There is a close correlation between conventional and digital subtraction angiocardiography for left ventricular end-diastolic and end-systolic volume as well as for left ventricular ejection fraction at rest and during exercise. The standard error of estimate of the mean LVA value was, however, slightly larger for the end-systolic than end-diastolic volume but was similar for the end-systolic volume and ejection fraction. Both observers had similar correlation coefficients and standard errors of estimate.

Regional left ventricular function parameters (Table 1 and Fig. 3)

There was a reasonably good correlation between conventional and digital subtraction angiocardiography for regional ejection fraction of the 3 superior and 3 inferior left ventricular regions at rest. However, the standard error of estimate was 27% of the mean LVA value for the 3 superior and 35% for the 3 inferior regions. During exercise the correlation coefficient remained good for the 3 superior regions but decreased from 0.74 at rest to 0.50 during exercise for the 3 inferior regions. The standard error of estimate amounted to 30% of the mean LVA value for the 3 superior and to 37% for the 3 inferior regions.

Left ventricular wall thickness and muscle mass (Table 1 and Fig. 4)

Both methods for left ventricular wall thickness and muscle mass determination showed good correlation coefficients between conventional and digital subtraction angiocardiography for data at rest and during exercise. Method 2 (planimetry) tended to have smaller standard errors of estimate than method 1 for both wall thickness and muscle mass. Exercise and resting data were similar and both observers had comparable correlation coefficients and standard errors of estimate.

Table 1. Correlation coefficients (r) and standard errors of estimate of the mean (SEE) for 20 patients at rest and 10 patients during exercise. The comparison is carried out between conventional and digital subtraction angiocardiography for LV end-diastolic (EDV; ml) and end-systolic volume (ESV; ml), LV ejection fraction (EF; %), regional ejection fraction (REF; %) of 3 superior (sup) and 3 inferior (inf) LV wall regions, LV wall thickness (Wth; cm) and LV muscle mass (LMM; g). All data are given for two observers (Ob1 and Ob2). LV wall thickness and muscle mass were determined by 2 methods: method 1 refers to the traditional Rackley technique and method 2 uses planimetry to obtain an average end-diastolic wall thickness (for further explanations see text). LV = left ventricular.

		EDV	ESV	EF	REF_{sup}	REF_{inf}	Wth_1	Wth_2	LMM_1	LMM_2
Rest										
n		20	20	20	60	60	17	17	17	17
r	Ob1	0.92	0.95	0.91	0.82	0.74	0.79	0.80	0.85	0.83
	Ob2	0.92	0.98	0.96	–	–	0.83	0.76	0.91	0.84
SEE	Ob1	10	18	12	27	35	13	9	16	12
	Ob2	10	11	8	–	–	9	9	11	11
Exercise										
n		10	10	10	30	30	7	7	7	7
r	Ob1	0.91	0.95	0.94	0.84	0.50	0.86	0.85	0.93	0.93
	Ob2	0.93	0.95	0.92	–	–	0.66	0.76	0.77	0.80
SEE	Ob1	10	13	13	30	37	8	6	11	7
	Ob2	8	13	13	–	–	13	9	17	13

LV VOLUME AND EJECTION FRACTION

REST

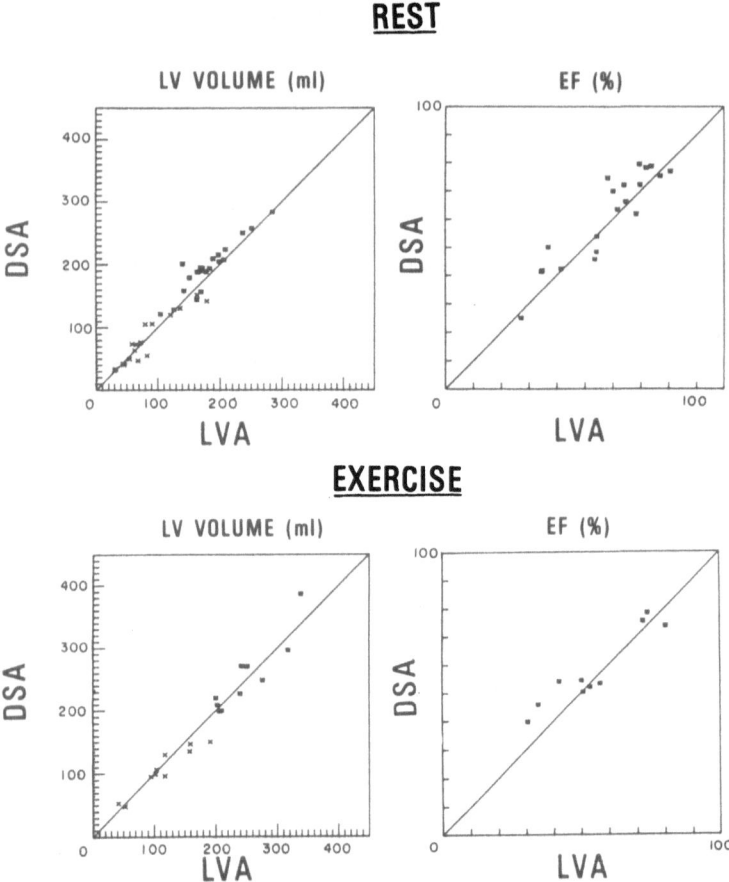

Fig. 2. Left ventricular (LV) volumes and ejection fraction at rest (upper panels) and during supine bicycle exercise (lower panels). The comparison between conventional (LVA) and digital subtraction angiocardiography (DSA) is shown for end-diastolic and end-systolic volumes (left hand panels) and for ejection fraction (EF; right hand panels). Both left ventricular volumes and ejection fraction show a good correlation between conventional and digital subtraction angiocardiography at rest and during exercise. For correlation coefficients and standard errors of estimate see Table 1.

REGIONAL EJECTION FRACTION
REST

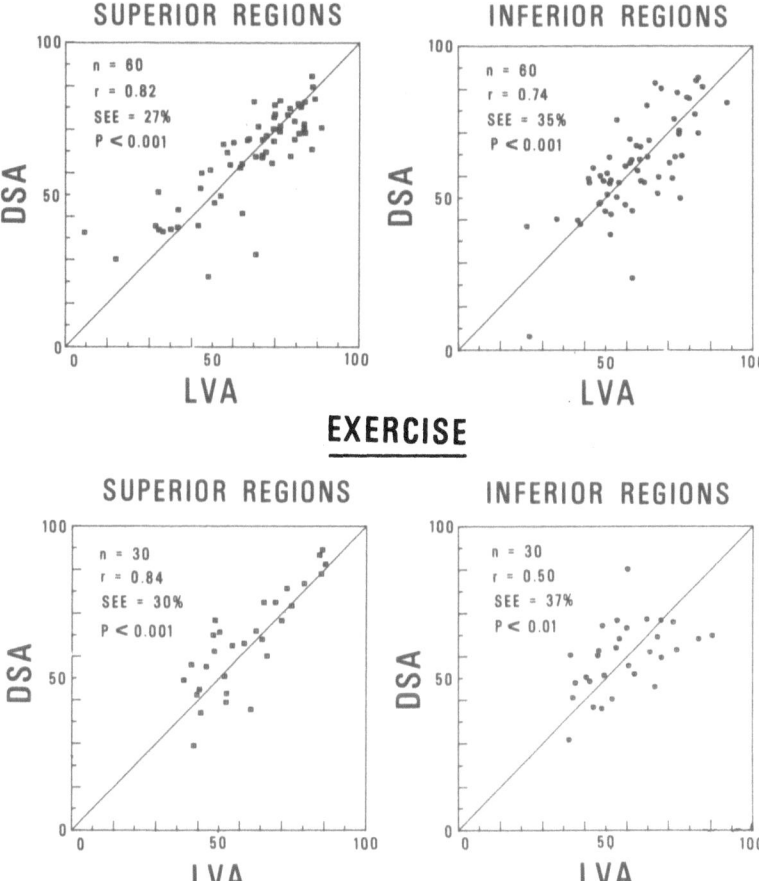

Fig. 3. Left ventricular regional ejection fraction at rest (upper panels) and during exercise (lower panels). The comparison between conventional (LVA) and digital subtraction angiocardiography (DSA) is shown for the 3 superior (left hand panels) and the 3 inferior (right hand panels) regions. The correlation between the two techniques is good for the 3 superior and 3 inferior regions at rest although the standard error of estimate of the mean LVA value is large for all regions. During exercise the correlation remains good for the 3 superior regions but is poor for the 3 inferior regions; the standard error of estimate of the mean LVA value is ≥ 30% for both superior and inferior regions during exercise. For correlation coefficients and standard errors of estimate see Table 1.

WALL THICKNESS AND MUSCLE MASS

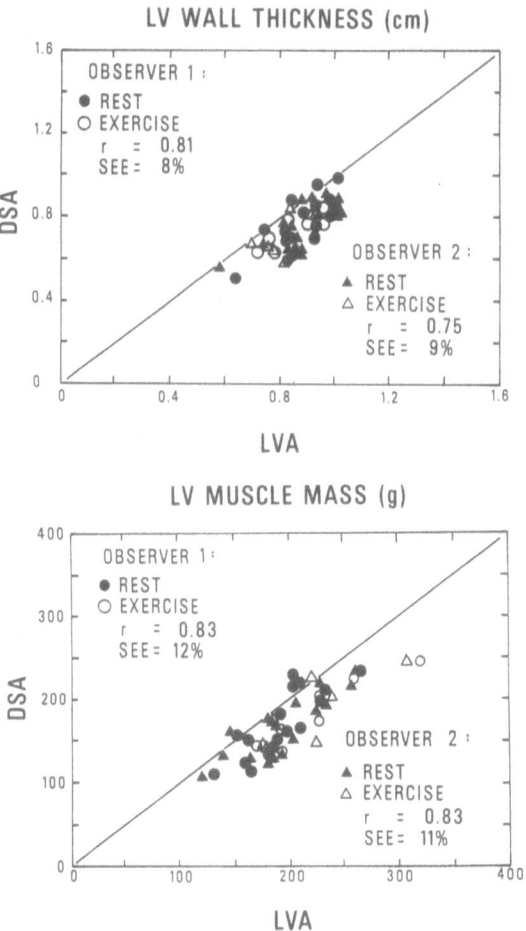

Fig. 4. Left ventricular (LV) end-diastolic wall thickness (upper panel) and muscle mass (lower panel) for data at rest (n = 17; closed symbols) and during exercise (n = 7; open symbols). Results of both observers (observer 1: circles; observer 2: triangles) are reported using method 2 (left ventricular wall thickness is determined by planimetry). The comparison between conventional (LVA) and digital subtraction angiocardiography (DSA) is shown for end-diastolic wall thickness and muscle mass. Correlation coefficients (r) and standard errors of estimate of the mean LVA value (SEE) are good although the standard error is larger for muscle mass than wall thickness.

Discussion

Digital subtraction angiocardiography is a reliable tool for the assessment of global left ventricular function at rest [1–3] and during supine exercise [3, 4]. Due to the semi-invasive nature of this technique digital subtraction angiocardiography has been used in ambulatory patients to study left ventricular function at rest and during exercise e.g., several years after aortic valve replacement [7]. The purpose of the present study was to evaluate the accuracy of digital subtraction angiocardiography for the assessment of global and regional left ventricular function as well as for the determination of left ventricular wall thickness and muscle mass. Conventional left ventricular angiocardiography was used as the reference method since both techniques are very similar in regard to data acquisition and data analysis. Digital subtraction angiocardiography was carried out with injection of contrast medium into the superior vena cava. Three different subtraction modes were used for quantitative analysis: mask mode subtraction, time interval difference subtraction and the combination of both subtraction modes were evaluated. The best results were obtained with the combined subtraction mode as it has been pointed out previously [3]. It is not surprising that a subtraction mode which relies on two different methods is better than a subtraction mode which relies only on one of the two methods. Thus, data are reported in the present study which were obtained by a combined subtraction mode using mask mode and time interval difference subtraction.

Cinefilm was used as a data carrier due to its high temporal and spatial resolution which is especially important under exercise conditions at high heart rates. Another advantage of cinefilm is related to its low cost and its simple and easy storage and re-analysis. In the literature, most authors have used video-recordings [1, 2, 4] due to its easy data acquisition directly from the image intensifier without the need for a photodiode camera (for digitization) and the possibility for on-line recordings and on-line data analysis.

The present evaluation of digital subtraction angiocardiography shows that this imaging technique is a reliable tool for the assessment of global left ventricular function not only at rest but also under exercise conditions. The assessment of regional left ventricular function is, however, associated with considerable variations especially during exercise. The correlation coefficient between conventional and digital subtraction angiocardiography was reasonably good for regional ejection fraction of the 3 superior regions at rest and during exercise but the standard error of estimate was in the range of 27 to 30% of the mean LVA value. The correlation coefficient was low for regional ejection fraction of the 3 inferior regions during exercise (Table 1) with a standard error of estimate of 37% of the mean LVA value. It is generally accepted that a reliable technique for the assessment of cardiac dimensions and shortening parameters should be associated with a standard error of estimate of the mean smaller than or equal to 10%. For example when left ventricuar end-diastolic volume is 150 ml and left ventricular ejection fraction 50%, the technique with a standard error of estimate of 10% measures left ventricular end-diastolic volume between 135 and 165 ml and left ventricular ejection fraction between 45 and 55%. A standard error of estimate of less than 10% is in the present study only fulfilled for the assessment of left ventricular end-diastolic volume and left ventricular wall thickness using method 2. The assessment of left ventricular ejection fraction and left ventricular muscle mass is associated with a slightly larger standard error of estimate than 10%. In contrast, the standard error of estimate of the mean is considerably larger than 10% for the assessment of systolic area reduction parameters of either region (superior or inferior) suggesting that these regional parameters can be estimated only with limitations using digital subtraction angiocardiography. The poor results for the inferior regions are clearly related to the superposition of the left ventricle and the diaphragm. Furthermore, it has to be realized that these regional function parameters are associated with considerable variations even in true normals [8]; mean standard deviation of the 3 superior regional ejection fraction amounted to 17% of the mean superior ejection fraction and to 20% of the mean inferior regional ejection fraction [8].

Left ventricular end-diastolic wall thickness can be determined with good accuracy by digital subtraction angiocardiography not only at rest but also during exercise. Method 2 which is based on the determination of left ventricular wall thickness by planimetry showed slightly better results than method 1 which is based on the original Rackley technique [6]. In some patients detection of left ventricular wall thickness was even easier in the subtracted images than in the conventional angiograms due to the fact that the epicardial border of the wall can be identified much better in the TID subtracted image than in the plain angiogram (Fig. 1).

In summary, we can conclude that digital subtraction angiocardiography is an accurate technique for the assessment of global left ventricular function not only at rest but also under exercise conditions. It must be realized, however, that regional left ventricular function can be evaluated only with limitations by digital subtraction angiocardiography due to the relatively large standard error of estimate. Left ventricular end-diastolic wall thickness and muscle mass can be determined accurately by digital subtraction angiocardiography due to the high resolution of the background subtracted images over the anterolateral border of the left ventricle.

Summary

The accuracy of digital subtraction angiocardiography (DSA) has been evaluated in 20 patients at rest and 10 during supine bicycle exercise for the assessment of left ventricular (LV) global and regional function. Conventional LV angiocardiography (LVA) served as the reference method and was carried out first. After a pause of 15 minutes DSA was performed with an injection of contrast medium into the superior vena cava. Both LVA and DSA were performed in the right anterior oblique (RA) projection using cinefilm as data carrier (50 frames/s). *Global* LV function was assessed from LV end-diastolic and end-systolic volume and LV ejection fraction. *Regional* LV function was evaluated from regional ejection fraction of 3 superior and 3 inferior LV regions defined by a radial axis system. *LV wall thickness* and *muscle mass* were determined according to the technique of Rackley and coworkers using two different methods.

Global LV function parameters showed excellent correlations between LVA and DSA (correlation coefficient $r \geq 0.91$ for end-diastolic volume, $r \geq 0.95$ for end-systolic volume and $r \geq 0.91$ for LV ejection fraction) at rest and during exercise. *Regional* LV function parameters showed good correlations between LVA and DSA for the 3 superior regions ($r \geq 0.82$ for regional ejection fraction) at rest and during exercise but only moderate correlations for the 3 inferior regions at rest ($r = 0.74$ for regional ejection fraction) and during exercise ($r = 0.50$). The standard error of estimate was considerably larger for regional ($\leq 37\%$ of mean LVA value) than for global LV function parameters ($\leq 18\%$ of mean LVA value). *LV wall thickness* and *muscle mass* showed good correlations between LVA and DSA at rest ($r \geq 0.76$ for wall thickness and $r \geq 0.83$ for muscle mass) and during exercise ($r \geq 0.66$ for wall thickness and $r \geq 0.77$ for muscle mass) with a standard error of estimate $\leq 17\%$ of mean LVA value. The standard error of estimate tended to be smaller for method 2 than 1.

It is concluded that digital subtraction angiocardiography is an accurate technique for the assessment of global LV function at rest but also during exercise. Regional LV funtion cannot be assessed reliably although correlation coefficients are satisfactory for regional ejection fraction of the superior regions but the standard error of estimate is larger than 20% of the mean LVA value. LV wall thickness and muscle mass are determined accurately by DSA.

References

1. Heintzen PH, Brennecke R, Bürsch JH: Computerized videoangiocardiography. In: Kaltenbach M, Lichtlen P, Balcon R, Bussmann WD (eds). Coronary heart disease; p. 116. Thieme Verlag, Stuttgart/New York, 1978.
2. Norris SL, Slutsky RA, Mancini J, Ashburn WL, Gregoratos G, Peterson KL, Higgins CB: Comparison of digital intravenous ventriculography with direct left ventriculography for quantitation of left ventricular volumes and ejection fractions. Am J Cardiol 1983; 51: 1399.
3. Birchler B, Hess OM, Murakami T, Niederer P, Anliker M, Krayenbühl HP: Comparison of intravenous digital subtraction cineangiocardiography with conventional ventriculography for the determination of left ventricular volume at rest and during exercise. Eur Heart J 1985; 6: 497.
4. Spiller P, Fischbach T, Jehle J, Lauber A, Pölitz B, Schmiel FK, Loogen F: Zuverlässigkeit der digitalen Subtraktionsangiographie zur Beurteilung der linksventrikulären Funktion unter körperlicher Belastung. Z Kardiol 1983; 72: 681.
5. Dodge HT, Sandler H, Baxley WA, Hawley RR: Usefulness and limitations of radiographic methods for determining left ventricular volume. Am J Cardiol 1966; 18: 10.
6. Rackley CE, Dodge HT, Coble YD, Hay RE: A method for determining left ventricular mass in man. Circulation 1964; 29: 666.
7. Monrad ES, Hess OM, Corin WD, Krayenbühl HP: Abnormal exercise hemodynamics late after aortic valve replacement (Abstract). Circulation (Suppl II) 1986;74: II–398.
8. Thüring Ch, Hess OM, Murakami T, Grimm J, Krayenbühl HP: Normwerte der linksventrikulären Funktion mittels biplaner Angiokardiographie. In preparation.

10. Assessment of Synchronism of Left Ventricular Wall Motion

P.-A. DORIOT, J.P. MELCHIOR, P. CHATELAIN &
W. RUTISHAUSER
Cardiology Center, University Hospital, Geneva, Switzerland

Introduction

Experienced cardiologists reviewing the RAO 30/ left ventricular angiogram of a patient will usually agree on normality or abnormality of the contraction/ relaxation pattern, and on the location of the abnormality if present. Thus, angiographic sequences really contain information allowing for an objective discrimination between normal and abnormal wall-motion. A great variety of quantification models have already been proposed to this purpose [1]. This, and the fact that consensus is still not obtained indicates that designing the most adequate model is not easy [2, 3]. Stating that each model has advantages, or deciding arbitrarily that realignment of the LV silhouettes is not worthy to be further investigated, may not be the right way to solve the problem. On the contrary, progress should still be achievable by improving basic concepts. The results presented in this contribution may be a step in this direction. They do not demonstrate the superiority of our model over existing ones since no cross-comparisons were performed. Our goal was rather to investigate with a new approach the old debated, but nevertheless important point: should the silhouettes of the left ventricle (LV) be realigned in order to compensate for the translation and rotation of the LV relatively to the imaging system, or should a good model include these 2 motion components, and thus quantify the overall motion (or overall displacement) of the left ventricular wall?

Theoretical considerations

The quality of a particular model is usually evaluated with reference to the subjective appreciations of experienced cardiologists. Consequently, the best model is in fact expected to simulate best what happens in the cardiologist's brain. It seems reasonable to assume that some kind of distinction between

P.H. Heintzen and J.H. Bürsch (eds), Progress in Digital Angiocardiography. ISBN 978-94-010-7093-5

movement and deformation of the LV cavity is mentally performed. A direct support to this point of view is that the intuitive concept according to which wall motion results from a translation/rotation of the enddiastolic silhouette and from a cyclic change of its size and shape is broadly accepted. Thus, necessity and modality of silhouette realignment may indeed be the important questions of wall motion analysis. Beside this somewhat philosophical aspect, there is also a plain physical reason justifying an investigation of necessity and modality of realignment: referring wall motion to the external system implies that a lot of forces transmitted to the left ventricular cavity will impinge strongly onto the results [4]. Sources of such forces are for instance the resistance of the blood column in the aorta, the truncs of the four great vessels, the heart mass, accelerated intra- or extracardiac blood masses, the surrounding lung structures, the diaphragm, etc. Focusing onto the size/shape deformation of the LV reduces most probably the impact of such forces because shape deformation of the LV is certainly less influenced by these forces than the overall movement of its interior wall.

Main features of the model

Conventional assessments of model performances by comparison with 'eyeball' evaluations of cardiologists having failed to achieve universal consensus on a proposed model, and being moreover subjective and time consuming, we chose to use a more objective criterion for investigating the effect of realignment. A criterion will be more valuable if it reflects a postulate well accepted by the community of cardiologists. Such a postulate states that ventricles of normal subjects contract and relax in a synchronous fashion, while functionally impaired LV are suspected to show some degradation in synchronism, especially at early diastole. The degree of synchronism of contraction/relaxation can be quantified using the 'phase analysis' technique [5]. Superiority of realignment over non-realignment with regard to the degree of synchronism can be demonstrated by showing that the former yields higher synchronism of contraction/relaxation in a group of patients presenting normal contraction/relaxation ('normal subjects') [6]. If realignment produces additionally a better differentiation between this control group and a group of patients with impaired left ventricular function, then the necessity and modality of realignment really deserve further investigation.

The wall motion model used by Ratib in its 'phase analysis' technique [5] was replaced first by the 'centerline' model of Sheehan [7]. However, this model produced often exotic apical segments (Fig. 1) and was therefore replaced by the model shown in Fig. 2. (The figure shows the realigning version, which is described in more detail in the next section.) Obviously, this solution does not

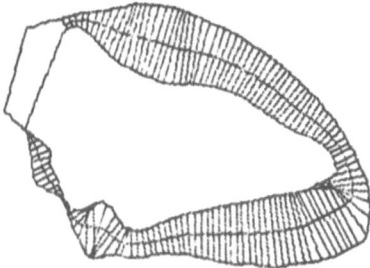

Fig. 1. Non-realigned pair of enddiastolic/endsystolic silhouettes with shortening segments generated by the 'centerline' model. This model was abandoned because of often unsatisfying apical
segments.

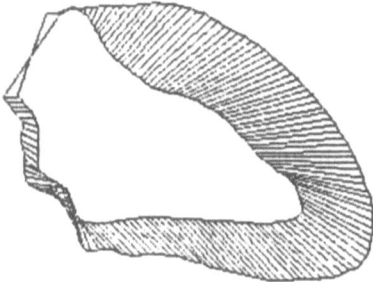

Fig. 2. Same pair of silhouettes as in Fig. 1, but after realignment and with new scheme of
segments.

differ essentially from the former. A problem specific to models of this type is
that absolute segment lengths are measured, instead of relative ones. Thus,
not only the actual left ventricular ejection fraction but also the size of the LV
has a direct impact onto the computed segments. This drawback was eliminated by normalizing the enddiastolic silhouette area of each patient to an
arbitrary constant value (a fixed number of pixels of our display). This value
was the same for all patients. The patient-dependent normalization factor was
applied to all involved silhouettes.

In order to create the realigning version of the model, compensation
schemes for the translation and the rotation had to be selected. Speculating
that the cardiologist perceives translation of the silhouette with respect to the
valvular area, superimposition of the mid-aortic points was selected. The
rotation was compensated by superimposing the (newly defined) long axes of
the silhouettes. Superimposition of the long axes was assumed to correspond
to the mental process of the cardiologist, and should moreover preserve or
even emphasize abnormalities in anterior and posterior regions of the LV [66].
Since the usual definition of the long axis by help of the 'farthest point of the

contour with regard to the mid-aortic point' results in some sensitivity to interobserver variability in contour tracing, our long axis was defined using an 'average' apical point (as explained in the next section).

Method

Beginning with the enddiastolic silhouette, the contours of all silhouettes of a selected cardiac cycle (25 images/s) are drawn on mask subtracted images and stored in a VAX-11/750 computer. These native contours are then area normalized (for the reason given previously) and divided by 2×64 equidistant points: 64 before and 64 after the usual apical point (anterior, respectively inferior region of the LV). Linking the 128 points of the first enddiastolic contour to the corresponding points of all following contours yields 128 time-shortening segments, as shown in Fig. 2 (for the realigned endsystolic silhouette). The realigned version is created by superimposing mid-aortic points and 'long axes' of the silhouettes. The 'long axis' of each silhouette is defined by the mid-aortic point and the already mentioned 'average' apical point. This point is obtained as follows: first the usual long-axis of the silhouette through the mid-aortic point and the farthest contour point is determined. Then a line perpendicular to this first axis is drawn at 95% of its length (measured from the mid-aortic point). The center of gravity of the small apical area delimited by this perpendicular line is defined as 'average' apical point. Figure 2 shows the endsystolic contour of Fig. 1 after realignment.

'Phase analysis' is performed on the selected cardiac cycle, in both model versions, as follows: the time-course of each segment is obtained by a 2-harmonics Fourier fit of its measured lengths in the course of cardiac cycle (Fig. 3). Cardiac cycle duration is normalized to 360/. The phase (Pha) of the first

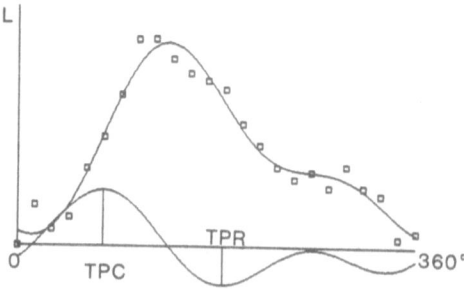

Fig. 3. Time-course of a shortening segment during the selected cardiac cycle. The parameters TPC and TPR are defined as 'time' of maximum and of minimum, respectively, of the first derivative of the time-course function.

harmonic is the first parameter obtained. Two other parameters, the 'time of peak contraction' (TPC) and the 'time of peak relaxation' (TPR) are defined as the times (in degrees) of the maximum and of the minimum value, respectively, of the first derivative of the fitted function (Fig. 3). Thus, 3 parameters expressed in degrees are assigned to each segment, each one reflecting an aspect of the time evolution of the segment during the cardiac cycle. The segments are color coded according to the value of the considered parameter and displayed at their respective location in the enddiastolic/endsystolic silhouettes pair. This yields 3 parametric images. The histogram of each parameter is also computed, with mean and standard deviation (SD).

Study on normal subjects and MI patients: results

Twenty normal subjects were studied without and with contour realignment. The means of the 3 histograms appeared to be useless. But the 3 SD, which reflect the degree of synchronism of the contraction or relaxation, show clearly that the postulated synchronism of left ventricular contraction/relaxation in normal subjects is better reflected if realignment is performed. The mean standard deviations ($\overline{SD}$) of the parameters TPC and TPR decreased by a factor 2 (Table 1). The standard deviations of these two $\overline{SD}$ decreased by a factor 4. This is in perfect agreement with the postulate of high synchronism in normal subjects.

Sixteen patients with proven myocardial infarction (MI) were also studied. All 3 SD appeared to be sensitive indicators of pathological states when

Table 1. Comparison of the mean standard deviations ($\overline{SD}$) of the parameters Pha, TPC and TPR before and after realignment in the control group of 20 normal subjects.

	$\overline{SD}$ of Pha	$\overline{SD}$ of TPC	$\overline{SD}$ of TPR
Before realignment	7.9 ± 3.8	12.0 ± 9.5	14.3 ± 10.0
After realignment	6.0 ± 2.7	5.5 ± 1.9	6.0 ± 2.3

Table 2. Comparison of the mean standard deviations ($\overline{SD}$) of the parameters Pha, TPC and TPR before and after realignment in the group of 16 MI patients.

	$\overline{SD}$ of Pha	$\overline{SD}$ of TPC	$\overline{SD}$ of TPR
Before realignment	23.3 ± 16.2	26.8 ± 16.1	33.4 ± 14.4
After realignment	13.9 ± 7.9	13.2 ± 7.5	23.8 ± 12.9

104

compared to the SD of normal subjects. The $\overline{SD}$ of all 3 parameters were also reduced by realignment (Table 2). However, unlike the case of normal subjects, this is rather regrettable. But the important result consists in the fact that realignment reduced also the overlap of the individual SD values between MI and control groups. Realignment allowed thus for a better differentiation of the MI patients from the normal subjects. The parameter TPR appeared thereby to be more sensitive for the detection of ischemic states than the two others, as expected. Regional amplitude of contraction was also studied in these 16 patients. After realignment hypokinesia was detected in the 16 infarcted territories corresponding to the occluded coronary artery. Without realignment hypokinesia was not detected in one patient and localized in a wrong territory (unrelated with the occluded vessel and the ECG Q-waves) in 2 patients.

Conclusion

Realignment of contours provides in control patients a higher homogeneity of all 3 parameters Pha, TPC and TPR, in agreement with the basic postulate that left ventricles of 'normal' patients contract and relax in a synchronous fashion. Realignment provided also more sensitivity in detection and localization of asynchronism, and reduced erroneous localization of hypokinesia. Thus, necessity and modality of realignment deserve further investigation. If automatic contouring of the LV silhouettes, offered now by some manufacturers of DSA equipment, proves to be reliable, quantification models including assessment of synchronism could become very attractive.

Summary

In order to investigate the effect of silhouette realignment on left ventricular wall motion analysis (RAO 30/ angiographic projection), a non-realigning contraction model and a realigning version of this model were created. The non-realigning version quantified overall wall-motion. The realigning version quantified wall motion after compensation of the translation/rotation of the silhouette in the images, so that contraction/relaxation of the left ventricle was considered as cyclic size/shape deformation of the silhouette. Both versions were used to assess the degree of synchronism of left ventricular contraction/ relaxation by help of the 'phase analysis' technique. Twenty patients presenting normal contraction/relaxation patterns were investigated. The results were compared to the values obtained similarly in a group of 16 MI patients (Myocardial Infarction). Realignment turned out to yield higher synchronism in both groups, a better differentiation between them, and a better localization of hypokinesia.

References

1. Sigwart U, Heintzen PH (eds): Ventricular wall motion. International Symposium Lausanne. Georg Thieme Verlag, New York, 1984.
2. Geldberg HJ, Brundage BH, Glantz S, Parmley WW: Quantitative left ventricular wall motion analysis. A comparison of area, chord and radial methods. Circulation 1979; 59 (5): 991–1000.
3. Bhargava V, Warren S, Vieweg WVR, Shabetai R: Quantitation of left ventricular wall motion in normal subjects: Comparison of various methods. Cath Cardiovasc Diagn 1980; 6: 7–16.
4. Heintzen PH: Erfassung der regionalen Motilität mit radiologischen Methoden. Nucl Med 1981; XX (4): 163–168.
5. Ratib O, Righetti A, Brandon G, Rasoamanambelo L: Usefulness of phase analysis for the evaluation of regional wall motion asynchrony from digitized contrast ventriculography. In: Sigwart U, Heintzen PH (eds) Ventricular wall motion. International Symposium Lausanne; pp 299–304 and color plates II to IV. Georg Thieme Verlag, New York, 1984.
6. Melchior JP, Chatelain P, Doriot P-A, Rutishauser W: Assessment of regional synchronism of regional left ventricular contraction and relaxation using realignment and 'phase analysis'. IEEE Proc Comp Cardiol 1986, IEEE Computer Society Press, pp 107–110.
7. Sheehan FH, Bolson EL, Dodge HT, Mitten S: Centerline method – Comparison with other methods for measuring regional left ventricular motion. In: Sigwart U, Heintzen PH (eds) Ventricular wall motion. International Symposium Lausanne; pp 139–149. Georg Thieme Verlag, New York, 1984.

11. Assessment of Left Ventricular Pressure–Volume Relationships Using an Automatic Computerized Videodensitometric Approach

R. SIMON, J. KOPP, I. AMENDE, W. QUANTE & P.R. LICHTLEN
Division of Cardiology, Department of Internal Medicine, Hannover Medical School, Hannover, FRG

Introduction

A detailed analysis of ventricular pump function in systole and diastole requires the reconstruction of the pressure–volume relationship. Computerized on-line processing of ventricular pressure data is a routine procedure in many laboratories today, whereas the assessment of volume data throughout the entire cardiac cycle is a tedious and time-consuming procedure. Even in case of computer assistance, ventricular silhouettes have to be outlined manually frame-by-frame, since a reliable method for an automatic border recognition is not at hand despite all efforts that have been undertaken in the last decade. Furthermore, technical problems such as low concentration of contrast medium and premature beats render this type of analysis often impossible in the clinical situation.

Roentgen videodensitometry has been shown to measure relative changes in ventricular volumes by assessing the content of contrast medium in individual heart chambers throughout the cardiac cycle during angiography [1–5]. The application of densitometric principles may have several advantages. Contrast medium densitometry can provide threedimensional information from single plane video recordings. Volume measurements are independent of heart chamber geometry, when contrast mass principles are applied [1]. More importantly, data can be acquired in a computerized on-line mode when appropriate regions of interest are chosen. It was the aim of the present study to investigate, whether videodensitometry might provide an automated acquisition of left ventricular volumes throughout the cardiac cycle, thus enabling a fast computerized reconstruction of pressure–volume diagrams during clinical heart catheterization.

P.H. Heintzen and J.H. Bürsch (eds), Progress in Digital Angiocardiography. ISBN 978-94-010-7093-5
© 1988, Kluwer Academic Publishers, Dordrecht

Patients and methods

Patients

This study was carried out in 17 patients, 15 men and 2 women, aged 42 to 64 years (mean age 54 ± 7 years), who underwent diagnostic catheterization in our laboratories because of suspected or known coronary disease. Fifteen patients had normal hemodynamics and normal left ventricular function as well as normal coronary arteries. The remaining 2 patients were studied 6 to 12 months after bypass surgery and proved to have normal ventricular function and patent grafts.

Methods and protocol

Following right and left heart catheterization, biplane left ventricular cine-angiocardiography was performed at mid-held inspiration of the patient in 30/RAO/60/LAO projection with an injection of 40 ml Urografin 76% at a rate of 20 to 25 ml/sec into the left ventricle. These angiograms were stored simultaneously on a videotape recorder (bandwidth 5 MHz) in a biplane fashion (split-mode) at 50 frames/sec for videodensitometric analysis. Modifications of the X-ray generator (OPTIMUS M 200, Philips, Eindhoven) and of the TV-circuitry in our laboratories enable a simultaneous and flickerless acquisition of cineangiograms and videoangiograms at stabilized radiation exposure and clamped video amplification. After ventriculography, selective coronary angiography was performed in all patients, and a subsequent interval of 20 minutes was allowed to re-establish baseline conditions.

For the assessment of ventricular volume throughout the cardiac cycle by videodensitometry, a second videoangiogram was then performed injecting 20 ml of Urografin 76% via a no. 8 French pigtail catheter into the pulmonary artery in order to avoid premature beats and to provide a sufficient mixing of contrast medium and blood before entering the left ventricle. This angiogram taken in 30/RAO projection at mid-held inspiration of the patient was recorded on videotape at 50 frames/sec. Simultaneously, the electrocardiogram and left ventricular pressure were stored on the audio channels of the videotape recorder using a frequency-modulated signal converter. Cardiac output was measured by the thermodilution technique immediately before the pulmonary videoangiogram, the final value representing the average of triplicate determinations.

Data analysis

Volume determination by videodensitometry. The system used for videodensi-

SYSTEM FOR X-RAY VIDEODENSITOMETRY AND MORPHOMETRY

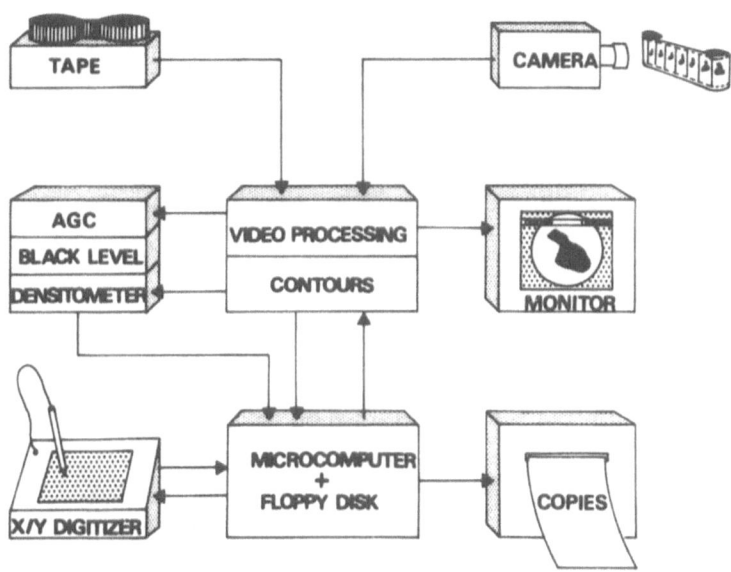

Fig. 1. System for X-ray-videodensitometry and morphometry. Tape: videotape recorder. Camera: videocamera for the conversion of cineangiograms to videoangiograms for morphometric analysis (not described in this paper). AGC, black level: automatic gain control and black level compensation in the videodensitometer (for further details see text).

tometric analysis is depicted in Fig. 1. The tape-stored videoangiograms are fed into a video-processing and contour unit that is coupled to the logarithmic videodensitometer and a microcomputer (CBM 8032). Regions of interest (ROI) of any desired size and shape can be defined by use of an x/y-digitizing graft pen interfaced to the microcomputer. The size and the position of these ROI is controlled on a videomonitor. During replay of the videotape, an ROI is outlined that covers the entire area of the left ventricle during contrast filling (Fig. 2). After compensation for undesired variations in roentgen intensity by an automated gain control circuitry (AGC, see [6]) and correction for radiation scattering and veiling glare in the image intensifier (black level; see [7, 8]), all video voltages in the ROI are converted logarithmically and integrated subsequently in the densitometer. The output signal of the densitometer is proportional to the dynamic changes in the content of contrast medium within the ROI [3, 9] and is fed into the microcomputer via a 10 bit AD-converter together with the electrocardiogram and left ventricular pressure (from tape audio channels). An example of a left ventricular densogram recorded with an ROI covering the entire area of the left ventricle after pulmonary injection of

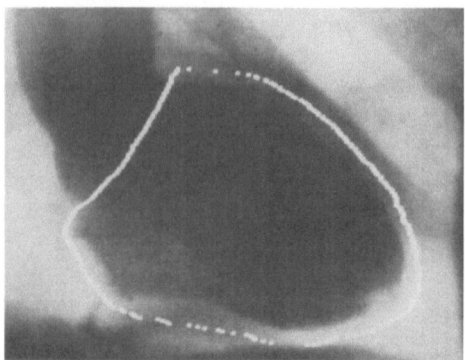

Fig. 2. Contours of a region of interest (ROI) covering the entire left ventricle.

20 ml of Urografin 76% and the simultaneously sampled electrocardiogram is given in Fig. 3.

All further steps in the evaluation are performed automatically by a computer program. The densogram is superimposed by cyclic undulations that are caused by variations in roentgen density due to the changes in volume and blood content of the heart during the cardiac cycle. In a first step of processing, the program derives a representative of this cyclic undulation ('background signal') by averaging 3 to 5 cycles in the late phase of the densogram after complete washout of contrast medium from the ventricle, using the electrocardiogram as a time reference. This average background signal is then subtracted from the entire densogram, again using the electrocardiogram as a time reference as suggested previously [10]. The result is a 'net' densogram that displays the dynamic change in the content of contrast medium within the left ventricle (Fig. 4). In the next step, ventricular residual fraction (end-systolic

LV DENSOGRAM : PA INJECTION (20 ML U-76), 12 SEC SAMPLING (50/SEC)

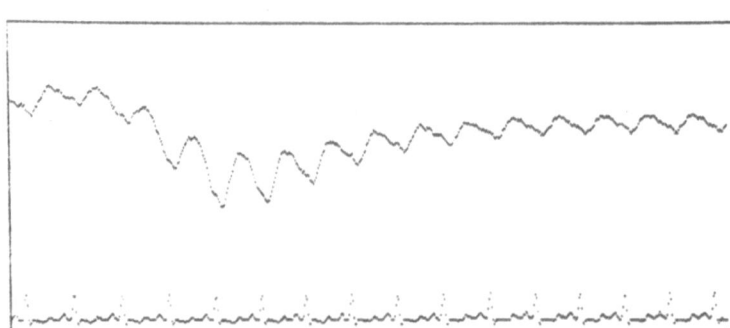

Fig. 3. Electrocardiogram (bottom) and videodensogram (top) of the left ventricle after injection of 20 ml contrast medium into the pulmonary artery.

LV DENSOGRAM AFTER PA INJECTION (20 ML U-76)

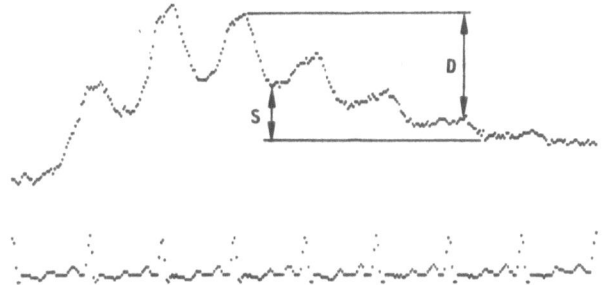

Fig. 4. Net videodensogram of the left ventricle after pulmonary injection of 20 ml contrast medium, compensated for background signal (see text). Increase in contrast medium content is displayed upwards in contrast to the raw densogram (Fig. 3). S: difference in end-systolic content of contrast medium between beat 3 and beat 6. D: end-diastolic difference in content of contrast medium between beat 3 and beat 6.

volume (ESV) divided by end-diastolic volume (EDV) is calculated. Assuming a constant concentration of contrast medium (c) in the left ventricle during systolic ejection yields

$$EDM = c \times EDV, \tag{1}$$
$$ESM = c \times ESV, \tag{2}$$

where EDM and ESM are the total mass of contrast medium in the chamber at end-diastole and end-systole, respectively. Residual fraction RF can then be calculated from the densogram as

$$RF = ESM/EDM. \tag{3}$$

There is, however, uncertainty about the baseline of the densogram due to contrast accumulation in the superimposing myocardium and tissue background [3, 9]. Therefore, a modified principle is applied that derives residual fraction from differences between several beats without taking the baseline into account. For beats a and b one can assume

$$ESMa = RF \times EDMa, \tag{4}$$
$$ESMb = RF \times EDMb, \tag{5}$$

resulting in

$$ESMa - ESMb = RF (EDMa - EDMb), \tag{6}$$
$$RF = (ESMa - ESMb) / (EDMa - EDMb), \tag{7}$$

which would equal S/D in Fig. 4.

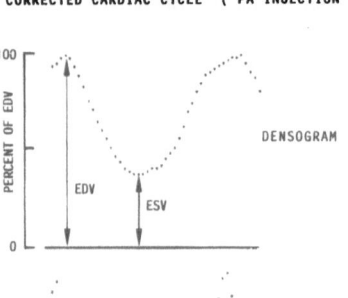

Fig. 5. Corrected cardiac cycle representing the relative change in left ventricular volume through-out one heart beat and electrocardiogram, derived from the beat of maximal contrast in Fig. 4.

The frame-by-frame change in ventricular volume throughout an entire cardiac cycle is assessed from the beat of maximal contrast during left ventricular opacification that is chosen to reduce the impact of background noise as much as possible. It is assumed that during systole the decrease in densitometric amplitude is proportional to the stroke volume ejected and thus proportional to the loss in ventricular volume. In analogy, the concentration of contrast medium within the blood entering the left ventricle from the left atrium during the next diastole is supposed to be constant, although not identical to that in the previous systole, thus rendering the diastolic change in densitometric amplitude proportional to the change in ventricular volume. The proportional expansion of the diastolic phase to the same height as the previous end-diastole leads to a corrected cardiac cycle that can be expressed in relative volume amplitudes using the residual fraction derived from the same densogram as described above (Fig. 5). In order to convert this relative volume curve to absolute volumes, the difference between end-diastolic and end-systolic volume was calibrated by stroke volume derived from the thermodilution cardiac output measurement that was performed immediately before the pulmonary videoangiogram in the present study. In the final step, the pressure-volume loop is constructed from the volume curve derived by densitometry and the left ventricular pressure data that had been sampled from the tape audio channel during replay.

Analysis of cineangiograms. The results of the computerized videodensito-metric volume determination were compared to a geometric volume analysis for a complete cardiac cycle derived from the biplane cineangiograms taken in RAO/LAO projection. Volumes over an entire cardiac cycle were analyzed on a computer-system (GRAFOMED, Philips, Eindhoven) using the biplane area-length method [11] and applying the regression equation suggested by Rogers and coworkers [12].

Results

Comparison of residual fraction

The comparison of left ventricular residual fraction derived from the pulmonary videoangiogram by videodensitometry and from biplane cineangiography by the area-length method revealed a slight overestimation by videodensitometry, but a good correlation between both measurements (Fig. 6). In an attempt to identify possible changes in ventricular function between cineangiography and the non-simultaneous pulmonary videoangiogram, residual fraction derived by densitometry from the pulmonary angiogram and the biplane videoangiogram that was stored simultaneously during cineangiography could be compared in 16 of the 17 patients. As shown in Fig. 7, both measurements were nearly identical rendering a major change in pump function unlikely.

Comparison of ventricular volumes

Left ventricular volumes derived from biplane cineangiography by the area-length method, and from pulmonary videoangiograms using the computerized densitometric technique in the same patient, are compared in Figs 8 and 9. The relation of all 640 volumes throughout all cardiac cycles analyzed in the entire group of 17 patients, is depicted in Fig. 10. There was a slight overestimation of

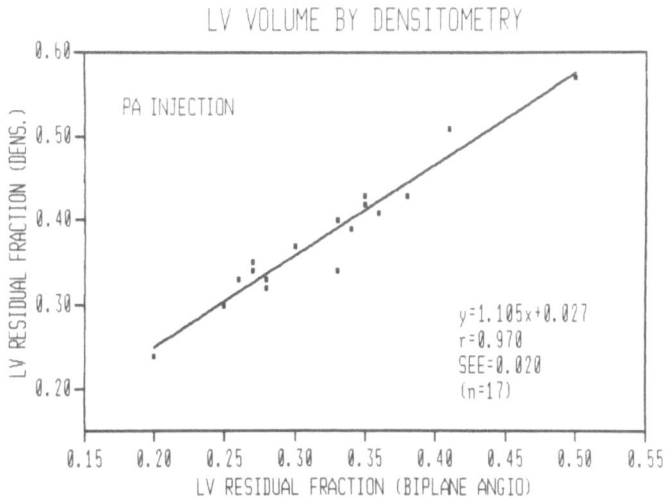

Fig. 6. Comparison of left ventricular residual fraction derived by computerized densitometry (ordinate) and biplane cineangiocardiography using the area-length method (abscissa).

114

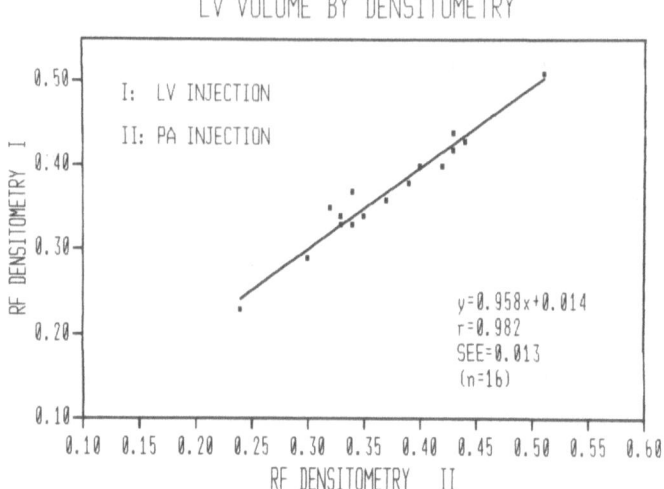

Fig. 7. Comparison of left ventricular residual fracton derived by computerized densitometry at the time of biplane cineangiocardiography (RF densitometry I) and of the pulmonary video-angiogram (RF densitometry II).

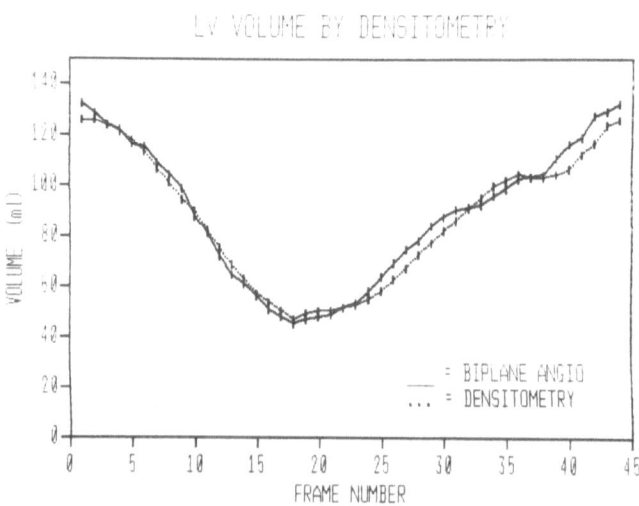

Fig. 8. Course of left ventricular volume throughout a cardiac cycle in a single patient, derived by the geometric area-length method (biplane angio) and computerized videodensitometry (densitometry). Abscissa: number of cineframes and videoframes, respectively. Ordinate: volume in ml.

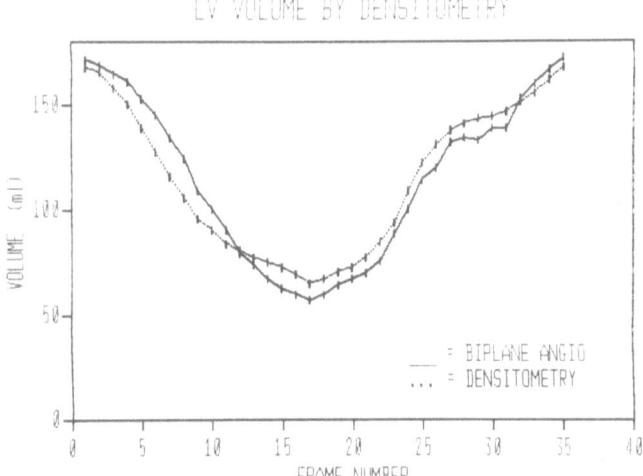

Fig. 9. Course of left ventricular volume throughout a cardiac cycle in a single patient, derived by the geometric area-length method (biplane angio) and computerized videodensitometry (densitometry). Abscissa: number of cineframes and videoframes, respectively. Ordinate: volume in ml.

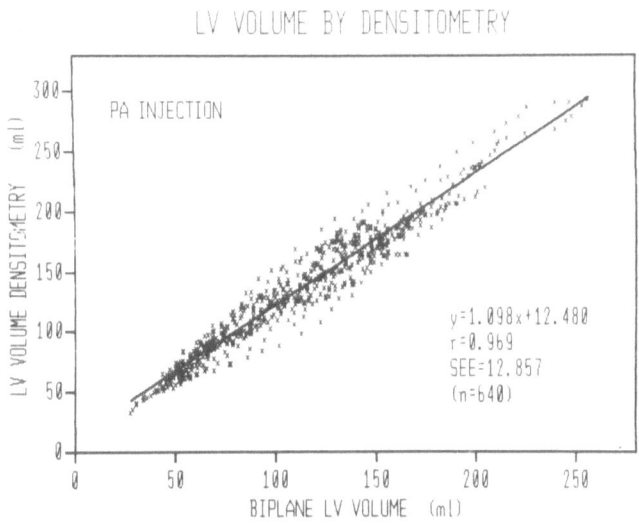

Fig. 10. Correlation of left ventricular volume determination by computerized videodensitometry (ordinate) and the biplane area-length method (abscissa) in 640 determinations in all 17 patients.

116

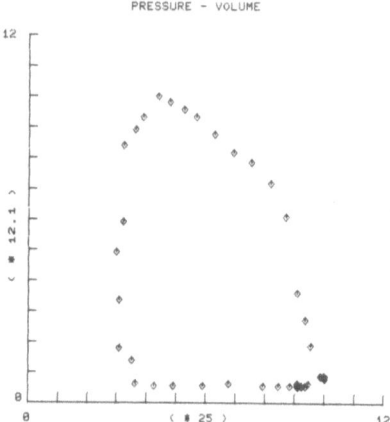

PRESSURE - VOLUME

Fig. 11. Original plot of a pressure–volume loop at 50 samples/sec. Volume data were derived automatically by computerized videodensitometry, sampled simultaneously with the audio channel-stored pressure data from videotape. Abscissa: left ventricular volume in multiples of 25 ml. Ordinate: left ventricular pressure in multiples of 12.1 mmHg.

ventricular volume by densitometry, but a sufficient correlation (r = 0.97), the standard error of estimate being about ± 13 ml for a range of 25 to 250 ml for ventricular volume.

Pressure–volume data

An example of a pressure–volume diagram that was derived automatically by computerized videodensitometry in a patient with normal cardiac function is given in Fig. 11.

Comment and implications

Our study may be subject to methodological criticism. The approach that has been applied is rather simplifying. For example, the use of a fixed ROI may not be appropriate in all cases since it does not take into account the movement of the valvular planes during the cardiac cycle. This may account for some of the scatter in the comparison of densitometry and cineventriculography. It is also conceivable that contrast medium accumulation in superimposing structures such as myocardial or lung tissue may not be compensated completely despite the use of a baseline-independent algorithm for the calculation of residual fraction. The non-simultaneous acquisition of cineventriculograms and densograms could have introduced additional errors. This, however, was unlikely since left ventricular pump function remained unchanged as shown by an unchanged residual fraction. Most of the deviations between both techniques in the present study seem to be due to problems inherent to the determination of stroke volume by the thermodilution method that has been used to calibrate the videoangiographic volume. A comparison of stroke volumes derived by angiography and the thermodilution technique revealed a correlation coefficient of only $r = 0.91$ between both methods.

Despite these considerations, our results are encouraging. Our data suggest that densitometric techniques may provide an automatic analysis of ventricular volumes throughout the cardiac cycle. The currently used technique allows the reconstruction of a pressure–volume diagram within minutes. The introduction of the principles described in this study to digital angiocardiography may widen the field of application in the future. Although we have used analog techniques for the videodensitometric measurements before AD-conversion, the results of our study are pertinent to digital angiocardiography. In a digital system, the transformation of the original angiogram to a ventricular volume curve is greatly facilitated by the primary digital storage of the angiographic raw data. All calculations described can be performed digitally on the stored data. ROI could be adjusted appropriately to the aortoventricular and atrioventricular borders throughout the cardiac cycle. Furthermore, digital contrast enhancement may provide sufficient opacification for an end-diastolic geometric volume calibration rendering an independent technique such as thermodilution unnecessary. We are currently investigating whether the entire analysis could be done from one digitally acquired angiogram after a pulmonary injection of about 20 ml of contrast medium. If this holds true, digital videodensitometry may, indeed, provide us with a fully automatic analysis of systolic as well as diastolic ventricular function throughout the entire cardiac cycle in an on-line fashion during the catheterization procedure.

Summary

In 17 patients with normal left ventricular function undergoing diagnostic heart catheterization, a densitometric technique was investigated supposed to enable a fast and objective assessment of complete left ventricular volume curves throughout the cardiac cycle. From videoangiograms with an injection of 20 ml of contrast medium (Urografin 76%) into the pulmonary artery and stored on a tape recorder, relative volume curves were derived automatically by computerized videodensitometry. These curves were calibrated to absolute ventricular volumes by comparing the stroke volume equivalent of the curve to actual stroke volume assessed by the thermodilution method.

A comparison to ventricular volumes measured from biplane cineangiocardiography (biplane area-length method) in the same patients revealed a good correlation (r = 0.97) and a standard deviation of ± 13 ml between both methods. Using this videodensitometric approach, a simple microcomputer system could display complete pressure–volume loops for a cardiac cycle (data rate: 50/sec) derived from videoangiograms and simultaneously sampled pressure curves within minutes. Although the method has still to be improved, our data support the contention that densitometric principles may allow a fully automatic assessment of ventricular volumes and pressure–volume relationships when applied to digital angiographic techniques.

References

1. Bürsch JH, Heintzen PH, Simon R: Videodensitometric studies by a new method of quantitating the amount of contrast medium. Eur J Cardiol 1974; 1: 437.
2. Simon R, Klebèr A, Rutishauser W, Grimm J: Assessment of mitral incompetence by videodensitometry. Animal experiments and results in patients. In: Heintzen PH, Bürsch JH (eds) Roentgen-video-techniques for dynamic studies of structure and function of the heart and circulation; p 85. Thieme, Stuttgart, 1978.
3. Grimm J, Simon R, Reimann A, Rutishauser W: Comparison of systolic left ventricular volume change obtained by videodensitometry and electromagnetically-measured aortic flow. A preliminary study. In: Heintzen PH, Bürsch JH (eds) Roentgen-video-techniques for dynamic studies of structure and function of the heart and circulation; p 101. Thieme, Stuttgart, 1978.
4. Kedem D, Kedem D, Rhea TC, Nelson JH, Graham TP, Brill AB: Left ventricular volume and ejection parameter-analysis by digital densitometry. In: Heintzen PH, Bürsch JH (eds) Roentgen-video-techniques for dynamic studies in structure and function of the heart and circulation; p 108. Thieme, Stuttgart, 1978.
5. Trenholm BG, Winter DA, Mymin D, Lansdown EL: Computer determination of left ventricular volume using videodensitometry. Med Biol Engin 1972; 10: 163.
6. Simon R, Ziegler K, Grimm J: Videodensitometer mit automatischer Regelung des Videoeingangs. Biomedizinische Technik 1979; 24 (Suppl): 156.
7. Brennecke R, Bürsch JH, Heintzen PH: Improvement in videodensitometric measurement techniques. In: Heintzen PH, Bürsch JH (eds) Roentgen-video-techniques for dynamic studies of structure and function of the heart and circulation; p 15. Thieme, Stuttgart, 1978.
8. Nalcioglu O, Seibert JA, Boone JM, Wang Y, Roeck WW, Henry WL, Tobis JM, Johnston WD: The effect of physical problems on the determination of ventricular ejection fraction by videodensitometry. In: Heintzen PH, Brennecke R (eds) Digital imaging in cardiovascular radiology; p 104. Thieme, Stuttgart, 1983.
9. Bürsch JH, Heintzen PH: Some principles for circulatory studies using videodensitometry. In: Heintzen PH, Bürsch JH (eds) Roentgen-video-techniques for dynamic studies of structure and function of the heart and circulation; p 2. Thieme, Stuttgart, 1978.
10. Smith HC, Sturm RE, Wood EH: Videodensitometric system for measurement of vessel blood flow, particularly in the coronary arteries, in man. Am J Cardiol 1973; 32: 144.
11. Dodge HT, Sandler H, Ballew DW, Lord JD: The use of biplane angiocardiography for the measurement of left ventricular volume in man. Am Heart J 1960; 60: 762.
12. Rogers WJ, Smith R, Hood WP, Mantle JA, Rackley CE, Russell RO: Effect of filming projection and interobserver variability on angiographic biplane left ventricular volume determination. Circulation 1979; 59: 96.

12. Computed Triple Orthogonal Projections for Optimal Radiological Imaging with Biplane Isocentric Multidirectional X-ray Systems

HELMUT WOLLSCHLÄGER, ANDREAS M. ZEIHER, PETER LEE, ULRICH SOLZBACH, TASSILO BONZEL & HANJÖRG JUST
Medical Clinic, Department of Cardiology, University of Freiburg, Freiburg, FRG

Introduction

One of the major objectives in angiocardiography is the visualization of anatomical details with projections perpendicular to the long axis of the anatomical structure. In addition, 'one of the most basic rules in radiology . . . is the need for at least two views of the object with the projections being perpendicular to each other' [1]. Thus, most useful informations can be derived from a radiological study if the concept of 'triple orthogonality' is applied: two projections perpendicular to the long axis of the anatomical object *and* perpendicular to each other.

Currently, repeated trials are necessary to approximate such desired projections empirically, if the axis of interest is oriented oblique relative to the long axis of the body. Then the radiological standard projections from the transerse plane (e.g. RAO and LAO) are not sufficient for an adequate visualization and hemiaxial views have to be applied.

Modern biplane isocentric multidirectional X-ray equipment with known geometrical properties allow spatial computations from two simultaneous views, independent of the angles of projection [2, 3, 4]. In addition, the algorithms for perpendicular positioning of the two X-ray stands have been developed, even if hemiaxial projections are used [5]. Thus, the mathematical prerequisites for the geometrical computation of distinct radiological projections are available.

Based on these algorithms, we have developed a new method for computer-assisted triple orthogonal adjustment of biplane X-ray systems.

Method

From any optional surveying simultaneous biplane views, the spatial orientation of the long axis of an object of interest – identifiable in the fields of view

P.H. Heintzen and J.H. Bürsch (eds), Progress in Digital Angiocardiography. ISBN 978-94-010-7093-5
© 1988, Kluwer Academic Publishers, Dordrecht

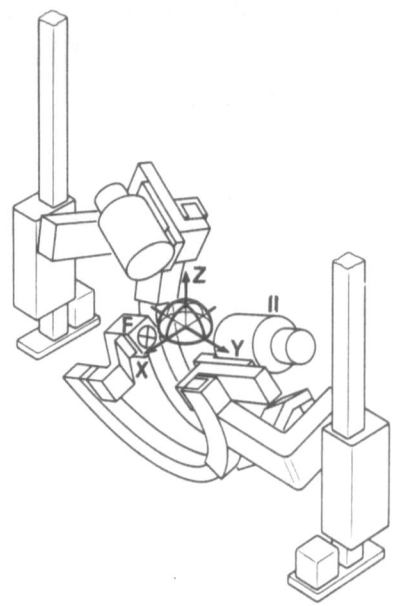

Fig. 1. Schematic representation of the 'global' coordinate system (, Y, Z) around the isocenter of a biplane multidirectional X-ray system (c-arm-L-arm-configuration, Bi-Angioskop C, Siemens AG, Erlangen, FRG). F: X-ray focus; II: image-intensifier.

of the two X-ray systems – can be defined as a vector in a three-dimensional Cartesian coordinate system. The origin of this patient-oriented 'global' coordinate system coincides with the constant isocenter of the X-ray systems (Fig. 1).

To calculate this spatial orientation of the axis (vector $\vec{v}$ in Fig. 2), the geometrical informations from 'local' two-dimensional coordinate systems on the surface of the image-intensifier entrance fields are used (Fig. 2): two subsidiary planes, enclosing the X-ray foci and the projections of the axis $\vec{v}$ on the two image-intensifier entrance fields (FA-A1-A2 and FB-B1-B2) are constructed. The calculated line of intersection of these two planes represents the spatial orientation of $\vec{v}$ in the 'global' coordinate system.

The informations necessary for the construction of the two subsidiary planes are:

1. the geometrical parameters of the portraying views of the two X-ray systems, and
2. the orientation of the projections of the axis within the two 'local' coordinate systems.

The latter can be determined by adjusting straight lines tangentially to the projections of the axis – V(A/B) in Fig. 3 – at well defined points C(A/B). The

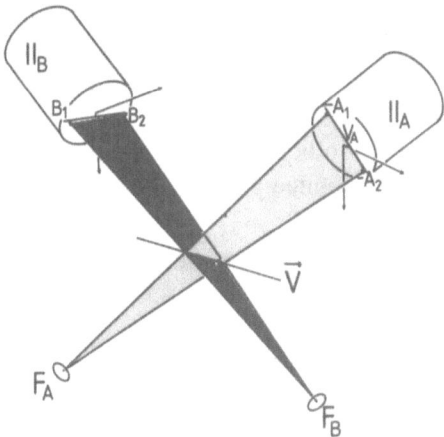

Fig. 2. Schematic representation of the determination of the spatial orientation of an axis (vector $\vec{v}$). F(A/B): X-ray foci; II(A/B): image-intensifiers; V(A/B): projections of the axis on the image-intensifier entrance fields with 'local' coordinate systems (indicated by arrows); A(1/2), B(1/2): subsidiary points on the projections of the axis V(A/B).

corresponding projections of the center of a coronary stenosis might serve as such well defined points – as indicated schematically in Fig. 3. The points A(1/2) and B(1/2) of the two planes can be defined from the zero-crossings of these tangential lines with horizontal axes of the local coordinate systems – Z(A/B) and the enclosed angles φ (A/B) (Fig. 3).

After the calculation of $\vec{v}$, one of the two X-ray systems is positioned perpendicular to the spatial orientation of $\vec{v}$ using an algorithm developed previously [5].

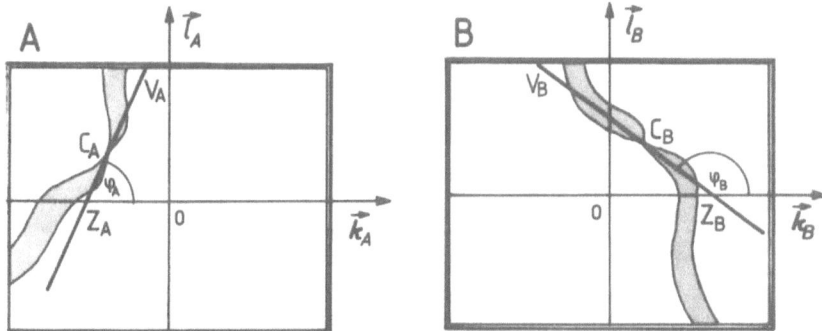

Fig. 3. Adjustment of tangential lines (V) at well defined points (C) to a schematic representation of a coronary artery segment in simultaneous biplane views (A and B). $\vec{k}$ and $\vec{l}$: axes of 'local' coordinate systems with origin 0. The tangential lines are mathematically defined by the zero-crossings with the horizontal axes (Z) and the included angles (φ).

122

For adjustment of the second X-ray system perpendicular to the first one as well as perpendicular to the axis, the vector product (vector of the central X-ray beam of the first system and vector $\vec{v}$ of the axis) is calculated, resulting in triple orthogonal projections.

The calculated angle of projection of 90/ is valid only for the central X-ray beam. Therefore, the well defined point of the axis (C) has to be shifted into the isocenter of the systems.

Verification

The algorithms were used for a laterally mounted C-arm-L-arm-configuration of a biplane isocentric X-ray equipment (Bi-Angioskop C with 7" image intensifiers, Siemens AG, Erlangen, FRG – see Fig. 1). Phantom studies were performed with a small disc, affixed between two screw nuts perpendicular to a little metal rod. This phantom was simultaneously visualized with randomly chosen multidirectional projections. The radiographic sequences were recorded on video-tape and filmed for documentation. Thereafter, two corresponding video-frames were analyzed and the mathematical calculations for obtaining triple orthogonal views were performed after input of one predetermined rotational parameter of one X-ray system (C-arm- or L-arm-rotation). Then the X-ray systems were readjusted according to the calculated results. After shifting the disc into the isocenter, the phantom was filmed again.

The phantom was fixed on the cradle in 10 different randomly chosen oblique positions. For each position, the calculations were performed and the X-ray systems readjusted. In case of impending system collision using the computed results, the rotational input parameter was changed and the calculations repeated.

Results

Visualization of the phantom with an angle of projection other than 90° results in an elliptical shape of the disc (Fig. 4). Only with an exact orthogonal view, the disc is projected as a straight line (Fig. 5).

After visualization of the phantom with computed readjustment of the systems, the projections of the disc were straight lines in both views, demonstrating exact triple orthogonality.

The Figs 4 and 5 not only demonstrate that exact triple orthogonal projections can be performed, in addition they show the usefulness of this approach for substantial improvement in image-information: the two screw nuts – not

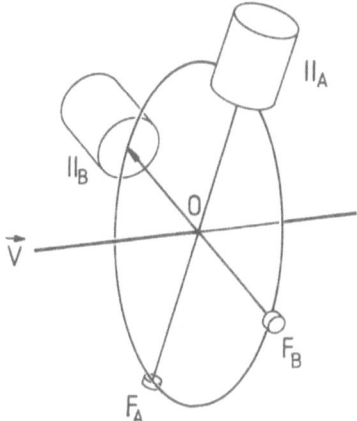

Fig. 4. Schematic representation of triple orthogonal projections. F: X-ray foci; II: image-intensifiers; O: isocenter of the two systems; $\vec{v}$: spatial orientation of the axis of interest. The central X-ray beams (F → II) are oriented perpendicular to $\vec{v}$ *and* perpendicular to each other.

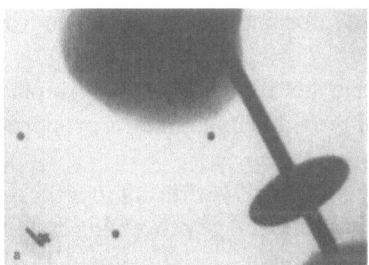
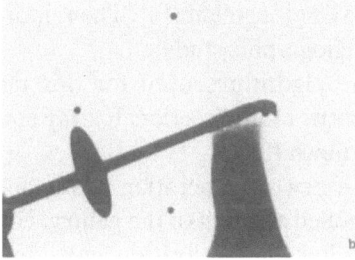

Fig. 5. Simultaneous biplane views of the phantom with randomly chosen projections. a: system A (C-arm-rotation +15/, L-arm-rotation −3/). b: system B (C-arm-rotation −73/, L-arm-rotation +90/). With an angle of view not equal to 90/ to the long axis of the phantom results in a projected elliptical shape of the disc.

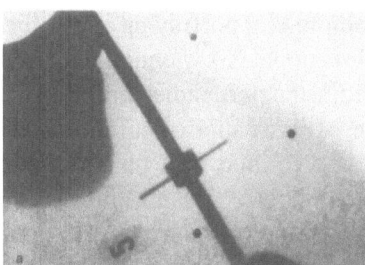
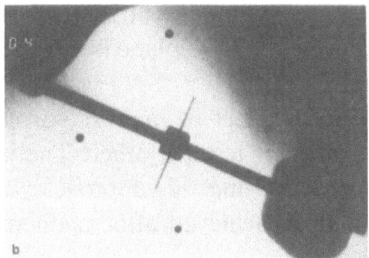

Fig. 6. Triple orthogonal projections: simultaneous biplane views of the phantom after computed readjustment of the two X-ray-systems. a: system A (C-arm-rotation +15/, L-arm-rotation −33/). b: system B (C-arm-rotation −55/, L-arm-rotation +34/). With an angle of view of exactly 90/ to the long axis of the phantom, the disc is projected as a straight line.

124

visible with oblique direction of the portraying X-ray beams – can be easily discerned after positioning the X-ray systems perpendicular to the axis of the phantom.

Discussion

The results of these studies demonstrate that exact triple orthogonal projections can mathematically be calculated from simultaneous biplane views. The method is applicable individually to any well definable axis independent of its spatial orientation.

The examples in our study clearly demonstrate the substantial improvement in image information from views being perpendicular to the long axis of the object: details not visible due to axis foreshortening of superposition of structures are clearly apparent after optimal radiological visualization.

In addition, this approach of individually adjusted perpendicular views will serve as prerequisite for reliable biplane densitometric reconstruction of coronary vessel segments [6]. Then, more precise informations can be drawn from an angiographic study.

The algorithms used for this method can be adapted to every biplane isocentric multidirectional X-ray equipment provided its geometric properties are known [3].

The newest generation of biplane X-ray systems [7] with microprocessor controlled steering of the gantry, coupled to on-line image processing systems will allow the realization individual triple orthogonal readjustment in the clinical setting.

Summary

A new method for exact triple orthogonal radiological portraying of an object was developed for biplane isocentric multidirectional X-ray equipment. With this method, the two X-ray systems can be adjusted perpendicular to the long axis of an object of interest – irrespective of its spatial orientation – *and* perpendicular to each other. The method was verified with phantom measurements. Using this approach, optimal radiological visualization can be individually achieved after mathematical computation of triple orthogonal projections.

References

1. Eldh P: Axial views. Cathet Cardiovasc Diagn 1976; 2: 315–317.
2. Taylor KW, McLoughlin MJ, Aldridge HE: Specification of angulated projections in coronary arteriography. Cathet Cardiovasc Diagn 1977; 3: 367–374.
3. Wollschläger H, Lee P, Zeiher A, Solzbach U, Bonzel T, Just H: Mathematical tools for spatial computations with biplane isocentric X-ray equipment. Biomed Techn 1986; 31: 101–106.
4. Wollschläger H, Lee P, Zeiher A, Solzbach U, Bonzel T, Just H: Derivation of spatial information from biplane multidirectional coronary angiograms. Med Progr Technol 1986; 11: 57–63.
5. Wollschläger H, Lee P, Bonzel T, Zeiher A, Just H: Biplane multidirectional angiocardiography: exact orthogonal positioning of the X-ray systems. Biomed Techn 1984; 29: 261–266.
6. Kenet R, Herrold E, Hill J, Waltman J, Diamond A, Fenster P, Barba J, Suardiaz M, Borer JS: Reconstruction of coronary-cross sections from two orthogonal digital angiograms. IEEE Proc Comp Cardiol, in press.
7. Wollschläger H, Haufe G: Biplane multidirectional angiocardiography with a new X-ray system. Electromedica 1986; 54: 114–118.

13. Clinical Applications of Cine Computed Tomography*

MELVIN L. MARCUS, JOHN A. RUMBERGER, STEVEN J. REITER,
WILLIAM STANFORD, CRAIG A. STARK & ANDREW J. FEIRING
*Departments of Medicine and Radiology and the Cardiovascular Center, University of Iowa
Hospitals, Iowa City, IA, USA*

Introduction

Standard computed tomographic scanners have limited applicability in cardiac studies due to a relatively long image acquisition time of 1 to 3 seconds. Since the heart contracts at frequencies that usually exceed one cycle/second, cardiac images obtained with standard tomographic instruments do not allow for discrimination of cardiac geometry at specific points of the cardiac cycle. Clinically useful images of the cardiac chambers can be obtained by employing prospective or retrospective gating of conventional computed tomographic images or utilizing specially designed computed tomographic instruments that obtain images in a fraction of a second. The first rapid computed tomographic scanner, the Dynamic Spatial Reconstructor, designed by Earl Wood and Eric Ritman at the Mayo Clinic, is able to obtain computed tomographic images in 10 msec. A more practical device for obtaining rapid computed tomographic images at 50 msec intervals has been developed by Boyd at the University of California, San Francisco. This device is commercially produced by the Imatron corporation (Imatron C-100). It employs an electron gun to generate an X-ray beam which can be guided around the patient with a magnetic field. In this brief review, we will describe two general cardiac applications of ultrafast computed tomography – studies of left and right ventricular function and size, and studies of vein bypass patency and flow reserve. All the data reported had been obtained with the Imatron C-100 scanner.

Studies of left ventricular function and geometry

To determine the accuracy whereby left ventricular mass can be quantitated using cine computed tomography (cine CT), we obtained cine CT images in

* Original studies reviewed in this manuscript were studied by the Ischemic SCOR HL 32295.

P.H. Heintzen and J.H. Bürsch (eds), Progress in Digital Angiocardiography. ISBN 978-94-010-7093-5

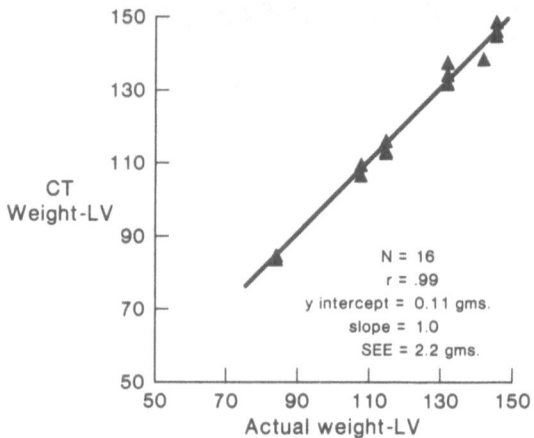

Fig. 1. Relationship between left ventricular mass obtained with cine computed tomography (CT) and anatomic measurements of left ventricular mass. These studies were performed in closed chest dogs during infusion of intravenous contrast. There is a close relationship between measurements of left ventricular mass with CT and anatomic measurements of left ventricular mass.

end-diastole of the left ventricles in closed chest dogs following an intravenous infusion of radiographic contrast media [1]. The serial tomographic images of the entire left ventricle from apex to base were obtained in a projection perpendicular to the long axis of the left ventricle. At the conclusion of the study, the anesthetized animals were killed, their hearts removed and the left ventricles weighed. The cine CT images of the left ventricle were analyzed by outlining the epicardial and endocardial border of each slice. Knowing slice thickness (0.8 cm) and the specific gravity of cardiac muscle allowed for determination of left ventricular mass using a modified Simpson's rule. Fig. 1 summarizes the results of this study. Left ventricular mass, calculated from the cine CT images, agreed with the actual weight of the left ventricle over a broad range. In other studies, we have demonstrated this approach is highly reproducible, and measurements of left ventricular mass can be obtained with similar accuracy even if tomographic images are obtained in projections which are no longer perpendicular to the long axis of the left ventricle [1]. Not only does this study demonstrate left ventricular mass can be accurately measured with cine CT, but this study confirms algorithms utilized in identifying the endocardial and epicardial borders of the left ventricle from the CT images must be accurate.

In an effort to determine whether end-systolic and end-diastolic volumes of the left ventricle can be accurately calculated, we obtained cine CT images of the left ventricle at multiple points of the cardiac cycle in dogs with chronically implanted flow meters on the ascending aorta. Flow meters of this type can be precisely calibrated and hence left ventricular stroke volume minus the small

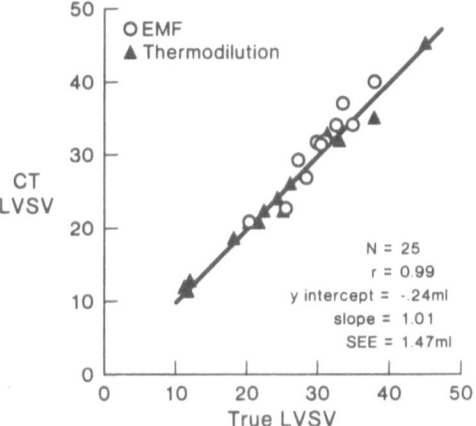

Fig. 2. Left ventricular stroke volume obtained with cine computed tomography (CT) and measurements of left ventricular stroke volume (LVSV) with a chronically implanted aortic flow meter (EMF) or multiple measurements of cardiac output with the thermodilution method. These studies were obtained in closed chest dogs given an intravenous infusion of a non-ionic contrast medium, Iohexol. There is a close relationship between stroke volume measurements obtained with these two methods. These data were originally presented by Reiter et al. and are reprinted with permission from the American Heart Association [2].

volume of blood that perfuses the coronary vessels can be accurately determined. Utilizing this animal preparation, we obtained multiple measurements of left ventricular stroke volume under a variety of conditions including changes in heart rate, left ventricular contractility (addition of positive or negative inotropic agents), volume overload (acute aortic insufficiency), and regional left ventricular dysfunction (occlusion of the proximal circumflex or left anterior descending coronary arteries) [2]. Under all of these conditions left ventricular stroke volumes, measured by the differences in cine CT end-diastolic and end-systolic tomographic volumes, agreed with stroke volumes measured with an electromagnetic flow meter or by multiple cardiac output determinations with the thermodilution method. From cardiac output measurements stroke volume could subsequently be calculated by dividing cardiac output by the animal's heart rate (Fig. 2) [2].

The accurate determination of ventricular stroke volumes by cine CT, when taken with the first study (determination of left ventricular mass), allows us to conclude that end-diastolic and end-systolic left ventricular volumes can be precisely measured even though in vivo validation studies of such measurements cannot be performed. It should be emphasized that precise measurements of cardiac chamber volumes can be obtained only if non-ionic contrast media are utilized, as was done in these studies [2].

To obtain clinical confirmation of these results, we measured left ventricular

130

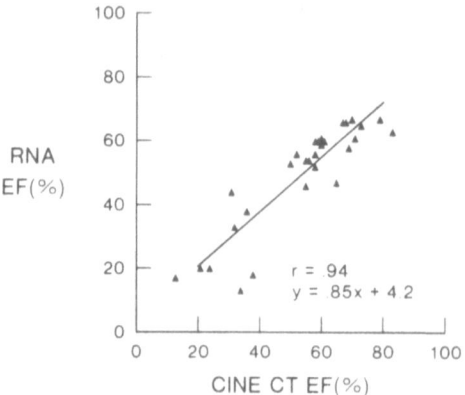

Fig. 3. Relationship between left ventricular ejection fraction calculated with cine computed tomography (cine CT EF) and left ventricular ejection fraction determined from equilibrium radionuclide ventriculograms (RNA, EF). These studies were performed in patients with a variety of heart diseases. The radionuclide and cine CT studies were performed within one or two weeks of each other without any clinical change in the patient's condition. The data demonstrate a reasonably close correlation between left ventricular ejection fraction obtained with these two methodologies. Since the cine CT information is dependent on border recognition and the radionuclide ejection fraction is independent of border definition, the close correlation suggests that the border recognition algorithm utilized for the cine CT is reasonably precise.

ejection fractions in normal patients and patients with a variety of cardiac diseases utilizing cine CT and compared the cine CT ejection fractions to those obtained in the same patients with the radionuclide ventriculogram. The radionuclide ventriculograms measured left ventricular ejection fraction from equilibrium studies employing the left anterior oblique projection in determining left ventricular ejection fraction. These clinical studies demonstrate that left ventricular ejection fraction measured with cine CT agrees reasonably well with measurements of left ventricular ejection fraction with radionuclide techniques (Fig. 3).

In other studies we have determined the normal range of values for left ventricular end-diastolic and end-systolic volumes, and left ventricular mass in normal volunteers [3]. We have also studied left ventricular diastolic and systolic function during an inotropic stress produced with intravenous infusion of dobutamine [4, 5], and various approaches to evaluating regional ventricular performance [6, 7].

Studies of right ventricular function

To evaluate cine CT's ability in assessing right ventricular geometry we obtained end-diastolic and end-systolic images of the right ventricle in anesthetized closed chest dogs and utilized the data to calculate right ventricular stroke volume. The right ventricular stroke volume measurements were compared to precise measurements of left ventricular stroke volume obtained with a chronically implanted flow probe on the ascending aorta, or with measurements of cardiac output determined with the thermodilution method. All measurements were obtained during suspended respiration in animals with normal hearts, and under these conditions the right and left ventricular stroke volumes are almost identical. Fig. 4 summarizes the results of these studies and demonstrates right ventricular stroke volumes can be measured accurately with cine computed tomography [2]. Again, precise measurements with cine CT can only be obtained if non-ionic contrast media are utilized to limit the hemodynamic effects that occur when standard contrast media are infused.

We have made near-simultaneous measurements of left and right ventricular stroke volumes in normal dogs during suspended respiration and demonstrated that under these conditions right and left ventricular stroke volume are nearly identical (Fig. 5) [2]. Subsequent studies in normal volunteers have also shown that during suspended respiration for 5–15 seconds, right and left ventricular stroke volumes are nearly identical [8].

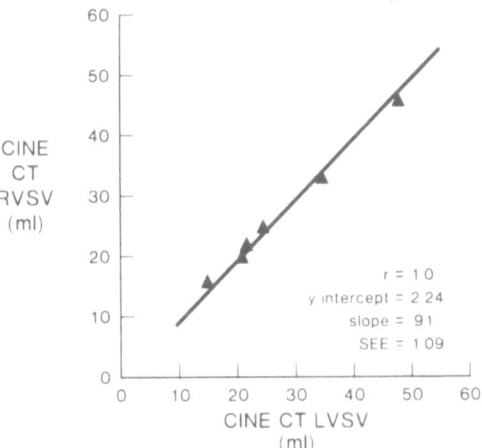

Fig. 4. Relationship between right ventricular stroke volume measured with cine computed tomography (cine CT) and right ventricular stroke volume measured with a chronically implanted aortic flow meter or thermodilution cardiac output/heart rate. There is a close relationship between measurements of right ventricular stroke volume with cine CT and the electromagnetic flow meter for cardiac output measurements.

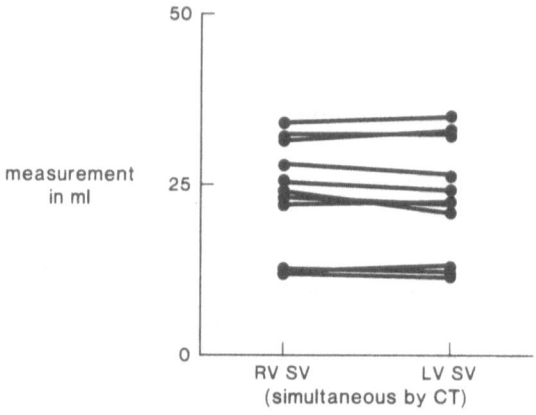

Fig. 5. Measurements of right and left ventricular stroke volume with cine computed tomography in dogs during suspended respiration. The right and left ventricular stroke volume measurements for each dog are connected by a line. It is notable that during suspended respiration differences between right and left ventricular stroke volume were negligible. These data were originally presented by Reiter et al. and are reprinted with permission of the American Heart Association [2].

With cine CT the epicardial surface of the right ventricle is not clearly seen and hence in normal right ventricles, right ventricular mass cannot be calculated. We have not compared cine CT measurements of right ventricular ejection fraction in normal patients to measurements of right ventricular ejection fraction using a radionuclide approach. Nonetheless, our results obtained thus far do suggest right ventricular geometry can be precisely defined with cine computed tomography.

Vein bypass graft patency and flow reserve

If a bolus of contrast is given through a peripheral vein and images of the thorax are obtained at fixed points in multiple cardiac cycles, it is possible to obtain a flow study with cine CT that allows us to define the arrival, peak and clearance of contrast in various vascular structures. Each thoracic structure has its own unique contrast appearance time and clearance curve which allow for separation of confounding structures such as pulmonary arteries and veins. It is even possible to differentiate saphenous vein bypass grafts from other structures and utilize cine CT in determining saphenous vein bypass graft patency.

Recently, a multicenter study involving five centers with C-100 scanners (University of Iowa, University of Illinois-Chicago, University of California-San Francisco, Deborah Hospital in New Jersey, and Cedars-Sinai Medical

Center in Los Angeles) has been completed [9]. This study analyzed the patency of 127 bypass grafts placed in 62 patients and demonstrated cine CT can determine bypass graft patency with an overall accuracy of 93%. This study also demonstrated the absolute number, location, type (internal mammary artery or vein bypass graft), and the presence of partial graft obstruction, did not influence the accuracy whereby cine CT could determine bypass graft patency. Other relatively non-invasive approaches of determining vein bypass graft patency (transcutaneous Doppler, intravenous infusion of contrast in association with digital subtraction angiography, and magnetic resonance imaging) cannot determine bypass graft patency with a similar degree of accuracy at this time.

In addition to assessing bypass graft patency, studies in anesthetized dogs indicate bypass graft flow reserve can also be assessed by comparing contrast clearance curves from bypass grafts obtained under control conditions and during maximal coronary dilation [10]. Although such experimental studies of vein bypass graft flow reserve have not yet been extended to the clinical arena, it is possible this approach can eventually permit measurements of vein bypass graft flow reserve in patients.

Future applications

In addition to the applications of cine CT which have been briefly described in this review, it should be noted cine CT can also be effectively employed to study pericardial effusion, pericardial thickening, aortic aneurysms, aortic dissection, periaortic masses and cardiac tumors of various types. It is possible that this technology in the future will be helpful in providing precise measurements of right and left atrial volumes and eventually regional myocardial perfusion.

Summary

Cine CT is a new exciting technology that allows for acquisition of high resolution tomographic images of cardiac structures allowing for precise measurements of global and regional cardiac function. This technology can be used in determining vein bypass graft patency and may be helpful in determining the flow reserve of bypass grafts and specific regions of the left ventricular myocardium. It is likely that information of this nature will be helpful in the care of patients with heart disease, and cine CT may find a place in the diagnostic evaluation of patients with cardiac disease.

References

1. Feiring AJ, Rumberger JA, Reiter SJ, Skorton DJ, Collins SM, Lipton MJ, Higgins CB, Ell S, Marcus ML: Determination of left ventricular mass in dogs with rapid acquisition cardiac CT scanning. Circulation 1985; 72: 1355–1364.
2. Reiter SJ, Rumberger JA, Feiring AJ, Stanford W, Marcus ML: Precision of right and left ventricular stroke volume measurements by rapid acquisition cine computed tomography. Circulation 1986; 74(4): 890–900.
3. Rumberger JA, Feiring AJ, Rees MR, Ell SR, Marcus ML: Quantitation of left ventricular mass and volumes in normal patients using cine computed tomography (Abstract). J Am Coll Cardiol 1986; 7(2): 173A.
4. Rumberger JA, Stark CA, Stanford W, Marcus ML: Heterogeneity of diastolic filling in normal patients as assessed by cine computed tomography (Abstract). J Am Coll Cardiol, in press.
5. Stark CA, Rumberger JA, Stanford W, Marcus ML: Dobutamine stress cine CT (Abstract). Clin Res 1986; 34(4): 902A.
6. Rumberger JA, Feiring AJ, Skorton DJ, Collins SM, Rees MR, Noel MP, Ell SR, Marcus ML: Patterns of segmental ejection fraction in normal adults within ventricular levels (Abstract). Circulation 1985; 72: III–130.
7. Feiring AJ, Rumberger JA, Reiter SJ, Rees MR, Ell SR, Marcus ML: Apex to base patterns of cavity ejection fraction in normal patients (Abstract). Circulation 1985; 72: III–367.
8. Stark CA, Rumberger JA, Reiter SJ, Marcus ML: Use of cine CT in assessing the severity of aortic regurgitation in patients (Abstract). Clin Res 1986; 34(4): 902A.
9. Stanford W, Brundage BH, McMillan R, Batemen TM, Chomka E, Lipton MJ, White CW, Wilson RF, Marcus ML: Sensitivity and specificity of assessing bypass graft patency with cine computed tomography: results of a multicenter study (Abstract). Circulation 1986; 74(4): II–41.
10. Rumberger JA, Feiring AJ, Hiratzka LE, Reiter SJ, Stanford W, Marcus ML: Determination of changes in coronary bypass graft flow rate using cine CT (Abstract). J Am Coll Cardiol 1986; 7(2): 155A.
11. Rumberger JA, Feiring AJ, Lipton MJ, Higgins CB, Marcus ML: Measurements of myocardial perfusion by ultrafast CT (Abstract). J Am Coll Cardiol 1985; 5(2): 500.

Part III: Digital Coronary Angiography

14. Morphologic and Densitometric Analysis of Coronary Arteries

JOHAN H.C. REIBER

Erasmus University Rotterdam, Rotterdam, The Netherlands

Introduction

The limitations in the visual interpretation of the morphology of coronary obstructions have been well documented in the literature. These are: the large intra- and interobserver variabilities, the fact that visually only relative per cent diameter and/or area stenosis can be estimated, and thirdly that the physiologic significance is very difficult, if not impossible, to assess. Moreover, the ever increasing application of recanalization techniques in the catheterization laboratory, such as PTCA [1–3], the use of thrombolytic agents [3–5], the introduction of the stent [6], and possibly in the near future laser [7] and/or spark erosion [8] techniques, the need to study the effects of vasoactive drugs [9, 10] and the interest in finding ways to achieve regression or nogrowth of coronary atherosclerosis [11], has stimulated the research and development towards computer-based techniques for the objective and reproducible quantitative analysis of the coronary morphology. Such techniques should provide, among others, absolute measurements on the minimal diameter, extent and asymmetry of the obstructions, relative per cent diameter and area stenosis, the roughness of the coronary arterial segment, as well as data on the mean diameters of non-obstructed coronary segments, assessed from multiple projections. By combining all stenosis measurements, the functional pressure-flow effects of the stenosis, as well as coronary flow reserve can be assessed [12]. In those situations, where the obstructions are very asymmetric, such as post-PTCA where dissections frequently occur, the computation of relative and absolute cross-sectional narrowing by densitometry seems the ultimate goal to achieve.

The majority of the applications of quantitative coronary cineangiography require the comparison of the arterial dimensions either in a control group versus those in a treated group, or pre- versus post-intervention and possibly with the data from some later control-angiogram. The sample size of the number of patients that need to be investigated to demonstrate a certain effect

P.H. Heintzen and J.H. Bürsch (eds), Progress in Digital Angiocardiography. ISBN 978-94-010-7093-5
© 1988, Kluwer Academic Publishers, Dordrecht

is proportional to the variability of the measurement technique divided by the number of years between the angiograms squared [13]. From a view point of the population size, duration and cost-effectiveness of a study, it is therefore of great importance to minimize the variability of the angiographic data acquisition and computer analysis procedures.

In general, the quantitative analysis of coronary obstructions is performed from 35 mm cinefilm. However, recent developments in digital cardiac imaging systems have been directed towards obtaining such measurements on-line during the catheterization procedure from video digitized images. With the present limitations in spatial resolution of these on-line digitized images, this approach is particularly of interest as a tool for diagnostic and/or therapeutic decision making during the catheterization procedure. However, with the use of modern small field-of-view (FOV) image intensifiers (4" and 5" FOV) and the increase in data transfer rates such that 1024^2 images at 30 frames/sec will become feasible, it may be possible in the near future to assess the effects of interventions on-line using the diameter and densitometric cross-sectional area measures mentioned above.

In this chapter an overview will be given of the different techniques that are now available for the quantitative morphologic and densitometric computer-aided analysis of the coronary obstructions [14, 15]. The majority of the techniques have been developed for cinefilm analysis; however, these are in the same or slightly modified format also applicable to the on-line digitally acquired data.

Image digitization

Because of its inherently high resolution, 35 mm cinefilm has continued to be the medium of choice for the registration of interventional coronary angiograms. For the digitization of selected cineframes, basically two approaches have been used:
1. a video camera based system with optical magnification [15, 16]; and
2. a CCD camera with a high resolution linear CCD-array that is mechanically scanned over the projected image [15, 17].

In our laboratory, a second generation video-based cine-digitizing system has recently been completed (Fig. 1). In this unit the cinefilm is mounted on a plateau with a film guiding system that can be moved under computer control left/right and upwards/downwards; the selected portion of the image is then projected onto a high resolution 1" Pasecon video camera. The camera and the projection lens can be moved independently from each other under computer control, allowing the selection of the appropriate optical magnification (ranging from 0.7 to 4 in steps of $\sqrt{2}$). The light source consists of three light

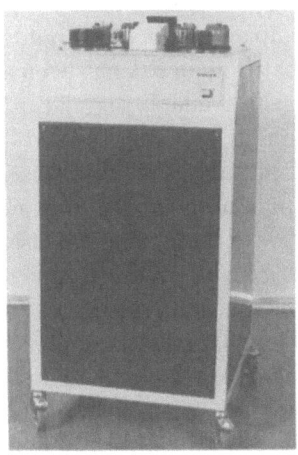

Fig. 1. Photograph of 2nd generation video-based cine-digitizing system.

emitting diodes (LEDs) with a narrow light spectrum; the emitted amount of light can be linearly adjusted. A user-controlled, motor-driven diaphragm and automated light control system further provide for optimal image quality in the selected region of interest. The resulting video signal is then digitized with a standard 15 MHz video A/D converter and the image data stored in an image processor. With a $2.0 \times$ optical magnification, the pixel size in the digitized image, referred to the original cineframe (18×24 mm) is 14.8μm. At the usual X-ray system settings of X-ray source and image intensifier (focus-isocenter = 70 cm, isocenter-image intensifier = 20 cm), a 7″ image intensifier and subtotal overframing of the cinefilm, the true object size of the original pixel at the isocenter is 71μm at this magnification. For a 5″ image intensifier the true pixel size would be 51μm.

The GE CAP 35 projector with video camera has also been used for cinefilm digitization; this projector uses a halogen light source for the illumination of the selected cineframe [18].

The CCD-camera cinefilm digitizer is a standard cineprojector (Tagarno 35 CX) with a field-installable modification package for high resolution digitization of a selected cineframe. This modification package consists of a film guiding system, a specially developed optical chain and a linear array (1728 elements) CCD camera; the array can be moved mechanically over a total of 2846 positions. The monochromatic light source consists of an array of LEDs optimally suitable for densitometric analysis of the cinefilm with the present optical chain. Any area of 6.9×6.9 mm in a selected cineframe (size 18×24 mm) can be digitized by the CCD-camera with a resolution of 512×512 pixels with 8 bits of grey levels. Effectively, this means that the

140

entire cineframe of size 18×24 mm can be digitized at a resolution of 1329×1772 pixels. A homogeneity in the brightness distribution over the entire digitized image of better than 5% has been achieved [19].

The currently commercially available digital cardiac imaging systems allow 512×512 matrix acquisitions at 30 frames/sec and 1024×1024 matrix acquisitions at max. 7 frames/sec, although the 30 frames/sec 1024^2 acquisitions have been announced already by a number of companies. In general, plumbicon video tubes with a $\gamma = 1$, with either interlaced or non-interlaced scanning systems have been used. For high resolution digitization non-interlaced (progressive) scanning should be used with preferably 10 bits of density resolution.

To compare the order of magnitude of the pixel sizes that can be achieved with a digital system with that from cinefilm digitization (71 μm at the isocenter with a 7″ image intensifier), we can make the following calculation. Assume again that a 7″ FOV image intensifier is used and that the 512^2 matrix precisely fits within the 7″ circle. With the heart positioned at the isocenter, and a distance from focus to isocenter of 70 cm and from isocenter to image intensifier of 20 cm, a pixel size of 188 μm is found at the isocenter. For a 5″ FOV image intensifier the true pixel size would be 134 μm. Of course, these pixel sizes should not be confused with the final resolution that one can obtain from these images; however, this simple calculation shows that the sampling density from cinefilm is a factor of 2.6 higher than from direct digital acquisition.

Calibration

To compute absolute sizes of the arterial segment analyzed, a calibration factor needs to be determined. Basically, two different approaches have been in use for the coronary arteries:
1. analytically from geometric X-ray system parameters;
2. on the basis of the known diameter of the contrast catheter.
Following the first approach, the size of an object in the plane through the center of rotation of the X-ray system (isocenter) and parallel to the image intensifier input screen can be determined from simple geometric principles from the height levels of X-ray tube and image intensifier. However, for objects above or below the center of rotation a slightly more complicated analysis must be carried out, requiring a second, preferably orthogonal view of the object. Wollschläger et al. have developed a method to calculate the exact radiological magnification factors for each point in the fields of view of biplane multidirectional isocentric X-ray equipment [20]. By this approach they avoid two error sources; contour detection of the catheter segment, and the differential magnification of the scaling device and the arterial segment.

If the catheter is used as a scaling device, the contours of a short segment of the tip or shaft may either be manually defined with a writing tablet, or contour detection techniques similar to those used for the coronary segments may be applied. In our routine practice, the catheter is magnified optically or electronically with a factor of $2\sqrt{2} : 1$ or $2 : 1$, respectively and a priori information is included in the iterative edge detection procedure, based on the fact that the selected part of the catheter is the projection of a cylindrical structure. It should be realized that the size of the catheter as given by the manufacturer, in general, will deviate from its true size, especially for disposable catheters. Therefore, for intervention studies it may be advisable to measure the size of the catheter following the catheterization procedure with a micrometer [21, 22].

If the known size of the catheter in a single angiographic view is used for calibration purposes, the computed calibration factor is only applicable to objects in the plane of the catheter parallel to the image intensifier input screen. The change in magnification for two objects located at different points along the X-ray beam axis is about 1.5% for each centimeter that separates the objects axially with the commonly used focus-image intensifier distances. For coronary segments lying in other planes corrections to the calibration factor can be assessed from other views.

From the above it is clear that for the measurement of truly absolute sizes of coronary segments, two views, preferably but not necessarily orthogonal to each other, are required. However, if one is only interested in the changes in sizes of coronary segments as a result of long- or short-term interventions, excellent results can be achieved from single plane views. For these situations one must make sure that for the repeat angiogram the X-ray system is positioned in exactly the same geometry as during the first angiogram. This requires registration of the angles and height levels of the X-ray system, preferably on-line with a microprocessor-based geometry read-out system [21]. Although the calibration factor used for a particular coronary arterial segment is then only an approximation of the true calibration factor, the same systematic error will be present for the first and repeat angiograms.

Pincushion distortion and correction

It is well-known that particularly the older types of image intensifiers introduce a geometric distortion, the so-called pincushion distortion. This results in selective magnification of an object near the edges of the image as compared to its size in the center of the field. These differences need to be corrected for, if absolute diameter measurements are to be derived from coronary angiograms. The standard procedure to assess the degree of distortion present is to film a cm grid, which is positioned against the input screen of the image intensifier. This needs to be done only once for a given image intensifier tube at each of the available magnification modes.

A number of approaches to correct for pincushion distortion have been implemented. Theoretically, pincushion distortion is radially symmetric about the central X-ray beam, because of the rotational symmetry of the curved image intensifiers input screen and its internal fields. The first approach makes the assumption that the distortion is indeed radially symmetric about the center of the image intensifier and that relative magnification can be determined from the distance of the pixel under consideration from the center of the image intensifier. An empirically determined analytical function of the radius is then used to correct for the distortion [23]. The second method is also based on radial symmetry, but relative magnification factors for a single radial line are stored in the memory of the computer system. The relative magnification for each distance was obtained by averaging the four values measured in the four quadrants of the cm-grid image. Hence, no analytical function is employed [16, 24]. The third method, which is in use in our center, makes no assumption about the geometrical distribution of the distortion and stores the relative magnifications of all the intersection points of the cm-grid [25]. We have developed a procedure that allows the fully automated detection of the wires and intersection points in the 1 : 1 projected cineframe. For a given point in the image which does not coincide with one of the displayed intersection positions, the correction vector is determined by means of bilinear interpolation between the correction vectors of the four neighboring intersection points.

In their digital cardiac system, LeFree et al. have implemented a somewhat similar approach, except for the fact that they correct the entire image by piecewise linear warping and not only the contour positions of the catheter and arterial segment [26]. For these purposes a 1 cm spaced orthogonal array of bronze ball bearings is imaged at the image intensifier input screen.

Contour detection coronary arterial segment

For the computer-assisted definition of the boundaries of a selected coronary segment, in general, the following steps can be distinguished:
1. definition global centerline of coronary segment;
2. edge enhancement;
3. contour definition.
The different implementations of these steps will be discussed in some more detail in the following paragraphs.

Definition global centerline

Edge positions of coronary segments in the digitized images can best be detected along scanlines perpendicular to the local centerline direction of the segment. For these purposes the first step in the contour detection algorithm requires the definition of the global trajectory of the centerline.

In general, two approaches have been advocated:
1. the user-definition of the global centerline; and
2. automated tracking of the centerline.

The user-interactive approach requires that the operator defines a midline estimate for the arterial segment to be analyzed by indicating a few center points along the vessel by means of a sonic pen or writing tablet [15, 27, 28]. This centerline is then smoothed and defines the scanlines perpendicular to the local centerline directions for the computation of the edge positions. Several groups have advocated to update this centerline by a new centerline computed from the contour positions once these have been detected and to repeat the contour detection procedure. By means of this iterative approach the influence of the user definition of the center points on the detected contour positions can be minimized.

Barth et al. have developed an automated tracking procedure for the centerline; the user only indicates a starting position and a flow direction within the arterial segment of interest [29, 30].

LeFree et al. also have developed an automated procedure for the definition of the centerline applied to digital cardiac images [26]. A polar coordinate search algorithm is used to identify the centerline of the artery following operator assignment of the approximate center of the lesion and the length of the arterial segment to be evaluated.

Edge enhancement

Edge enhancement of the digitized data is usually based on the application of first or second derivative functions or a combination of these two. In general, these derivative functions are applied to the individual scanlines perpendicular to the local centerline directions and the edge positions are subsequently defined on the basis of a given contour definition criterion. To simplify and speed up the edge enhancement and contour definition procedures both Barth et al. and Kooijman et al. resample the digital data along the scanlines, resulting in a stretched version of the arterial segment [15, 25, 29, 30]. In this resampled matrix the centerline has become a straight vertical line, whereas the scanlines are oriented horizontally. Edge enhancement can now easily be achieved by applying simple one-dimensional gradient functions along the

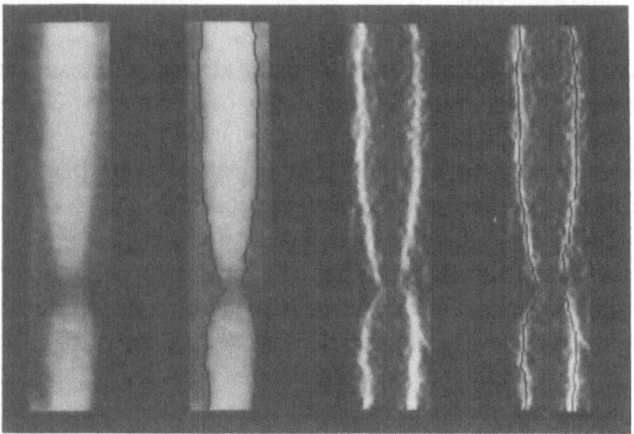

Fig. 2. Minimal cost contour detection procedure (a–d is from left to right). a: transformed intensity matrix; b: transformed intensity matrix with contours superimposed; c: cost matrix; d: cost matrix with contours superimposed.

horizontal lines. Second derivative values can be obtained by applying the gradient function to the first-derivative matrix. In Fig. 2a the resampled intensity matrix of a coronary arterial segment is shown; Fig. 2d is the cost matrix of this example where the intensity value of a pixel is a measure for the inverse value of the weighted sum of the first- and second-derivative values for that pixel.

Contour definition

To date there does not seem to be a generally accepted contour detection technique; each research group has developed and used their own algorithm. A number of these techniques will be described briefly in the following paragraphs in alphabetic order of the authors. In general, one can distinguish between local and global edge definition procedures. With the local procedure the edge points are defined on a scanline-by-scanline basis, possibly using expectation windows or the like to limit the search regions. With the global procedures, all the intensity and/or derivative information along the arterial segment are taken into account in the definition of the arterial contour.

Barth et al. use a correlation technique using 18 to 27 pixels wide edge models, one for the left edge and one for the right edge, to find the positions along the scanlines which correlate best with this model [29, 30]. The contour positions essentially correspond with the maximal 2nd derivative response of the model.

In the global approach described by Kooijman et al. the left and right contours are obtained by searching in a cost matrix from top to bottom for a minimal cost path (satisfying some connectivity constraints) to the left and right of the center column, respectively [25]. Fig. 2d shows these minimal cost contours superimposed in the cost matrix, while these contours are shown superimposed in the stretched arterial matrix in Fig. 2b. The great advantage of this minimum cost contour detection algorithm is the fact that the edge positions are not determined per individual scanline, but that information gathered from all the other scanlines is also taken into account. As a result, this approach is less sensitive to intervening structures such as branches and overlying structures than the local approach. The contour detection procedure is performed iteratively; following the first iteration of the contour detection and possibly the manual correction of erroneous contour points, a new center-line is computed as the midline of the detected points and the contour detection procedure is repeated, resulting in the final arterial contours.

In the technique described by LeFree et al. automatic edge detection is accomplished in two passes over the scanlines [26]. During the first pass the edge points are chosen between the locations defined by the extrema of the first (inflection point) and second (base point) derivatives of the arterial profile, such that the brightness level of the edge point equals 75% of the brightness difference at the inflection and base points, above the brightness level at the base point. Those initial edge points with a distance from neighboring edge points greater than an empirically determined distance are marked as not falling on the true arterial edge contour. During the second pass the threshold values for the profiles corresponding to these spurious edge points are discarded and replaced by linear interpolation from the intensities at neighboring valid edge points. The final edge points thus use local gradient and intensity information.

In the approach described by Kirkeeide et al. the derivative function along a scanline is computed according to a least squares convolution technique [31]. Two parameters of the edge detection algorithm are important: the convolution kernel size and the edge threshold level in the derivative function. They have shown that the errors in the diameter detection are hyperbolically related to the kernel size, which can be corrected for by simple empirical formulas.

Sanders et al. determine the positions with maximal first derivative response along lines perpendicular to manually traced margins to improve on these manually determined positions [16, 24].

Selzer et al. search for positions with maximal first derivative response along scanlines perpendicular to the local direction of the earlier defined centerline [27, 28]. These positions correspond with the inflection points of the brightness profiles along the scanlines. It has been our experience that such positions fit the arterial segments too tightly; if only the 1st derivative response is used, certain correction factors should be employed such that the final contour positions are shifted towards the base of the brightness profiles.

Smith et al. do not employ 1st or 2nd derivative operators to determine the arterial contours; their approach is based on the selection of a global threshold level following background subtraction [32]. The varying background in the image is removed by sliding a large sphere underneath the surface of the image. If the diameter of the sphere is chosen to be larger than the diameter of the artery, only the background signal will be located by the transformation. This signal is then subtracted to provide a background normalized image. As a final step, a threshold level is determined from this background normalized image that locates the contours of the artery.

In most publications no mention is made of particular procedures to eliminate extraneous detected positions. Experience from our earlier work made clear that certain precautions need to be taken if the contours are determined on a line-to-line basis. That means that one should define, for example, an expectation window for a certain scanline based on the detected position(s) on the previous scanline(s).

Following contour definition, a smoothing procedure is usually applied to each of the detected contour paths, which may consist of a least-squares error first degree polynomial fit through a number of nearest points on each side of the edge point under consideration. On the basis of these smoothed contours, quantitative data about the arterial dimensions can be obtained in the contour analysis phase.

Contour analysis

From the contours of the analyzed arterial segment, following pincushion correction and calibration, a diameter function can be determined by computing the distances between the left and right edges. From these data a number of parameters may be calculated such as:
1. minimal obstruction diameter;
2. extent of the obstruction;
3. percentage diameter stenosis;
4. percentage area stenosis (assuming circular cross sections);
5. hemodynamic parameters of the obstruction [12]; and
6. mean diameter of a non-obstructive coronary segment.
Particularly the minimal obstruction diameter is of great importance as it is present to the inverse fourth power in the formulas describing the pressure loss over a coronary obstruction. Moreover, to determine the effect of interventions on the severity of coronary obstructions, one should compute the changes in minimal obstruction diameter and not those in percentage diameter

narrowing, as the reference position in general will also be affected by the intervention.

However, as cardiologists have been trained to express the severity and also the changes in severity of an obstruction in terms of percentage diameter narrowing, these values are mostly included in quantitative reports. The usual way to determine percentage diameter stenosis of a coronary obstruction, requires the user to indicate a reference position. A reference diameter is then usually computed as the average value of a number of diameter values in a symmetric region with center at the user-defined reference position. It is clear that this computed %-D narrowing of an obstruction depends heavily on the selected reference position. In arteries with a focal obstructive lesion and a clearly normal proximal arterial segment, the choice of the reference region is straightforward and simple. However, in cases where the proximal part of the arterial segment shows combinations of stenotic and ectatic areas, the choice may be very difficult. To minimize these variations, alternative methods have been developed which are not dependent on a user-defined reference region [15, 25, 27, 28]. By these methods an estimate of the normal or pre-disease arterial size and luminal wall location is obtained on the basis of the computed centerline and the 90th percentile of the diameter values [27, 28], or on the basis of a first degree polynomial computed through the diameter values of the proximal and distal centerline segments followed by a translation to the 80th percentile level (reference diameter function) [15, 25]; tapering of the vessel to account for a decrease in arterial caliber associated with branches is taken care of. The reference diameter is now taken as the value of the reference diameter function at the location of the minimal obstruction diameter. The interpolated or computer-defined percentage diameter stenosis is computed by comparing the minimal diameter value at the obstruction with the corresponding value of the reference diameter. An example of our technique is shown in Fig. 3 for an obstruction in the proximal portion of the LAD in the RAO-projection. The actual contours of the arterial segment are superimposed in the image as well as the estimated pre-disease reference contours. The difference in area between the reference and the detected luminal contours is marked over the obstructive lesion; this area is a measure for the atherosclerotic plaque in this particular angiographic view. The upper function is the diameter function with the straight line being the reference diameter function; the lower function is the densitometric area function (see section Densitometry).

In addition, this interpolated or computer-defined reference diameter technique allows the assessment of the symmetry or asymmetry of the lesion in a given view with respect to a reconstructed centerline. Vessel midpoints for the proximal and distal 'normal' portions are found by averaging the coordinates of the left and right contour points. However, for the obstructive region the vessel midpoints are obtained by interpolation between the proximal and

148

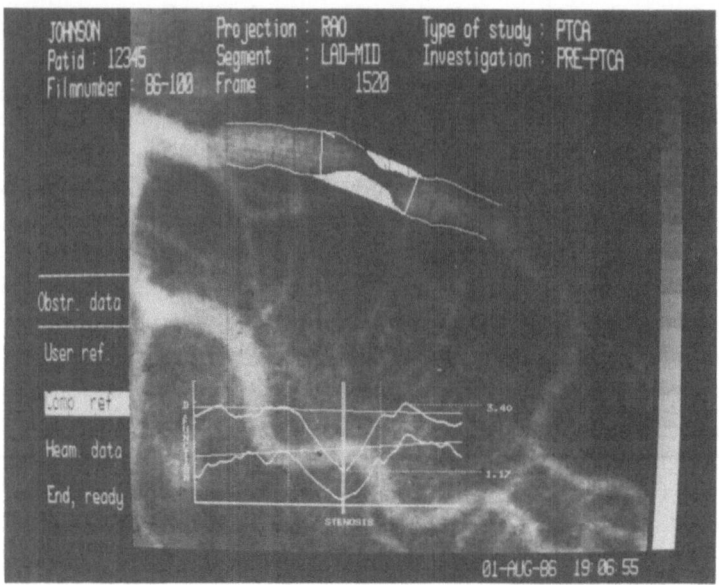

Fig. 3. Example of the automatically detected luminal boundaries of the proximal LAD-segment and the estimated pre-disease dimensions of the vessel at the site of the obstruction (reference edges). The upper function is the diameter function with the straight line through it being the reference diameter function; the lower function is the densitometric area function.

distal vessel midpoints with a second degree polynomial. The symmetry measure is given as a value between 0 and 1, with 1 representing a concentric lesion and 0 the most severe case of asymmetry or eccentricity. The extent of the obstruction is determined from the diameter function on the basis of significant maxima in curvature using variable degrees of smoothing. In addition to the fact that the interpolated technique provides data about the area of the atherosclerotic plaque and the lesion's symmetry in a given view, there is another very practical advantage. By this technique, knowledge about the exact location of a reference, either proximal or distal to the stenosis, is not required for the analysis of repeated angiograms.

From the available morphological data of the obstruction, the Poisseuille and turbulent resistances at different flows and thus the resulting transstenotic pressure gradients can be computed on the basis of the well-known fluid-dynamic equations [12, 15].

For the example of Fig. 3, the following quantitative measurements were obtained:
- extent obstruction : 7.51 mm
- reference diameter : 3.16 mm
- obstruction diameter : 1.17 mm

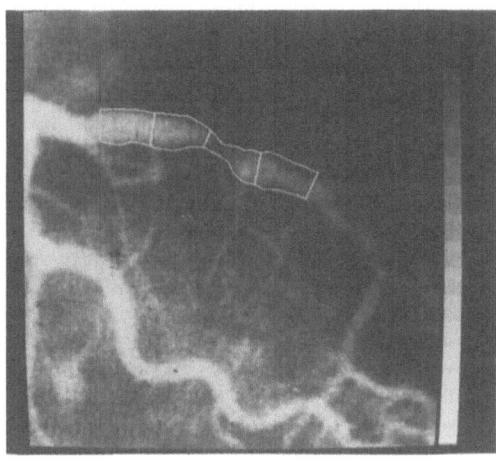

*Fig. 4.*To obtain information about the 'roughness' (irregularities) of the arterial segment, the segment is subdivided into an integer number of subsegments with lengths of approximately 5 mm and for each subsegment the standard deviation with respect to the mean value is computed. The subsegmental data for this example are presented in Table 1.

- reference area (assuming circular cross-sections) : $7.86 \, \text{mm}^2$
- obstruction area (densitometric) : $0.84 \, \text{mm}^2$
- area atherosclerotic plaque : $9.90 \, \text{mm}^2$
- symmetry measure : 0.53
- diameter stenosis : 63.1%
- area stenosis (densitometric) : 89.4%
- transstenotic pressure gradient at mean flow of 1 ml/s : $3.04 \, \text{mm Hg}$.

The mean diameter of a nonobstructive coronary segment can easily be determined from the diameter data by requesting the user to indicate with a writing tablet, lightpen or similar device the proximal and distal boundaries of the desired segment; the length of the segment in mm is usually also provided. For intervention studies coronary branch points may be used to define the boundaries of the segment, as these can be determined fairly reproducible.

Information about the 'roughness' of the arterial segment and thus about diffuse coronary artery disease may be obtained by subdividing the coronary segment into an integer number of subsegments with a length of about 5 mm and calculating for each subsegment the minimal, maximal, mean diameter and the standard deviation of the diameter values. The standard deviation possibly is a measure for diffuse atherosclerosis; clinical validation procedures need to be carried out to determine the true value of this parameter. On the basis of the quotient of the standard deviation value and the difference between minimal and maximal diameter, it can be determined whether a subsegment is focally or diffusely diseased, or normal. Figure 4 shows the four

Table 1. Subsegmental data for the example of Fig. 4. Segment no. 1 is the most proximal segment.

	Segment			
	1	2	3	4
Length (mm)	5.51	5.51	5.51	5.51
Minimal diameter (mm)	2.92	1.74	1.17	2.68
Maximal diameter (mm)	3.29	3.27	3.03	3.40
Mean diameter (mm)	3.04	2.85	2.02	2.99
Standard deviation (mm)	0.12	0.48	0.69	0.24
Focal or diffuse disease	no	yes	yes	no

subsegments for the example of Fig. 3; the derived subsegmental data are given in Table 1.

Densitometry

Since the luminal cross-section at a coronary obstruction is frequently irregular in shape, percentage diameter reduction measured in a single angiographic view is of limited diagnostic value. The hemodynamic resistance of an obstruction is determined to a great extent by the minimal cross-sectional area. Computation of this cross-sectional area reduction from the percentage diameter reduction measured in a single view requires the assumption of, e.g., circular cross-sections, an assumption which hardly ever holds. The resulting error may be reduced by incorporating two orthogonal projections and computing elliptical cross-sections. However, with the often occurring eccentric lesions even this last approach may yield inaccurate results.

The edge detection techniques described above, in general are based on the measurement of changes in the brightness profiles along scanlines perpendicular to local centerline segments. However, if one could constitute the relationship between the path lengths of the X-rays through the artery and the absolute brightness values in the digitized image, one would obtain the information required to compute the cross-sectional areas from a single view (Fig. 5). It is clear that a homogeneous mixing of the contrast agent with the blood must be assumed for the measurement to have any meaning.

A simplified block diagram of a complete X-ray/cine acquisition and analysis system is shown in Fig. 6. In a digital cardiac system the cinefilm components are absent and the video camera at the output screen of the image intensifier (not shown in Fig. 6) is connected directly to the A/D-converter.

Constitution of the relationship between path length and brightness values requires detailed analysis of the complete imaging system. In a simplified

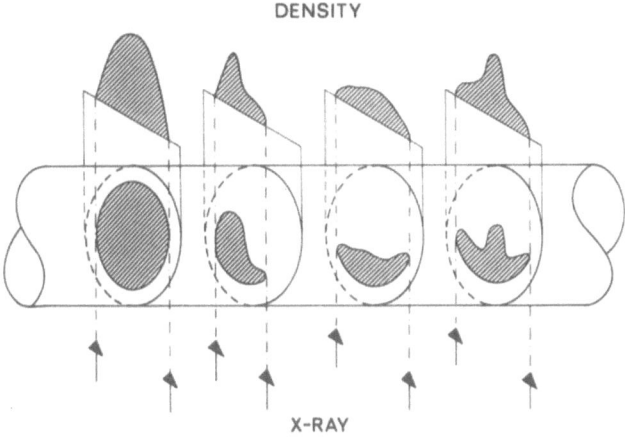

DENSITY

X-RAY

Fig. 5. Schematic illustration of the relationship between the irradiated object thickness and the brightness level in the digitized angiographic image.

approach, we are only interested in the static properties of the system. Analysis of the static transfer function of each link in the chain reveals that computation of the complete transfer function is very difficult. There is a large number of parameters involved, many of which are spatially variant [15, 33]. A few different approaches towards densitometric analysis of selected coronary arterial segments have been published and will be described briefly in the following paragraphs.

Most authors assume that the X-ray absorption process, comprising the first part of the imaging chain from X-ray source to the image intensifier input screen, can be described by the Lambert-Beer law. Despite many potential sources of errors in the absorption process (non-monochromatic X-ray spectrum, beam hardening, scattering, etc.) it has indeed been demonstrated by Bürsch and Heintzen that by the use of appropriate filters and scatter grids the Lambert-Beer law is applicable for densitometric measurements in clinical studies with a sufficient degree of accuracy [34, 35].

On the other hand, Doriot et al. have indicated that the Lambert-Beer absorption law cannot account for the non-linear relationship beween densitometric signal and logarithmic X-ray transmission through the lumen of an opacified coronary artery [36, 37]. Therefore, they have developed a physical model which takes the polychromasy and scattered radiation into account and have shown that this relation can be approximated by a 2nd order polynomial. The coefficients of this polynomial depend primarily on the voltage applied to the X-ray tube and on the iodine concentration of the injected contrast medium. For a particular X-ray system the coefficients of the polynomial can simply be obtained once by means of a linear wedge filled with contrast material.

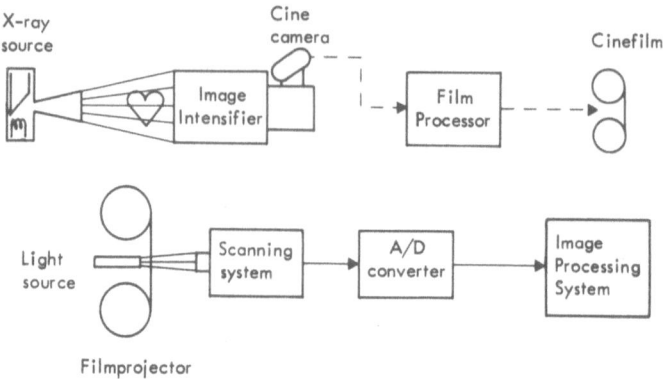

Fig. 6. Block diagram of an X-ray/cine acquisition and analysis system.

However, in general, for the remaining subsystems of the cinefilm imaging chain comprising the image intensifier, the cinefilm exposure and development process, and the film sampling process which may be achieved via video and A/D conversion, with a CCD camera or other device, simplified formulas relating measured brightness levels with the irradiated object thicknesses are used neglecting the influence of spatially non-homogeneous responses [29, 38]. By this approach the response of film exposure, the density D versus log (exposure) curve, is being linearized (linear transfer function).

We have implemented a more complicated approach in an attempt to correct for the non-linearities in the D versus log (E) plot and for the daily variations in the cinefilm processing [15, 33]. For this purpose, a special sensitometer has been developed which allows 21 full cineframes covering the entire densitometric range of the film to be exposed on each film cassette before it is mounted on the image intensifier of the X-ray system (Fig. 7). The color temperature of the light source is the same as the one from the output screen of the image intensifier. The analysis procedure of a coronary cineangiogram therefore starts with the digitization of these 21 sensitometric frames, allowing the assessment of a non-linear transfer function.

By means of this calibration procedure many non-linear, and temporally and spatially variant effects in the film-processing and the film-video or film-CCD camera system are taken into account. It has indeed been shown that this sensitometric approach improves the accuracy of measurement of cross-sectional area measurements as compared to the linear approach [39].

In a digital cardiac system, the transfer function from the output of the image intensifier up to the digitized image can be assumed to be a linear function.

The basic steps in the densitometric procedure to compute percentage cross-sectional area reduction of a selected lesion can be summarized as

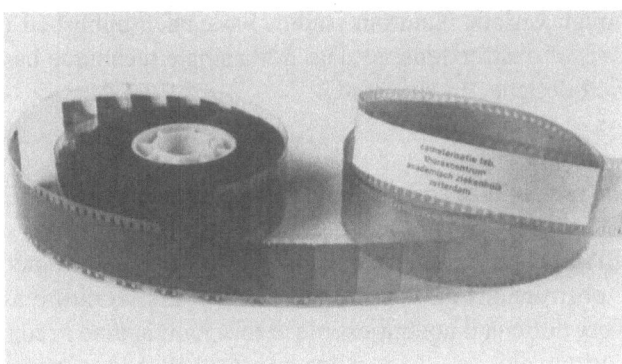

Fig. 7. Example of cinefilm with sensitometric strip of 21 homogeneously exposed cineframes.

follows. The contours of a selected arterial segment are detected as described before. On each scanline perpendicular to the centerline, a profile of brightness values is measured. This profile is transformed into an absorption profile by means of the computed transfer functions (linear or non-linear depending on the technique used). The background contribution is estimated by computing the linear regression line through the background points directly left and right of the detected contours. Subtraction of this background portion from the absorption profile within the arterial contours yields the net cross-sectional absorption profile. Integration of this function results in a measure for the cross-sectional area at the particular scanline. By repeating this procedure for all the scanlines, the cross-sectional area function $A(i)$ is obtained. Percentage area reduction of an obstruction is determined by comparing the minimal area value at the obstruction with the mean value at a selected reference position. The earlier mentioned interpolated approach can also be applied for the estimation of the pre-disease area values. If we assume that the cross-section at the reference position is circular, absolute cross-sectional values (in mm^2) for the arterial segments and thus for the minimal cross-section can be obtained.

The lower function in the example of Fig. 3 is the densitometric area function for the segment. A percentage densitometric cross-sectional area reduction of 89.4% was found, indicating that the obstruction is slightly more severe than one would estimate by assuming circular cross-sections (86% area reduction).

It will be clear that the densitometric analysis of coronary arterial segments is a difficult problem because of all the potential problems that may arise. In addition to all the possible error sources mentioned above, another important aspect is the orientation of the vessel of interest with respect to the X-ray beam [40]. In addition, sidebranches or branches lying very close to the arterial segment to be analyzed will cause errors in the background correction tech-

nique. Although various phantom studies have been published on densitometric analysis of obstructions, to date not a single technique has been validated in a well-designed in vivo study.

Measurement variabilities and validation procedures

Although different approaches on the morphologic and densitometric analysis
of coronary obstructions have been published in the literature as described
above, it is very difficult if not impossible at this point in time to compare these
systems quantitatively, i.e. the question how well all these systems work with
routinely obtained coronary angiograms cannot be answered. Data about the
accuracy and precision of the edge detection and analysis procedures, the
success scores under different image qualities, computation time, etc. are
usually not provided in the publications; if they are provided different parameters to describe the validation results have been used making comparisons very
difficult. Recently, discussions among several groups active in this field have
taken place in an attempt to define commonly accepted validation procedures
for the quantitative coronary angiography analysis systems. In my opinion the
following validation procedures should be carried out:

1. *Assessment accuracy edge detection and densitometric techniques.*
   - Phantom studies of coronary obstructions with dimensions from 0.5 to
     5.0 mm under different imaging conditions (various concentrations of the
     contrast agent, different kV-levels covering the routinely used range)
     and under static and dynamic flow conditions.
   - In vivo animal studies with hollow plastic cylinders of various luminal
     shapes and sizes inserted in the coronary arteries [41, 42].
   - For densitometric studies the results should be independent of the angio-
     graphic views in which these studies were acquired.
2. *Reproducibility.* Repeated analysis of a set of clinical coronary angiograms
   obtained under various imaging conditions to assess inter- and intra-observer variabilities.
3. *Parameters describing the validation results.* It is suggested to describe the
   results from the validation studies in terms of the mean differences and the
   standard deviations of the differences (measurement 1 – measurement 2;
   not absolute differences) between the true and measured values or between
   the values from repeated measurements.

Approaches towards standardization in angiographic data acquisition and analysis

It has been shown that the variabilities in the arterial measurements can be decreased by standardizing on the angiographic data acquisition and analysis procedures [21, 43]. In summary, the following measures have been proposed:

1. precise registration of the angulations of the X-ray system for the different angiographic views, so that the repeat angiographies can be performed in the same views;
2. administration of vasodilative drug immediately prior to angiographic investigations;
3. use of modern isoviscous and iso-osmolar contrast agents;
4. administration of contrast medium preferably by ECG-triggered injector;
5. selection of contrast catheter constructed of such material that high quality image results (high angiographic image contrast and edge gradient);
6. measurement of actual size catheter with micrometer following catheterization procedure.

Summary

There is an increasing demand for the objective and reproducible assessment of coronary arterial dimensions to study the efficacy of new recanalization techniques in the catheterization laboratory, to study new approaches to achieve regression or no-growth of coronary atherosclerosis and also as a means for diagnostic and therapeutic decision making during the cardiac catheterization. This last application requires the use of digital cardiac imaging systems with the capability to store the images on-line on real-time disks; at the present time, the other applications are usually evaluated off-line from 35 mm cinefilm.

In this chapter an overview is presented on the different techniques that have been developed for the quantitative analysis of the size and shape of coronary arterial segments, and in particular of coronary obstructions. The first approaches have been directed towards the (semi-)automated boundary detection of the arterial segments and the subsequent computation of the relative and absolute length and width dimensions; later approaches have attempted to determine the cross-sectional narrowing of obstructions from a single angiographic view by densitometry. In general, the algorithms are applicable to both digitized cineframes and the on-line acquired digital images, possibly requiring slight modifications from the one medium to the other.

Acknowledgements

The author wishes to thank Mrs S.M. Spierdijk and Mrs M.J. Kanters-Stam for their secretarial assistance in the preparation of this manuscript.

References

1. Serruys PW, Reiber JHC, Wijns W, Brand M van den, Kooijman CJ, Katen HJ ten, Hugenholtz PG: Assessment of percutaneous transluminal coronary angioplasty by quantitative coronary angiography: diameter versus densitometric area measurements. Am J Cardiol 1984; 54: 482–488.
2. Serruys PW, Geuskens R, Feyter P de, Brand M van den, Deckers J, Katen H ten, Reiber H: Incidence of restenosis 30 and 60 days after successful PTCA: A quantitative coronary angiographic study in 200 consecutive patients (Abstract). Circulation 1985; 72 (Suppl III): III-140.
3. Serruys PW, Wijns W, Brand M van den, Ribeiro V, Fioretti P, Simoons ML, Kooijman CJ, Reiber JHC, Hugenholtz PG: Is transluminal coronary angioplasty mandatory after successful thrombolysis? A quantitative coronary angiographic study. Br Heart J 1983; 50: 257–265.
4. Serruys PW, Arnold AER, Brower RW, Bono DP de, Rutsch W, Uebis R, Vahanian A: Quantitative assessment of the effect of continued rt-PA infusion on the residual stenosis after initial recanalisation in acute myocardial infarction (Abstract). Circulation 1986; 74: II-368.
5. Serruys PW, Arnold AER, Brower RW, Bono DP de, Bokslag M, Lubsen J, Reiber JHC, Rutsch W, Uebis R, Vahanian A, Verstraete M: Effect of continued rt-PA administration on the residual stenosis after initially successful recanalization in acute myocardial infarction – a quantitative coronary angiography study of a randomized trial. Eur Heart J 1987; 8 (in press).
6. Sigwart U, Puel J, Mirkovitch V, Joffre F, Kappenberger L: Intravascular stents to prevent occlusion and restenosis after transluminal angioplasty. N Engl J Med 1987; 316: 701–706.
7. Isner JM, Clarke RH: Laser angioplasty: unraveling the Gordian Knot. J Am Coll Cardiol 1986; 7: 705–708.
8. Slager CJ, Essed CA, Schuurbiers JCH, Bom N, Serruys PW, Meester GT: Vaporization of atherosclerotic plaques by spark erosion. J Am Coll Cardiol 1985; 5: 1382–1386.
9. Serruys PW, Lablanche JM, Reiber JHC, Bertrand ME, Hugenholtz PG: Contribution of dynamic vascular wall thickening to luminal narrowing during coronary arterial vasomotion. Z Kardiol 1983; 72: 116–123.
10. Deckers JW, Reiber JHC, Serruys PW: Long-lasting vasodilatory effect of intracoronary administration of Molsidomine metabolite SIN-1. In: Bing RJ, Stauch M (eds) Ischemic heart disease and heart failure. Advances in treatment with Molsidomine; pp 80–85. Urban and Schwarzenberg, Munich/Vienne/Baltimore, 1986.
11. Arntzenius AC, Kromhout D, Barth JD, Reiber JHC, Bruschke AVG, Buis B, Gent CM van, Kempen-Voogd N, Strikwerda S, Velda EA van der: Diet, lipoproteins, and the progression of coronary atherosclerosis. The Leiden Intervention Trial. N Engl J Med 1985; 312: 805–811.
12. Gould KL, Kirkeeide RL: Assessment of stenosis severity. In: Reiber JHC, Serruys PW (eds) State of the art in quantitative coronary arteriography; pp 209–228. Martinus Nijhoff Publishers, Dordrecht/Boston/Lancaster, 1986.
13. Blankenhorn DH, Brooks SH: Angiographic trials of lipid-lowering therapy. Arteriosclerosis 1981; 1: 242–249.
14. Reiber JHC, Kooijman CJ, Slager CJ, Gerbrands JJ, Schuurbiers JCH, Boer A den, Wijns

W, Serruys PW: Computer-assisted analysis of the severity of obstruction from coronary cineangiograms: a methodological review. Automedica 1984; 5: 219–238.

15. Reiber JHC, Serruys PW, Slager CJ: Quantitative coronary and left ventricular cineangiography; methodology and clinical applications. Martinus Nijhoff Publishers, Boston/Dordrecht/ Lancaster, 1986.

16. Sanders WJ, Alderman EL, Harrison DC: Coronary artery quantitation using digital image processing techniques. Comp Cardiol 1979; 15–20.

17. Reiber JHC, Kooijman CJ, Slager CJ, Ree EJB van, Kalberg RJN, Tijdens FO, Plas J van der, Frankenhuyzen J van, Claessen WCH: Taking a quantitative approach to cine-angiogram analysis. Diagnostic Imaging, April 1985; 87–89.

18. Selzer RH, Shircore A, Lee PL, Hemphill L, Blankenhorn DH: A second look at quantitative coronary angiography: some unexpected problems. In: Reiber JHC, Serruys PW (eds) State of the art in quantitative coronary arteriography; pp 125–143. Martinus Nijhoff Publishers, Dordrecht/Boston/Lancaster, 1986.

19. Kooijman CJ, Kalberg R, Slager CJ, Tijdens FO, Plas J van der, Reiber JHC: Densitometric analysis of coronary arteries. In: Young IT, Biemond J, Duin RPW, Gerbrands JJ (eds) Signal processing III: theories and applications; pp 1405–1408. North Holland, Amsterdam/ New York/Oxford/Tokyo, 1986.

20. Wollschläger H, Lee P, Zeiher A, Solzbach U, Bonzel T, Just H: Improvement of quantitative angiography by exact calculation of radiological magnification factors. Comp Cardiol 1985; 483–486.

21. Reiber JHC, Serruys PW, Kooijman CJ, Slager CJ, Schuurbiers JCH, Boer A den: Approaches towards standardization in acquisition and quantitation of arterial dimensions from cineangiograms. In: Reiber JHC, Serruys PW (eds) State of the art in quantitative coronary arteriography; pp 145–172. Martinus Nijhoff Publishers, Dordrecht/Boston/Lancaster, 1986.

22. Reiber JHC, Kooijman CJ, Boer A den, Serruys PW: Assessment of dimensions and image quality of coronary contrast catheters from cineangiograms. Cath Cardiovasc Diagn 1985; 11: 521–531.

23. Brown BG, Bolson E, Frimer M, Dodge HT: Quantitative coronary arteriography. Estimation of dimensions, hemodynamic resistance, and atheroma mass of coronary artery lesion using the arteriograms and digital computation. Circulation 1977; 55: 329–337.

24. Alderman EL, Berte LE, Harrison DC, Sanders W: Quantitation of coronary artery dimensions using digital imaging processing. In: Brody WR (ed) Digital radiography; pp 273–278. SPIE 314, 1982.

25. Kooijman CJ, Reiber JHC, Gerbrands JJ, Schuurbiers JCH, Slager CJ, Boer A den, Serruys PW: Computer-aided quantitation of the severity of coronary obstructions from single view cineangiograms. First IEEE Comp Soc Int Symp on Medical imaging and image interpretation. IEEE Cat No 82 CH1804-4, 1982; 59–64.

26. LeFree M, Simon SB, Lewis RJ, Bates ER, Vogel RA: Digital radiographic coronary artery quantification. Comp Cardiol 1985; 99–102.

27. Selzer RH, Blankenhorn DH, Crawford DW, Brooks SH, Barndt R: Computer analysis of cardiovascular imagery. Proceedings of the Caltech/JPL Conference on Image processing technology, data sources and software for commercial and scientific applications, Pasadena, 1976; 1–20.

28. Ledbetter DC, Selzer RH, Gordon RM, Blankenhorn DH, Sanmarco ME: Computer quantitation of coronary angiograms. In: Miller HA, Schmidt EV, Harrison DC (eds) Noninvasive cardiovascular measurements; pp 17–20. SPIE 167, 1978.

29. Barth K, Epple E, Irion KM, Faust U, Decker D: Quantifizierung von Stenosen der Herzkranzgefässe durch Digitale Bildauswertung. Erg Bd Biomed Technik 1981; 26.

30. Barth K, Faust U, Both A, Wedekind K: A critical examination of angiographic stenosis

quantitation by digital image processing. First IEEE Comp Soc Int Symp on Medical imaging and image interpretation, IEEE Cat No 82 CH1804-4, 1982; 71–76.

31. Kirkeeide RL, Fung P, Smalling RW, Gould KL: Automated evaluation of vessel diameter from arteriograms. Comp Cardiol 1982; 215–218.

32. Smith DN, Colfer H, Brymer JF, Pitt B, Kliman SH: A semiautomatic computer technique for processing coronary angiograms. Comp Cardiol 1982; 325–328.

33. Reiber JHC, Slager CJ, Schuurbiers JCH, Boer A den, Gerbrands JJ, Troost GJ, Scholts B, Kooijman CJ, Serruys PW: Transfer functions of the X-ray-cine-video chain applied to digital processing of coronary cineangiograms. In: Heintzen PH, Brennecke R (eds) Digital imaging in cardiovascular radiology; pp 89–104. Georg Thieme Verlag, Stuttgart, 1983.

34. Bürsch J, Johs R, Heintzen P: Validity of Lambert-Beer's law in roentgendensitometry of contrast material (Urografin) using continuous radiation. In: Heintzen PH (ed) Roentgen-, cine- and videodensitometry: fundamentals and applications for blood flow and heart volume determinations; pp 81–84. Georg Thieme Verlag, Stuttgart, 1971.

35. Heintzen P, Moldenhauer M: X-ray absorption by contrast material using pulsed radiation. In: Heintzen PH (ed) Roentgen-, cine- and videodensitometry: fundamentals and applications for blood flow and heart volume determinations; pp 73–81. Georg Thieme Verlag, Stuttgart, 1971.

36. Doriot P-A, Pochon Y, Rasoamanambelo L, Chatelain P, Welz R, Rutishauser W: Densitometry of coronary arteries – an improved physical model. Comp Cardiol 1985; 91–94.

37. Doriot P-A, Pochon Y, Welz R, Rutishauser W: Non-linearity by densitometric measurements of coronary arteries. In this volume, pp. 171–178.

38. Sandor T, Als AV, Paulin S: Cine-densitometric measurement of coronary arterial stenoses. Cath Cardiovasc Diagn 1979; 5: 229–245.

39. Reiber JHC, Kooijman CJ, Slager CJ, Boer A den, Serruys PW: Improved densitometric assessment % area-stenosis from coronary cineangiograms (Abstract). X World Congress of Cardiology, Washington, 1986; 39.

40. Parker DL, Pope DL, Petersen JC, Clayton PD, Gustafson DE: Quantitation in cardiac video-densitometry. Comp Cardiol 1984; 119–122.

41. Block M, Bove AA, Ritman EL: Coronary angiographic examination with the dynamic spatial reconstructor. Circulation 1984; 70: 209–216.

42. Mancini GBJ, Vogel RA: Coronary arteriography, stress test and coronary flow reserve measurements: comparative studies. In this volume, p. 293–303.

43. Reiber JHC, Serruys PW, Kooijman CJ, Wijns W, Slager CJ, Gerbrands JJ, Schuurbiers JCH, Boer A den, Hugenholtz PG: Assessment of short-, medium- and long-term variations in arterial dimensions from computer-assisted quantitation of coronary cineangiograms. Circulation 1985; 71: 280–288.

15. Comparison of 35 mm Cine Film and Digital Radiographic Image Imaging for Quantitative Coronary Arteriography

ROBERT A. VOGEL, MICHAEL T. LEFREE &
G.B. JOHN MANCINI
Cardiology Section, Veterans Administration Medical Center, Department of Internal Medicine, University of Michigan Medical School, Ann Arbor, MI, USA

Visual interpretation of coronary stenosis severity is complicated by the irregular geometry and unknown orientation of the vessel, and the presence of adjacent or superimposed structures [1]. These problems combine to contribute to imprecision and observer variability [2, 3]. This problem has given rise to the development of several computerized quantitative arteriographic techniques [4–26]. Methods employing computer analysis of manual tracings of the borders of magnified cine film projections of coronary artery segments were first reported by Brown and co-workers [4]. Quantitative arteriography has now progressed through the efforts of many investigators to the point of requiring little operator intervention due to the use of automated edge detection computer algorithms [10, 15–19]. This reduces variability by removing the subjectivity of manual tracing of arterial borders. Most approaches determine the absolute geometric extent of a lesion by edge detection and relative cross-sectional area by densitometry within the detected edges.

To this point, 35 mm cine film remains the standard image storage medium for this type of analysis. Within the last few years digital radiographic imaging has become widely available [18, 27]. This new technology has the ability to directly digitize and store the angiographic video output in real time (30 frames/sec) without the use of film. This achievement has raised the question of whether cine film or digital storage is optimum for quantitation coronary arteriography. Tobis and co-workers have clinically addressed this issue by comparing visual assessment and manual caliper quantitation of cine film and 512×512 pixel digital radiographic coronary arteriography [28]. They reported no significant difference between the two image recording methods. In spite of this work, routine clinical application of digital radiography of the coronary arteries has been hampered because of the hypothesis that the usable spatial resolution of digital imaging at 512×512 pixel resolution is reduced relative to that of standard 35 mm cine film. Recently, 1024×1024 pixel digital radiographic imaging has been developed to overcome this problem. In view of the latter developments, it has become important to determine which imaging

P.H. Heintzen and J.H. Bürsch (eds), Progress in Digital Angiocardiography. ISBN 978-94-010-7093-5
© 1988, Kluwer Academic Publishers, Dordrecht

method best supports automated quantitative arteriography. The use of digital radiographic imaging quantitation would be especially desirable in the setting of interventional procedures such as percutaneous transluminal coronary angioplasty, which are hampered by the delay of film development.

The purpose of this study was to compare quantitative arteriography based on 35 mm cine film and 512×512 and 1024×1024 pixel digital imaging of a radiographic arterial phantom. This comparison uses a new fully automated computer program which quantitates arterial dimensions both geometrically and densitometrically.

Image acquisition

An arterial radiographic phantom was designed and constructed consisting of a 1.0 cm thick plate of lucite precision-drilled with holes ranging from 0.5 mm to 5.0 mm in diameter. These holes were grouped in seven 'arterial' segments, providing fourteen lesions ranging from 17% to 87% diameter stenosis. This phantom was filled with a 100% concentration of iodine contrast medium (Renografin 76, E.R. Squibb and Sons), oriented with the axes of the arterial models perpendicular to the X-ray beam, and imaged with both 35 mm cine film (VARI-X, 400u) and a commercially available digital radiography system (ADAC Laboratories, DPS-4100C). Efforts were made to mimic actual clinical imaging conditions by including 15 cm depth of water as a scattering medium, an object-detector distance of 15 cm, a 0.6 mm focal spot size, and 2.5 mm aluminium equivalent filtration. X-ray beam energies of 70–80 kVp with a standard cineangiographic exposure rate of 25 micro-Roentgens per frame were employed with both imaging techniques using a Siemens Pandoros biplane angiographic X-ray system. In all cases a 12.5 cm diameter field-of-view was utilized.

In the case of digital radiography, single-frame progressively scanned video images at both $512 \times 512 \times 8$ bit and $1024 \times 1024 \times 8$ bit resolution were directly digitized and analyzed. The digital radiographic system uses a video camera with a 1000:1 signal-to-noise ratio lead-oxide vidicon. After development in a standard cine film processor (Jamieson, Model 54), the 35 mm cine film images were projected on a cine projector (Vanguard Instruments XR-15) which has optical coupling to a video camera (of the same type as the digital radiographic camera) via a 10:1 beam splitter. Using 4:1 optical magnification, the resulting video signal was digitized at $512 \times 512 \times 8$ bit resolution into the digital radiographic system for storage and analysis. The video noise of this method of film digitization was reduced by averaging four successive video frames prior to storage. At that magnification, sub-frame film images were analyzed at the actual resolution of 2048×2048 pixels. Digital radiographic images were subjected to digital magnification to an effective full-frame resolution of 2048 × 2048 pixels using bi-linear interpolation (4X magnification for 512 × 512 images, and 2X magnification for 1024 × 1024 images). In order to provide as direct comparison as possible with the 35 mm images digitized in this manner, the digital radiographic images were subjected to digital magnification to an effective full-frame resolution of 2048 × 2048 pixels using bi-linear interpolation (4X magnification for 512 × 512 images, and 2X magnification for 1024 × 1024 images).

Image pre-processing

Both film and digital images were subjected to pre-processing prior to quantitative analysis. Both had gray-scale modification after magnification to linearly expand their individual dynamic ranges to the full 8-bits of the digital radiographic system. No subtraction techniques were employed with either film or digital images.

Image analysis

Our quantitation program uses image analysis techniques similar to several previous efforts [15], but was specifically designed to provide rapid results with minimal operator interaction [18, 19]. The operator chooses a circular region of analysis by first positioning a light-pen cursor over the arterial lesion itself and then adjusting the size of the circular region to encompass the desired segment of artery to be analyzed. The software then proceeds without further operator intervention. The centerline of the arterial segment within the analysis region is determined by analyzing circular profiles of decreasing radius. After the centerline is determined, linear density profiles perpendicular to the arterial centerline are extracted at intervals of approximately 0.25 mm over the length of the arterial segment. Automatic edge detection is accomplished in two passes over these linear density profiles. On the first pass, initial edge points are found by noting the gray-scale densities of points at the extrema of the first (inflection) and second (base) derivatives of each perpendicular density profile. A local threshold is calculated to fall between the densities at the base and inflection points on either side of the artery. Initial edge points are defined as those points which fall at an empirically determined value of 75% of the difference between the densities at these derivative extrema. This percentage was determined experimentally to yield the best combination of regression statistics.

Due to radiographic, subtraction, or film noise, and adjacent structures, these gradient-determined initial edge points sometimes fail to form a continuous edge contour. To avoid this, spurious edge points are discarded with application of a spatial continuity criterion. During a second edge detection pass, the threshold values at non-continuous locations are replaced by linear interpolation from the densities at neighboring valid edge points. Processed in this manner, the final edge contour is found using both local gradient and density information. The program is therefore able to account for varying background densities along each side independently.

Densitometric relative cross-sectional area is also calculated from the perpendicular density profiles following the method of Kruger *et al.* [23]. In this calculation, the edge positions along each density profile establish the limits for the integration of the individual density profiles. We employ background compensation which uses the densities at the edge points to either side of the artery to provide base points to construct a linearly interpolated approximation for the superimposed background densities. The integral of densities under the resulting background density compensation curve is simply subtracted from the integral of the actual density curve. Per cent diameter and cross-sectional area stenoses are calculated from comparison of stenotic and normal region data. The operator is able to interact with the final display by guiding a graphics cursor along the arterial centerline to extract the quantitative information at any location along the arterial segment. Cursors simultaneously display the cursor location on a straightened, stylized artery at the top of the display and the corresponding position along the diameter and area plots. Calculated values for diameter and area per cent stenosis are also displayed. The computer program is able to complete the analysis of a single lesion in approximately thirty seconds. In order to characterize the accuracy and precision of this analysis for the three imaging techniques, this quantitation was performed over an approximately 1.0 cm long segment of each diameter of the arterial phantom. Program output was modified to include the printout of the mean geometric diameter, mean densitometic relative cross-sectional area, and standard deviation of diameter measurements at all points along the length analyzed. Since the arterial phantom consists of cylindrical holes, the standard deviation of projected geometric diameter was included as a measure of the variability of single diameter measurements. Per cent diameter stenosis and per cent area stenosis were calculated from the mean diameter and relative cross-sectional area data. Data for projected geometric diameter, per cent diameter stenosis, densitometric relative cross-sectional area, and per cent area stenosis were subjected to linear regression analysis to calculate the slope, y-intercept, coefficient of correlation, and standard error of the estimate of measured versus actual values for these parameters.

The inter- and intra-observer reproducibility of the technique was measured by linear regression analysis of blinded observations by two operators using identical data sets and by multiple observations by a single observer.

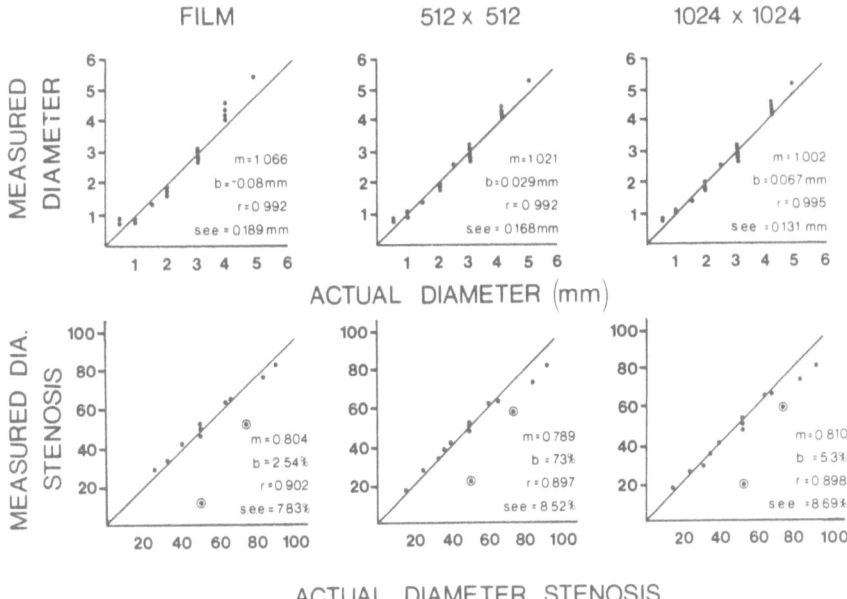

Fig. 1. Projected geometric diameter and per cent diameter stenosis linear regression results for cine film, 512 × 512 and 1024 × 1024 digital radiography. R is the coefficient of correlation, m is the regression slope, b is the regression intercept, and s_e is the standard error of the estimate.

Results

The linear regression results are summarized in Figs 1 and 2. These figures show linear regression plots and statistics for projected geometric diameter, per cent diameter stenosis (Fig. 1), and for densitometric relative cross-sectional area, and per cent area stenosis (Fig. 2), for 35 mm cine film as well as 512 × 512 and 1024 × 1024 pixel digital radiographic imaging techniques. Also shown in Fig. 1 are average values for the diameter variability measurement for each imaging technique.

Reproduction tests showed that paired multiple observations of projected geometric diameter or densitometric relative cross-sectional area by a single observer or comparing blinded results by two different operators never yielded linear regression results with a coefficient of correlation less than r = 0.997.

The corresponding regression plots for diameter stenosis were again similar, although the coefficient of correlation for film (r = 0.902) was reduced relative to those of both direct digital methods (512 × 512, r = 0.897, and 1024 × 1024, r = 0.898). The standard error of the estimate of film diameter stenosis (s_e = 13.42%) was greater than those of 512 × 512 (s_e = 8.53%) or 1024 × 1024 imaging (s_e = 8.70%), although the electronic imaging methods were only

164

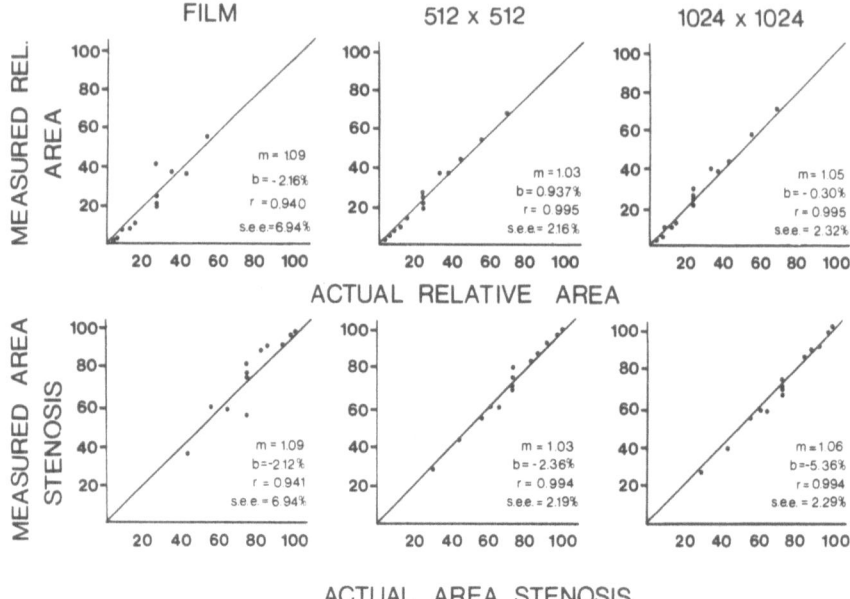

nearly significantly superior to film (512 × 512, p = 0.054; 1024 × 1024, p = 0.062). The regression slopes (on the order of 0.80) and intercepts (5.32%–7.26%) were not significantly different than 1.0 and 0.0, respectively. No method had slopes or intercepts superior to another. Points with tight (below 1.0 mm) stenoses showed marked underestimation of per cent diameter stenosis (note the circled points).

Densitometric relative cross-sectional area regression analysis revealed coefficients of correlation for digital radiographic methods (r = 0.995) to be somewhat greater than that for film (r = 0.940). Standard errors of the estimates for the electronic imaging media were superior to that of film (512 × 512 and 1024 × 1024, p<0.0001). The slopes and intercepts were not significantly different from 1.0 and 0.0, respectively, for all three methods, and the analysis of covariance showed no significant differences between the regression slopes and intercepts for the different methods.

Per cent area stenosis analysis showed results similar to relative cross-sectional area data.

Reproducibility tests showed that paired multiple observations of geometric diameter or densitometric relative cross-sectional area by a single observer or comparing blinded results by two different operators did not yield linear regression results with coefficients of correlation under r = 0.9997.

Discussion

The results of this experiment must be interpreted within the confines of its experimental design. This experiment was intended to be a direct comparison of the basic intrinsic properties of 35 mm cine film and digitized video as imaging media for coronary quantitation. There are two clinically relevant factors which were not addressed, namely: non-circular lesional cross-sectionality and arterial projection. In addition, certain physical phenomena known to effect the clinical accuracy of the method were not corrected for in order to more effectively delineate the differences between the three imaging methods. In order to calculate absolute arterial dimensions, correction for geometric magnification is necessary. In clinical practice, the operator has the option of using the known diameter of the catheter or an orthogonal grid imaged in the same geometry as the artery to achieve pixel calibration for magnification correction. In the case of catheter calibration, the same edge detection algorithm is employed over a small segment of the catheter, the pixel linear correction factor is calculated, and the operator may then proceed with arterial analysis as described above. When using the grid calibration method, a rectangular area of known dimension is determined. Magnification correction using an external reference object can itself cause significant variation in the results [29]. Therefore, for the purpose of this study, we chose to employ an internal magnification in order to eliminate this source of variability. Magnification correction was achieved by averaging the six 3.0 mm diameter lumena pixel dimensions. Additionally, in clinical use, images are corrected for pincushion distortion by the application of a geometric transformation which maps the distorted coordinates of an 1.0 cm spaced orthogonal grid of small bronze ball bearings as imaged onto an ideally spaced undistorted grid [30]. The image intensifier is not the only source of geometric distortion in an angioscopic image chain. Both cine film and video cameras view the output of the image intensifier through a main objective lens in the image distributor as well as their own individual lenses. Each stage of optics contributes to the geometric distortion in resulting images. The electron optics of video pickup tubes are under the subjective control of the calibration engineer and also have inherent distortions. The cine film digitization process also uses a video camera. For these reasons, images used for the data presented here were not corrected for geometric distortion in order to include distortion as a variable.

Another important phenomenon was not corrected for, and was therefore included as a study variable. It is well known that film has a very non-linear density response. Although video cameras are tuned for maximum linearity of density response, the logarithmic correction for Lambert-Beers X-ray absorption which is used in digital radiography can result in a non-linear system density response as well. For these reasons, the densitometry of the two imaging methods was left uncorrected, with any non-linearities due to density response being reflected in the final results.

Projected geometric diameter

The most striking finding of this study is the comparison of projected geometric diameter results obtained from film and digital radiographic imaging. As mentioned above, it has been hypothesized that 35 mm cine film possesses greater usable spatial resolution than does direct digital imaging. Another hypothesis is that 1024×1024 imaging should yield superior resolving power over 512×512 digital imaging. The results of projected geometric diameter analysis in this experiment do not support either of these hypotheses. All three imaging techniques exhibited regression results that show no significant difference from each other in measuring the diameter of arterial lumena. The slopes, y-intercepts, coefficients of correlation, and standard errors of the estimates are virtually identical. In addition, single diameter variability measured as the average standard deviation of projected geometric diameter measurements along the length of the lumena showed insignificant differences. An important observation of this experiment is not obvious from reviewing the regression coefficients in the overestimation of lumena with diameters less than 1.0 mm. All three imaging techniques exhibited very similar overestimation of diameters in this range. This was also found by Kirkeeide *et al.* [17].

Explanation for the similar projected geometric diameter results of film and both digital radiographic imaging methods is required. The key concept in this issue is *usable* spatial resolution. As an image receptor, a 1000 line video camera is not capable of transferring as much spatial information as an equivalent area of 35 mm cine film. Depending on its speed, film is capable of recording approximately 50 line pairs per mm, at least twice the theoretical resolution at the target of a 2.54 cm, 1000 line plumbicon [31, 32]. Unfortunately, the spatial resolution of today's cesium iodide image intensifiers is limited to approximately 4–5 line pairs per mm (exposed at the input, measured at the output [27, 33]), so that the full spatial resolution of cine film cannot be exploited. The spatial resolution of film after the image intensifier and image distributor is approximately 2.0–2.5 line pairs per mm [33], the degradation from the image intensifier resolution being due to the main objective lens in the image distributor and cine camera optics. This is comparable to the spatial resolution of a high quality 500 line video pickup tube which can exceed 2.0 line pairs per mm when viewing an image-intensified scene [23].

We also must address the question of why the 1024×1024 digital images did not surpass the ability of 512×512 imaging in estimating the diameter of lumena under 1.0 mm. There are physical restrictions which limit the spatial resolution of 1000 line video pickup tubes. Among the most significant is the size of the electron beam which sweeps the video tube target to read the charge pattern of the stored image. This limits the resolution capacity of one-inch video pickup tubes typically used in radiography to somewhat under 1000 lines [32]. Quantum mottle is also a more significant problem with 1024×1024 images, compared to 512×512 images acquired with the same X-ray dose, since 1024×1024 images contain four times the number of pixels. Since coronary arteriographic images are typically quantum-limited, this is a significant factor in the utilization of 1024×1024 digital radiographic images for quantitative coronary arteriography.

There is another factor which is not taken into account when a cineangiographic system's spatial resolution is measured using standard techniques. The resolving power of a system as measured using tungsten wires or lead strips does not adequately reflect the system's ability to image small absorbers with more realistic object contrast. The object contrast of the X-ray attenuation due to a high atomic number material such as tungsten in a background of attenuation due to a lower atomic number material such as flesh or water is not anatomically relevant. When a phantom such as the one employed in this experiment is used to characterize spatial resolution, results which are more analogous to clinical imaging are obtained. For this reason, the results of standard resolution measurements are not readily extrapolated to the clinical imaging situation.

Per cent diameter stenosis

The major finding of this experiment with regard to per cent diameter stenosis is the scattering of the results as reflected by the reduced coefficients of correlation compared with projected geometric diameter measurements (film, $r = 0.902$; 512×512, $r = 0.897$; 1024×1024, $r = 0.898$). On first examination it would seem that the excellent correlation of projected diameter measurements would lead to similarly high coefficient of correlation values in the per cent diameter stenosis calculation. Unfortunately, the problem of the overestimation of lumena under $1.0 \, \text{mm}$ in diameter leads to the underestimation of the severity of very small diameter lesions, and is the cause of the reduced correlation. Again, the response is very similar with all three imaging methods. In each case, the points which correspond to the 'lesions' with the $0.5 \, \text{mm}$ lumena show a significant underestimation of per cent diameter stenosis (note the circled points in the appropriate regression plots, Fig. 1).

Densitometric relative cross-sectional area

It is in the comparison of densitometric relative cross-sectional area measurements that significant differences between the cine film and digital imaging methods become apparent. Both 512×512 and 1024×1024 digital techniques yield similar findings. They exhibit very high coefficients of correlation, slopes very close to 1.0, small y-intercepts, and acceptable standard errors of the estimate which are not significantly different from each other. Film, on the other hand, shows a reduction in the quality of the regression results. The reduction in quality of regression statistics is thought to be due to the high degree of non-linearity in the densitometric curve of film.

Per cent area stenosis

Not unexpectedly, the per cent area stenosis regression results show findings similar to these of densitometric relative cross-sectional area analysis. The results of film analysis show reduced coefficients of correlation and an increased standard error of the estimated compared with either digital method.

Limitations of this experiment

This phantom study does not address a multitude of issues having to do with the clinical utilization of quantitative coronary arteriography. For example, we used undiluted contrast medium in a static environment. The effects of such phenomena as contrast mixing and streaming are not taken into account. The experimental apparatus did not include a spatially varying distribution of background attenuation, such as is found in the chest. Other factors such as rotational variation, imaging lumena not parallel to the image intensifier, testing the response for non-circular cross-section lumena, and more complex arterial structures are also beyond the scope of this work. These and other clinically relevant issues were deliberately avoided in the experimental design in order to restrict the number of variables and yet allow the comparison of the intrinsic performance of cine film and digitized video as image receptors. The data in this paper were obtained from a single angiographic system and cannot, therefore, be extended to all radiographic and digital systems and cine films. The purpose of this paper was not, however, to provide an inter-system comparison or a comprehensive evaluation of film types.

Lastly, one of the great difficulties with phantom expriments such as this is that one must always question the accuracy and precision of the phantom itself. Various construction methods were tested, and a number of phantoms were discarded before this phantom was made.

Summary

Based on the results of this experiment, we conclude first that the three imaging methods yield equivalent ability to measure the diameter of arterial lumena. They all overestimated lumena below 1.0 mm in diameter, giving rise to the underestimation of per cent diameter stenosis for arteries with lumena having diameters in this range. The hypothesized spatial resolution advantage of film over digital methods or of 1024×1024 images compared with 512×512 images is not substantiated by this experiment. Secondly, densitometric relative cross-sectional area analysis does not suffer from similar problems of overestimation of small lumena or underestimation of high-grade stenoses. Thirdly, digital techniques are more precise than film in the application of densitometric methods for estimating the relative cross-sectional area of lumena in the diameter range tested. In light of these results, we conclude that direct digital imaging provides an attractive alternative to standard 35 mm cine film analysis.

References

1. Robbins SL, Rodriguez FL: Problems in the quantitation of coronary arteriosclerosis. Am J Cardiol 1966; 18: 153.
2. Fisher LD, Judkins MP, Lesperance J, Cameron A, Swaye P, Tyan T, Maynard C, Bourassa M: Reproducibility of coronary arteriographic reading in the coronary artery surgery study (CASS). Cathet Cardiovasc Diagn 1982; 8: 565.
3. Zir LM, Miller SW, Dinsmore RE, Gilbert JP, Harthorne JW: Interobserver variability in coronary angiography. Circulation 1976; 53: 627.
4. Gensini GG, Kelly AE, Da Costa BCB, Huntington PP: Quantitative angiography: the measurement of coronary vasomobility in the intact animal and man. Chest 1971; 60: 552.
5. Brown BG, Bolson E, Frimer M, Dodge HT: Quantitative coronary arteriography: Estimation of dimensions, hemodynamic resistance, and atheroma mass of coronary artery lesions using the arteriogram and digital computation. Circulation 1977; 55: 329.
6. Reiber JHC, Booman F, Tan HS, Slager GJ, Schuurbiers JCH, Gerbrands JJ, Meester GT: A cardiac image analysis system objective quantitative processing of angiocardiograms. Comput Cardiol 1978; 239.
7. Booman F, Reiber JHC, Gerbrands JJ, Slager CJ, Schuurbiers JCH, Meester GT: Quantitative analysis of coronary occlusions from coronary cine-angiorams. Comput Cardiol 1979; 177.
8. Raffenbeul W, Smith LR, Rogers WJ, Mantle JA, Rackley CE, Russell RO: Quantitative coronary arteiography: coronary arnatomy of patients with unstable angina pectoris reexamined 1 year after optimal medical therapy. Am J Cardiol 1979; 43: 699.
9. Wijk van, Brievingh RP van, Heethaar RM, Werf T van der: Determination of coronary artery diameter and contrast medium concentration from angiograms – possibilities and limitations. J Biomed Eng 1981; 3: 57.
10. Sanders WJ, Alderman EL, Harrison DC: Coronary artery quantitation using digital image processing techniques. Comput Cardiol 1979; 15.

170

11. Smith DN, Colfer H, Brymer JF, Pitt B, Kliman SH: A semi-automatic computer technique for processing coronary angiograms. Comput Cardiol 1982; 325.
12. Gould KL, Kelley KO,Bolson EL: Experimental validation of quantitative coronary arteriography for determining pressure-flow characteristics of coronary stenosis. Circulation 1982; 66: 930.
13. Brown BG, Peterson RB, Pierce CD, Bolson EL, Dodge HT: Arteriographic assessment of coronary disease: Advantages, limitations, and clinical uses of a computer-assisted method. In: Rappaport E, Kouchoukos NT, Oparil S, Pitt B, Popp RL, Scheinman MM (eds) Cardiology update; p. 67. Elsevier Biomedical, New York, 1982.
14. Spears JR, Sandor T, Als AV, Malagold M, Markie JE, Grossman W, Serur JR, Paulin S: Computerized image analysis for quantitative measurement of vessel diameter from cineangiograms. Circulation 1983; 68: 453.
15. eiber JHC, Kooijman CJ, Slager CJ, Gerbrands JJ, Schuurbiers JCH, Boer A den, Wijns W, Serruys PW: Computer-assisted analysis of the severity of obstructions from coronary cineangiograms: a methodological review. Automedica 1984; 5: 219.
16. Reiber JHC, Serruys PW, Kooijman CJ, Wijns W, Slager CJ, Gerbrands JJ, Schuurbiers JH, Boer A den, Hugenholtz PG: Assessment of short-, medium-, and long-term variations in arterial dimensions from computer-asssisted quantitation of coronary cineangiograms. Circulation 1985; 71: 280.
17. Kirkeeide RL, Fung P, Smalling RW, Gould KL: Automated evaluation of vessel diameter from arteriograms. Comput Cardiol 1982; 215.
18. LeFree MT, Simon SB, Lewis RJ, Bates ER, Vogel RA: Digital radiographic coronary artery quantitation. Comput Cardiol 1985.
19. LeFree MT, Simon SB, Mancini GBJ, Vogel RA: Digital radiographic assessment of coronary arterial geometric diameter and videodensitometric cross-sectional area. Proc SPIE 626, 1986 (in press).
20. Sandor T, Sridhar B, Paulin S: Remote densitometric analysis of stenotic lesions. Int J Bio-Med Comput 1979; 10: 15.
21. Sandor T, Als AV, Paulin S: Cine-densitometric measurement of coronary arterial stenoses. Cathet Cardiovasc Diagn 1979; 5: 229.
22. Spears JR: Rotating step-wedge technique for extraction of luminal cross-sectional area information from single plane coronary cineangiograms. Acta Radiol (Diagn) 1981; 22: 217.
23. Kruger RA: Estimation of the diameter of an iodine concentration within blood vessels using digital radiographic devices. Med Physics 1981; 8: 652.
24. Nichols AB, Gabrieli CFO, Fenoglio JJ, Esser PD: Quantification of relative coronary arterial stenosis by cinevideodensitometric analysis of coronary arteriograms. Circulation 1984; 69: 512.
25. Harrison DG, White CW, Hiratzka LF, Doty DB, Barnes DH, Eastham CL, Marcus ML: The value of lesion cross-secctional area determined by quantitative coronary angiography in assessing the physiologic significance of proximal left anterior descending coronary artery stenoses. Circulation 1984; 69: 1111.
26. Serruys PW, Reiber JHC, Wijns W, Brand MVD, Kooijman CJ, Brand M van den, Katten HJ ten, Hugenholtz PG: Assessment of percutaneous transluminal coronary angioplasty by quantitative coronary arteriography: diameter vs densitometric area measurements. Am J Cardiol 1984; 54: 482.
27. Mistretta CA, Crummy AB, Strother CM, Sackett JF (eds): Digital subtraction arteriography: an application of computerized fluoroscopy; p 16. Year Book Medical Publishers, Chicago, 1982.
28. Tobis J, Nalcioglu O, Iseri L, Johnston WD, Roeck W, Castleman E, Bauer B, Montelli S, Henry WL: Detection and quantitation of coronary artery stenoses from digital subtraction

angiograms with 35-millimeter film cineangiograms. Am J Cardiol 1984; 54: 489.

29. Seibes M, Selzer RH: How accurate is the catheter as reference for arterial dimensions in quantitative coronary angiography? Comput Cardiol 1985.

30. LeFree MT, Mulvaney JA, Vogel RA: Image corrections for digital radiographic geometric and videodensitometric distortions (Abstract). Radiology 1985; 157: 36.

31. Theris NA: Imaging systems requirements and film for fluorography. In: Haus AG (ed) The physics of medical imaging: recording system measurements and techniques; p 216. American Institute of Physics, New York, 1979.

32. Sandrik JM: The video camera for medical imaging. In: Fullerton GD, Hendee WR, Lasher JC, Properzio WS (eds) Electronic imaging in medicine; p 145. American Institute of Physics, New York, 1983.

33. Mistretta CA: X-ray image intensifiers. In: Haus AG (ed) The physics of medical imaging: recording system measurements and techniques; p 182. American Institute of Physics, New York, 1979.

16. Nonlinearity by Densitometric Measurements of Coronary Arteries

P.-A. DORIOT, Y. POCHON[1], R. WELZ & W. RUTISHAUSER

Cardiology Center, University Hospital, Geneva, Switzerland; [1] Institute of Applied Physics, Department of Physics, Swiss Federal Institute of Technology, Lausanne, Switzerland

Introduction

Lambert-Beer's absorption law (LB-law), often assumed to be the adequate basis for densitometry of coronary arteries, predicts proportionality between a layer of thickness t of contrast medium inside the artery and the resulting logarithmic attenuation of the concerned X-ray beam element:

$$\log [I_{incident}] - \log [I_{transmitted}(t)] = \text{const.} \times t; \tag{1}$$

I is the intensity of the beam element. Experiments on phantoms show, however, that the actual relationship is not linear. This can also be expected from former investigations performed by Bürsch and coworkers [1]. A direct consequence of non-linearity is that conventional densitometry of coronary arteries is not only inaccurate, but also dependent (for instance) on the diameter of the artery, on the size and shape of the stenotic lumen and on its orientation with regard to the X-rays, contrarily to frequently encountered statements (the 'orientation' is here the rotational position of the stenotic lumen around the axis of the stenotic vessel segment, which is itself assumed perpendicular to the relevant X-rays). The dependence on orientation is demonstrated by the degrees of stenosis obtained on the two 'half-moon' stenoses of the phantom depicted in Fig. 1 ('uncorrected' and 'HD-corrected' degrees of stenosis).

The aim of this study was to assess the errors of degrees of stenosis and residual lumen areas measured by conventional densitometry (the residual area is obtained from the inaccurate degree of stenosis and the area of the intact lumen, determined by diameter measurement).

Method

The logarithmic attenuation of the X-ray beam element X_P due to a layer

P.H. Heintzen and J.H. Bürsch (eds), Progress in Digital Angiocardiography. ISBN 978-94-010-7093-5

thickness $t(P)$ of contrast medium inside the coronary artery is reflected by the 'luminance contrast' $c_{lum}[t(P)]$ of the concerned pixel P on the output plate of the image intensifier, the luminance contrast being defined relatively to the vessel surrounding background:

$$c_{lum}(t) = \log L[Q] - \log L[t(P)]. \tag{2}$$

$L[t(P)]$ is the luminance (brightness) of pixel P (on the vessel shadow) and $L(Q)$ the luminance of a pixel (or region) representative of the background.

A mathematical/physical model taking polychromasy of the X-ray beam and scattered radiation into account [2,3] leads to the non-linear relation:

$$c_{lum}[t(P)] = A_1(P)\ t(P) + A_3(P)\ t^2(P) + \text{terms of higher order}. \tag{3}$$

The terms of higher order can be neglected by coronary arteries filled with a usual contrast medium if their diameter does not exceed 6 mm. It can be shown that the coefficients A_1 and A_3 depend primarily on the actual X-ray tube voltage (kV) regulated automatically by the angiocardiographic unit to match the patient's attenuation (by constant tube current and pulse duration), and on the iodine concentration c_I of the selectively injected contrast medium (total filling of the vessel is assumed). We have thus $A_1 = A_1(kV,c_I)$ and $A_3 = A_3$ (kV,c_I). A third summand $A_2(kV,c_I)m(P)t(P)$ appears when background inhomogeneities are also taken into account, $m(P)$ being then a local modulation factor.

The unknown functions $A_1(kV,c_I)$ and $A_3(kV,c_I)$ were determined experimentally on our angiocardiographic unit [3] with the help of linear wedges of contrast medium of different concentrations. The wedges were filmed successively on homogeneous backgrounds $[m(P) = 0]$ provided by paraffine plates embedding the wedge. Various patient attenuations and scatterings were simulated by varying the number of paraffine plates or adding a 0.2 mm copper sheet to the stack; this produced voltages of 55 to 100 kV. All other conditions of routine coronary angiography were best possibly respected. Values for the coefficient functions $A_1(kV,c_I)$ and $A_3(kV,c_i)$ were obtained pairwise as coefficients of second order polynoms fitted through the obtained HD-corrected contrast curves.

Mathematical transformation of equation 3 yields:

$$A_1(kV,c_I)t(P) = \frac{-1 + \sqrt{1 + 4\ [A_3(kV,c_I)/A_1^2(kV,c_I)]\ c_{lum}[t(P)]}}{2\ [A_3(kV,c_I)/A_1^2(kV),c_I)]}. \tag{4}$$

$A_1(kV,c_I)t(P)$ can be viewed as a 'corrected' (fictive) contrast $c_{cor}[t(P)]$ proportional to $t(P)$. Since A_1 and A_3 depend primarily on only two parameters (kV and c_I), whereby one of the two is the same in each examination (c_I), equation 4 allows to transform the real contrast $c_{lum}[t(P)]$ in each pixel into its associated value $c_{cor}[t(P)]$.

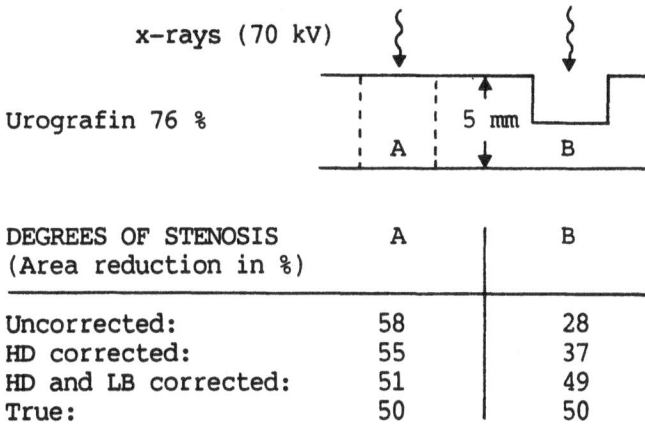

DEGREES OF STENOSIS (Area reduction in %)	A	B
Uncorrected:	58	28
HD corrected:	55	37
HD and LB corrected:	51	49
True:	50	50

Fig. 1. Phantom presenting two 'half-moon' stenoses rotated 90 degrees against each other. The incident X-rays are parallel to the drawing plane. 'Uncorrected', respectively 'HD corrected', means 'before', respectively 'after', compensation of the non-linearity due to the *H*urter-*D*riffield transfer function of the 35 mm cinefilm. 'HD and LB corrected' means 'after pixel by pixel correction of the luminance contrast'.

As can be seen in Fig. 1, use of the obtained numerical values $A_1(kV,c_I)$ and $A_3(kV,c_I)$ in equation 4 yields degrees of stenosis close to the expected ones. ('HD and LB corrected' degrees of stenosis. The 'true' values are themselves only accurate to a few percents for machining reasons.)

The quotient function $A_3(kV,c_I)/A_1(kV,c_I)$, which reflects the degree of non-linearity, decreases with increasing tube voltage (Fig. 2). This function allows to calculate analytically, or numerically if necessary, the errors of hypothetical, uncorrected degrees of stenosis and the resulting error of the derived residual areas. The involved parameters are thereby:

1. the size and shape of the intact and residual lumens,
2. their respective orientation relatively to the X-rays,
3. the tube voltage (kV),
4. the iodine concentration c_I.

Assuming a circular intact lumen, the greatest possible errors can be found for given tube voltage and iodine concentration by choosing the particular form of residual lumen depicted in gray in Fig. 3, and the two particular indicated orientations with respect to the incident X-rays. These errors define boundaries of domains of errors. Domains of errors for the degree of stenosis and for the corresponding stenotic area have been calculated for a 3 mm and a 5 mm coronary artery filled with Urografin76%. The assumed voltages were 60, 80 and 100 kV.

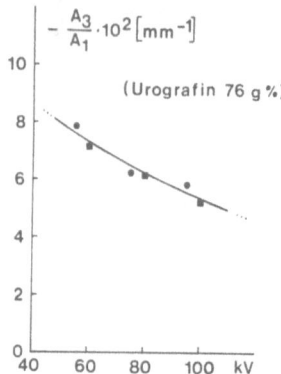

Fig. 2. Quotient function $A_3(kV, c_I)/A_1(kV, c_I)$ obtained from the wedge measurements. The voltages 60, 80 and 100 kV (square dots) were obtained from the voltages 55, respectively 75 and 95 kV by adding a 0.2 mm copper sheet to the paraffine plates. The copper sheet had obviously no specific effect.

Results and discussion

Figure 3 shows the 3 domains of errors of the degree of stenosis of each artery. The X-axis represents the true degree of stenosis (area reduction percentage). The ordinate is also labelled in percents of area reduction, that means in the same percents as the X-axis. The degree of stenosis can be overestimated (upper lobes) or underestimated (lower lobes) according to the particular shape, size and orientation of the residual lumen. The magnitude of errors decrease with increasing voltage. The difference in area between upper and lower lobes suggests that underestimation is more probable than overestimation. This trend has been confirmed by the experimental results obtained on real stenoses and shown in Fig. 5. Mid-range stenoses are obviously more sensitive than benign or severe ones. The dashed curved lines represent the location of errors at 60 kV if the residual lumen is circular. The position of these lines well inside the 60 kV domains reveals that phantoms presenting circular residual cross-sections are not the best appropriate ones for testing the performances of a densitometer for coronary artery measurement. The best shape of residual lumen to this purpose is obviously the one used here to find the limits of the domains since it yields the greatest error when adequately oriented. The location of errors for the functionally important residual area of 1 mm^2 is the vertical dashed line at 86% area reduction (3 mm artery), respectively at 95% area reduction (5 mm artery). Since perfect accuracy of the degree of stenosis is represented by a line (the X-axis), one can say that conventionally measured degrees of stenosis are always inaccurate!

Figure 4 shows the domains of errors of the residual area at 60 and 100 kV.

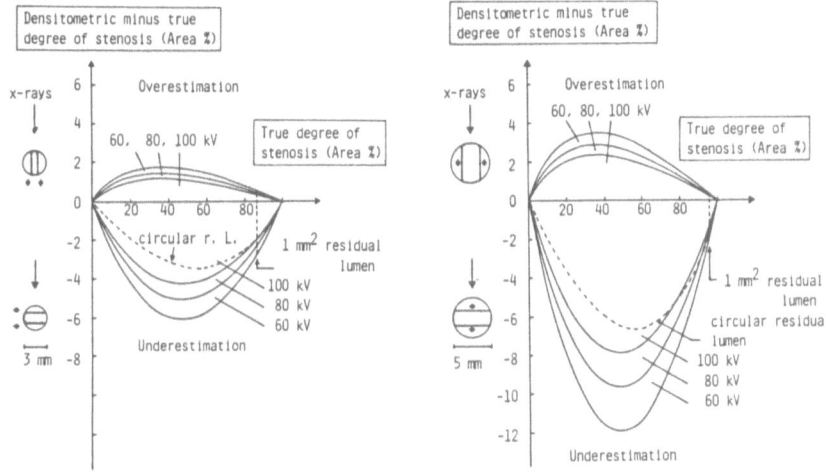

Fig. 3. Domains of errors of the degree of stenosis for a 3 mm and a 5 mm artery filled with Urografin 76%, at 60, 80 and 100 kV. The greatest one (60 kV) includes the two others. The ordinate is labelled in percent area reduction.

The left ordinate scale gives the ratio of densitometric residual area S'_s over true residual area S_s. S_s has been made equal to the densitometric residual area one would obtain if the contrast were proportional to the layer thickness of contrast medium with proportionality constant 1 (the proportionality constant has been arbitrarily chosen equal to 1 for simplicity). For instance (Fig. 4), the true residual area S_s of the 3 mm artery at 0% area reduction, and thus also the true area S_p of the prestenotic lumen, are densitometrically underestimated (S'_s, respectively S'_p) by 19% at 60 kV. Underestimation of the residual lumen decreases toward zero with increasing true degree of stenosis if the greater symmetry axis of the stenotic lumen is perpendicular to the incident X-rays. If it is parallel, underestimation increases further to 23%.

The right ordinate scale gives the over-, respectively underestimation of the true residual area S_s calculated from the erroneous degree of stenosis ($1-S'_s/S'_p$) × 100 and the true area S_p of the intact circular lumen (obtained from its diameter). The residual lumen area of the 3 mm artery can be maximally underestimated by 5% or overestimated by 23% at 60 kV. A residual area of 1 mm² can be underestimated by 5% or overestimated by 20%, according to its actual shape and orientation with respect to the incident X-rays (vertical dashed line in Fig. 4).

Since perfect accuracy of the derived residual area (right scale) is represented by a line (the horizontal line through the domains of errors), one can say again that conventionally measured residual areas are always inaccurate.

The calculated domains of errors reflect only the inaccuracy resulting from

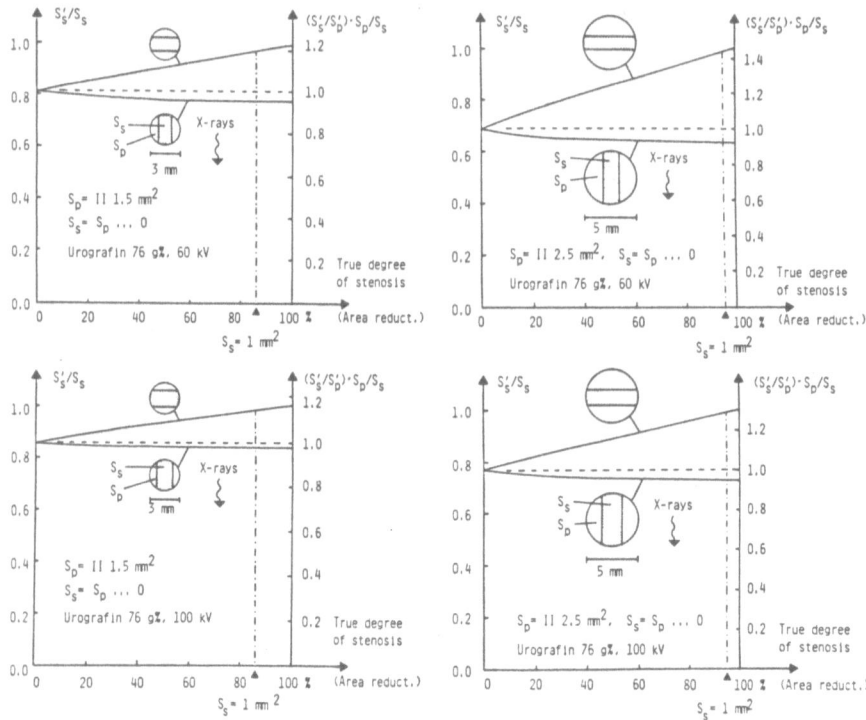

Fig. 4. Domains of errors of the residual area. The left ordinate scale gives the ratio of densitometric residual area S'$_s$ over true residual area S$_s$. The right scale gives the ratio of residual area obtained from the erroneous degree of stenosis and the true area of the intact lumen over true residual area.

non-linearity between t and corresponding luminance contrast. They do not include other sources of inaccuracy such as transfer function of the cinefilm, inaccurate diameter determination (or even excentricity) of the intact lumen, inadequate orientation of the axis of intact and stenotic vessel segments or inhomogeneous vessel background.

It should also be kept in mind that the determined coefficients $A_1(kV,c_I)$ and $A_3(kV,c_I)$ may be somewhat specific to the actual angiocardiographic unit, and that they are only approximations of the exact, local coefficients $A_1(P)$ and $A_3(P)$ which depend on nearly every thinkable parameter of coronary angiography. Nevertheless, the calculated domains of errors are certainly representative of the impact of non-linearity.

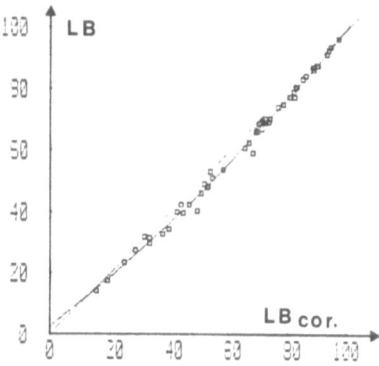

Fig. 5. Degrees of stenosis (in area reduction percents) obtained from routine coronary angiograms of several patients. As expected, conventional densitometry (LB) underestimates in
average the true degree of stenosis, approximated here by the degrees of stenosis obtained
densitometrically using the correction formula 4. Because the actual voltages were not available, a
voltage of 80 kV was assumed, so that the resulting underestimation is itself somewhat underestimated.

Conclusion

Conventional densitometry is wrongly believed to be independent of size,
shape and orientation (in the previously defined sense) of intact and residual
lumens. This dependence produces erroneous degrees of stenosis, and considerable errors of the derived residual area, especially by severe stenoses and
despite the fact that the measured degree of stenosis may be accurate to a few
per cents. Using equation 4 to correct the luminance contrast produces more
accurate degrees of stenosis and associated residual areas. Since other sources
of inaccuracy were neglected in the calculation of the domains of errors, real
errors are in fact greater. Therefore, correction of the contrast values according to equation 4 should be performed (an analogous equation allows to
correct the native cinefilm contrast). Even if the actual tube voltage is not
available, assuming an adequate average voltage (for instance 80 kV) will
generally improve measurements.

Summary

Phantom experiments show that Lambert-Beer's absorption law is not an
adequate physical model for densitometry of coronary arteries. Layer thickness t(P) of contrast medium inside the artery and resulting 'luminance'
contrast $c_{lum}[t(P)]$ of the concerned image pixel P on the vessel shadow are in

fact not linearly related. A model taking beam-polychromasy and scattered radiation into account leads to the polynomial relation $c_{lum}[t(P)] = A_1(P)t(P) + A_3t^2(P)$, where the coefficients $A_1(P)$ and $A_3(P)$ depend primarily on the voltage of the X-ray tube (kV) and on the iodine concentration c_I of the (vessel filling) contrast medium: $A_1 = A_1(kV,c_I)$, $A_3 = A_3(kV,c_I)$. A supplementary term $A_2(kV,c_I)m(P)t(P)$ appears when inhomogeneities of the vessel background are also taken into account. The quotient function $A_3(kV,c_I)/A_1(kV,c_I)$ has been determined experimentally. It allows to predict the error of hypothetical, conventionally measured degrees of stenosis and derived stenotic lumen areas in function of shape, size and orientation (with respect to the X-rays) of the intact and stenotic lumens, of the kV and of c_I. Assuming a circular intact lumen and a particular shape of the stenotic lumen, the domains of errors of the degree of stenosis and of the residual area have been determined for a 3 mm and a 5 mm artery filled with Urografin 76%, at 60, 80 and 100 kV.

References

1. Bürsch J, Johs R, Heintzen P: Validity of Lambert-Beer's law in Roentgendensitometry of contrast material (Urografin) using continuous radiation. In: Heintzen PH (ed) Roentgen-, cine and videodensitometry; pp 81–84. Georg Thieme Verlag, Stuttgart, 1971.
2. Pochon Y: Critères objectifs de qualité des images radiologiques. Thèse No 479. Ecole polytechnique fédérale, Lausanne, 1983.
3. Doriot P-A, Pochon Y, Rasoamanambelo L, Chatelain P, Welz R, Rutishauser WJ: Densitometry of coronary arteries – An improved physical model. IEEE Proc Comp Cardiol 85; pp 91–94. Computer Society Press, Washington DC, 1986.

17. Three-dimensional Reconstruction and Cross-section Measurements of Coronary Arteries using ECG-Correlated Digital Coronary Arteriography

DENNIS L. PARKER, DAVID L. POPE, RUDY E. VAN BREE &
HIRAM MARSHALL
Department of Medical Informatics, LDS Hospital/University of Utah, Salt Lake City, UT, USA

Introduction

The advent of digital image processing has facilitated accurate quantitative analysis of coronary artery morphology [1–7]. To optimally utilize the morphological information available in multi-view cine-angiography and potentially completely replace inaccurate visual determinations of lesion severity [8–13], it is desirable to consolidate the information available into a single densitometric analysis of the arterial tree. In recent years the problem of three-dimensional reconstruction of vascular beds from multi-view angiography has been addressed by several research groups [14–20]. Methodology utilized include the centerline reconstruction methods of Potel et al. [15] and Kim [16], circular reconstructions of Mol et al. [18], the morphologic cross-section reconstructions of Reiber et al. [17] and other multi-view tomographic techniques such as those of Kruger [19] and Mawko [20].

All three-dimensional arterial reconstruction methods require tight tolerances in geometric accuracy. For example, geometric inconsistencies will generally cause lines from the same point in two views to not intersect upon back-projection. This non-intersection will result in severe streak artifacts in systems based upon geometric reconstruction techniques such as those of Kruger and Mawko. Distortions will occur in other techniques to the extent that the geometric inconsistencies are not handled properly.

In this paper we review the methodology utilized [21–23] and present some validation studies of a system that performs three-dimensional reconstruction of the coronary arteries at multiple points in the cardiac cycle. Although similar in some respects to techniques of others [14–20], there are several unique aspects which contribute to the simplicity, stability and potential accuracy of the algorithm:
1. The arterial bed is represented by a hierarchal tree structure with the same primary structure in each of the projections as well as the final 3D representation.

P.H. Heintzen and J.H. Bürsch (eds), Progress in Digital Angiocardiography. ISBN 978-94-010-7093-5

2. Dynamic programming is used to refine vessel centerline and edge locations.
3. Point matching for the 3D reconstruction is based on a constrained minimization technique which is relatively insensitive to geometric distortions.
4. Orientation-corrected densitometric measurements are used for the vessel
cross-section reconstruction.
5. Densitometric cross-section measurements obtained throughout the cardiac cycle are averaged to obtain a single more precise measurement for
each point along each vessel segment.

Although operator interaction is required in establishing the original hierarchy
and in establishing the correspondence of node or branch points between
views, the determination of vessel centerlines and edges is an automated
process which proceeds through all images in each view without operator
interaction. Upon completion of the automated process, the results can be
reviewed and corrected interactively if necessary.

In the following sections we first review the methodology of the algorithm
and then give some examples of the results on phantoms and human coronary
arteries.

Reconstruction method

The steps involved in the reconstruction process have been presented previously [16] and can be segmented into two general categories:
1. the determination of the projection of the arterial bed in each image of each
view; and
2. the combining of information from each projection image in generating a
three-dimensional representation of the arterial bed.

For algorithmic convenience we combine the information from the projection
of the arterial bed into a data structure referred to as the 'plane-tree', Y.
Likewise, the reconstructed arterial bed is found in a data structure representation called the '3D-tree', ψ. In the current 2 view implementation of the
algorithms, these structures are defined:

$Y\{$	plane tree structure
Projection geometry	relative to the 3D coordinate system
Branch {	plane tree branch structure
Hierarchy	interconnection for this branch
Element {	plane tree element data structure
u	x-coordinate of the vessel centerline
v	y-coordinate of the vessel centerline
r	radius of the vessel at point (u, v) in pixels

a	sum of densities across this profile
d_{max}	maximum density value on this profile
A	densitometric area of the vessel
β	3D vessel projection angle

} } }

ψ {	3D tree structure
Branch {	3D tree branch structure
Hierarchy	interconnection of this branch
Element {	3D tree element structure
x	vessel centerline position
θ	polar angle of centerline
φ	axial angle of centerline
R	average radius of vessel at (x)

} } }

Plane tree determination

Computer generation of the plane tree structure is basically a semi-automated procedure requiring an operator-entered target structure which specifies the vessel branching structure and the approximate vessel positions. The operator also specifies the approximate vessel size. Except for the densitometric area measurement, A, and the 3D projection angle, all of the information in a plane tree structure is required for this target. It is thus convenient and logical to use the plane tree structure as the target structure. This has the distinct advantage of allowing a plane tree determined from a previous image to serve as a target for a subsequent image.

Given the target specification, automated techniques are then used to locate the vessel centerline and edges [24–27]. Because the basic data structure of each branch is identical, each branch of the target is considered separately. An extracted matrix is generated, the rows of which consist of image values extracted along lines orthogonal to the elements of the branch. A shape-specific matched filter is used to enhance the vessel centerline or edges. Dynamic programming is then used to search this enhanced matrix for the optimal path, giving the desired centerline or edge. In addition to the normal continuity constraint of dynamic programming, the algorithm also includes simple geometric constraints (e.g. centerlines and edges do not cross). Subsequent operator correction is simply accomplished by allowing the operator to indicate a point on the true path, storing an impossibly large value at the corresponding point in the enhanced matrix, and researching the matrix.

The geometrically determined edges (i.e. the edges found using the dynamic programming algorithm described above) are used to delineate the region for densitometric measurements. Several points external to the geometric edge are averaged to find a background level for each side of the vessel. Linear interpolation of these two values is used to determine the background value to be subtracted from the profile:

$$d_{ij} = d'_{ij} - d_{bj}, \qquad (1)$$

where d' is the value before background correction, and i and j are the indices along and perpendicular to the vessel respectively.

The densitometric area is defined as the sum of the density values after background correction:

$$a_i = \sum_j d_{ij}. \qquad (2)$$

This area, a_i, as well as the maximum density value, d_{max} is stored in the plane tree structure for determination of absolute area during the computation of the 3D tree.

Plane tree structures are obtained from subsequent images using the same procedure. In principle, it is possible to use the plane tree from the previous image as the target structure for an image. We have found, however, that the reconstruction algorithm is very sensitive to node placement. For this reason, nodes are entered on all images in a view during the operator interactive target generation procedure. The target centerlines are not re-entered after the first image of each view, but are warped for each image based upon the node movements from the original image. This procedure is relatively fast, requiring about 20 minutes for 32 images (16 images in 2 views). For target entry on the images of the second view, nodes are constrained to occur along lines specified by the X-ray paths through the nodes of the first view [23].

3D tree determination

The 3D centerline is obtained from the two plane tree centerlines based upon a constrained minimization technique. In the absence of geometric distortion, a line representing the X-ray path through a point in one view should intersect a line representing the X-ray path through the same point in another view. Geometric distortions in the imaging system as well as movements between views will cause the lines to not intersect. If the lines are nearly orthogonal, the error made in choosing the point of intersection as the point closest to both lines is of the same magnitude as the geometric distortion. The more parallel the lines, the greater the magnification of the error in the direction of the lines.

Implicit in the reconstruction process is the matching of points (elements of each plane tree) between views. The node points are matched between views at the time of target entry. The elements along corresponding branches are matched based upon the relative nearness to intersection of the X-ray path lines. The algorithm chooses the set of matched pairs such that adjacent points along the vessel in each view are connected and the total squared distance between matched lines is minimized.

Once the three-dimensional centerline of the arterial bed is determined, the vessel cross-sectional area is then obtained from orientation-corrected densitometric plane tree measurements. To convert the area, a, into true vessel area, it is necessary to correct for magnification as well as the iodine density/imaging system gain:

$$A_i = \frac{a_i}{g\,\mu_I\varrho_I}\,\Delta x_i = k\,a_i\Delta x_i\,,\tag{3}$$

where g is the system gain, μ_I is the mass attenuation coefficient and ϱ_I is the iodine density. Δx converts the distance measurement from pixels to distance, and includes the correction for magnification obtained from the 3D centerline reconstruction. The constant, k, only depends on the imaging system and the iodine density. It is assumed that after an extended (2–3 second) injection of iodine, the concentration of iodine in the arteries has reached a relatively uniform, steady state distribution. The constant, k, is then the same throughout the arteries of interest in each image of each view. Kruger has demonstrated that, for a circular vessel whose long axis is parallel to the imaging plane:

$$k = \frac{4}{\pi}\,\frac{a}{d_{max}^2}\,.\tag{4}$$

If the vessel is at a small angle, β, with respect to the imaging plane, and if the vessel segment does not change dimensions rapidly near the region of interest, then the constant, k, can still be determined from the angle-corrected densitometric measurements:

$$k = \frac{4}{\pi}\,\frac{a}{d_{max}^2\,\cos\beta}\,.\tag{5}$$

The absolute cross-sectional area, corrected for orientation and iodine density, then becomes:

$$A = k\,a\,\cos\beta\,\Delta x\,.\tag{6}$$

For those regions in the plane tree projection where the angle of inclination, β, is too large or where the algorithm recognizes that vessels have overlapped in the view, the area measurement is disregarded in the reconstruction. With two views, most points in the arterial bed are clearly visualized in at least one view. For those points where this is not the case, linear interpolation from neighboring visible regions is used to specify the cross-sectional area. Additional views would help to eliminate such problems.

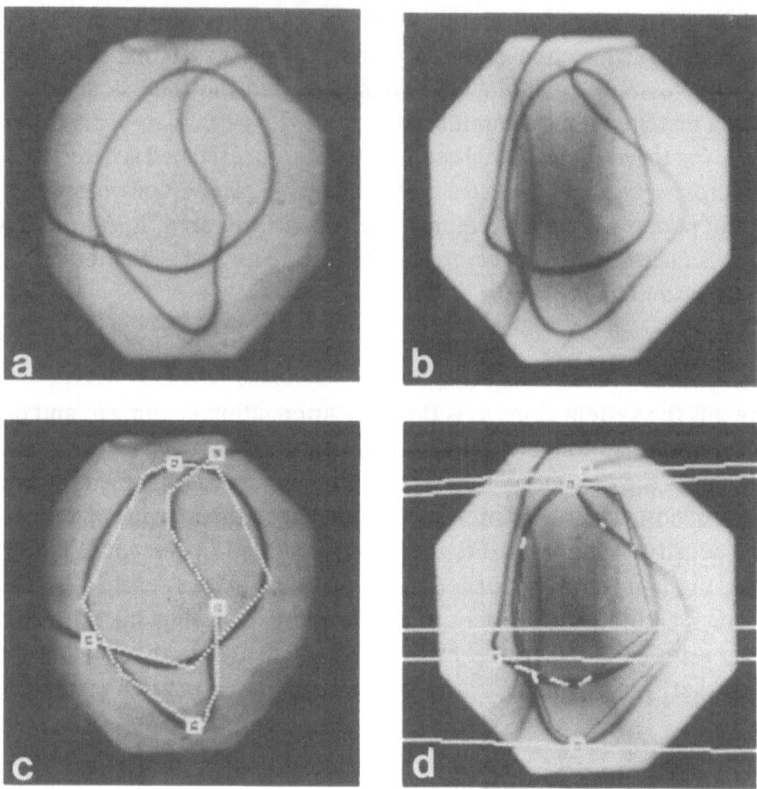

Fig. 1. a and b. Two unsubtracted views of a flow phantom consisting of plastic tubing attached to the vertices of a pyramid. Wire loops have been attached to points around the plastic tubing to provide points for node entry in both views. c. The target structure is entered on the image of the first view. d. The nodes are constrained to be along lines representing the projected X-ray paths from the view in part a.

Phantom studies

At this point in time, some initial experience in evaluating the accuracy of the reconstruction algorithm has been obtained. Two static objects have been reconstructed. The first consisted of 3.18 mm diameter plastic tubing rigidly attached to the vertices of a pyramid. To provide node points for target entry, 3 small wire loops were wrapped around the tubing in various positions. The original images shown in Fig. 1 were used for target entry. The constrained selection of nodes in the second view is shown in Fig. 1b. The subtracted images of Fig. 2 were then used for determination of the vessel centerlines, edges and densitometric measurements of the plane tree structure. After obtaining the plane tree structure in both views, the 3D tree was reconstructed.

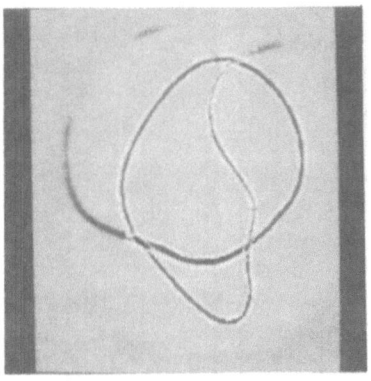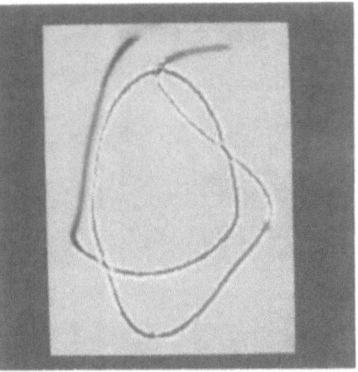

Fig. 2. Edges determined and displayed on the subtracted images from Fig.1.

A test of the accuracy of the 3D centerline reconstruction can be performed by reprojecting the centerline onto a third view. Using a reconstruction obtained from two views separated by about 42° the reconstruction of Fig. 3 is obtained. Although it appears correct, when the centerline is projected onto a third view (Fig. 3b) it is seen that the reconstruction matches well everywhere except for one branch that is significantly wrong. This problem is corrected by using a larger angle between views. Some shaded surface renderings of the corrected 3D reconstruction are shown in Fig. 4.

Given a good centerline reconstruction the densitometric cross-section is obtained and compared with the expected value (Fig. 5). Although not evident from this figure, the greatest errors have occurred where the projections of the vessels of this phantom cross or overlap within a view. Although the algorithm does well, further work is needed to correct this error source.

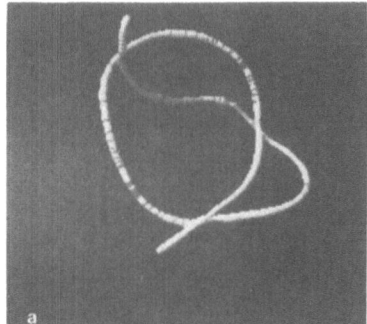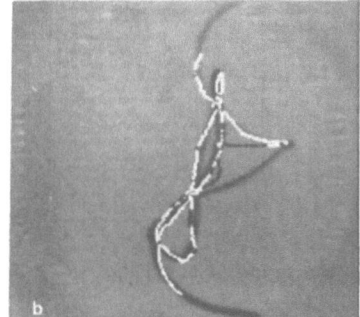

Fig. 3. a. Shaded surface display of reconstructed flow phantom obtained from views separated by 42°. b. Reprojection of reconstruction onto a 3rd view illustrating that while most branches are accurate, the branch extending to the right is significantly in error.

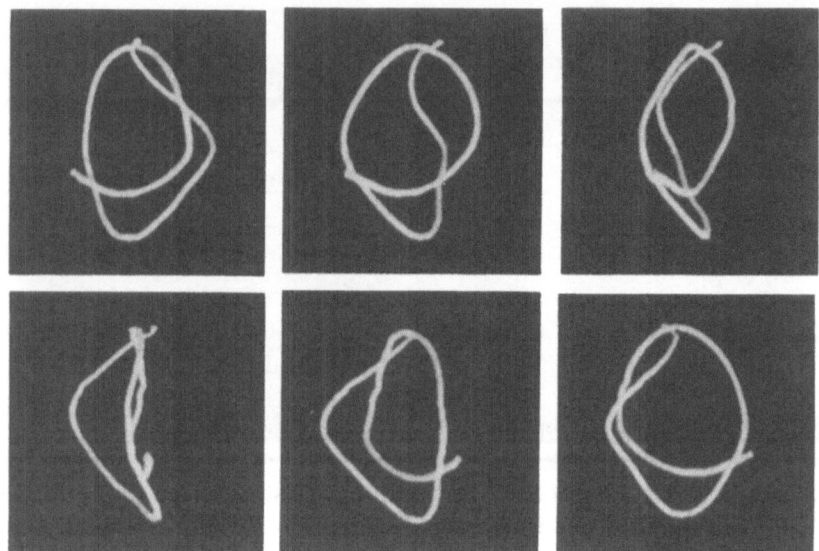

Fig. 4. Shaded surface display of reconstructed flow phantom from various orientations. This reconstruction was obtained from 2 views separated by 57°. The error indicated in Fig. 3b is corrected.

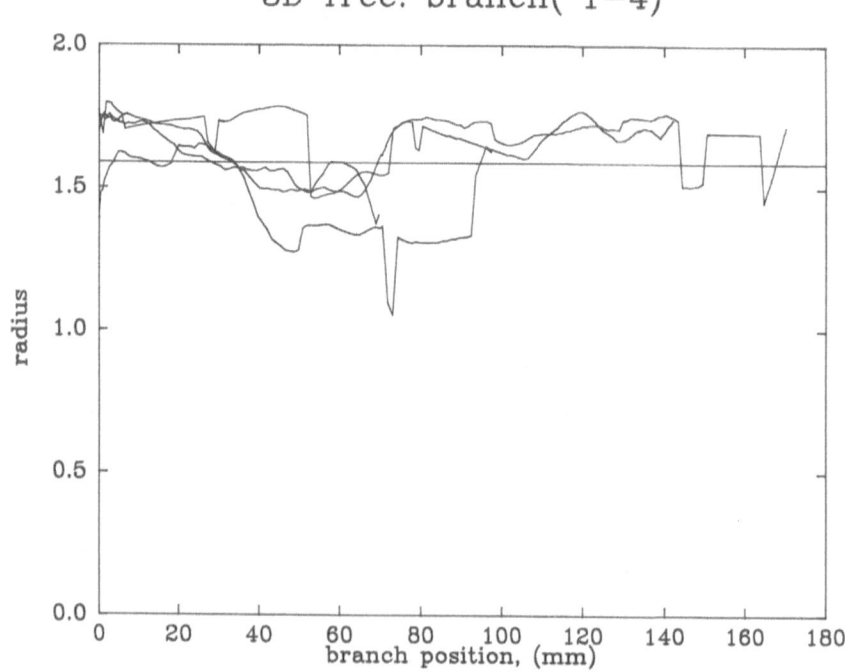

Fig. 5. Plot of densitometric measurements of radius of the plastic tubing determined from the densitometric cross-sectional area.

DENSITOMETRIC MEASUREMENTS

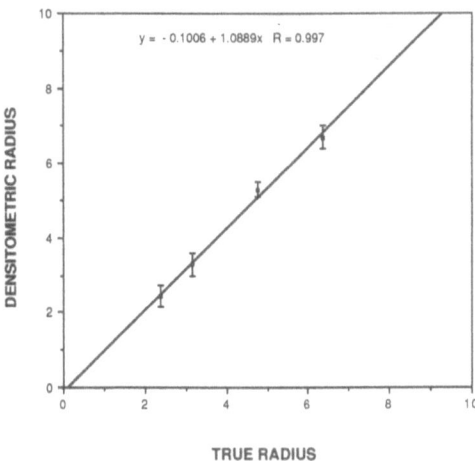

$$y = -0.1006 + 1.0889x \quad R = 0.997$$

Fig. 6. Plot of radii determined for a phantom consisting of teflon rods of 4 different sizes. The teflon was imaged in air with no scattering material.

The second phantom studied consisted of teflon rods of known diameters imaged in air. This lack of X-ray scattering material provides an indication of the accuracy of the algorithm when scatter has been properly corrected. Veiling glare and X-ray focal spot blurring are still a problem, but the dimensions of the phantom were such that these effects were minor. The results are plotted in Fig. 6.

Clinical results

To date, only one patient reconstruction has been performed. For this study images were acquired digitally in a 512×512 matrix at 15 frames per second for two separate injections of contrast media. The two views were separated by approximately 96°. Subtraction masks were selected on a frame-by-frame basis for each image with contrast. A set of 16 images representing an ECG-correlated cycle from late in the injection of each view was selected for processing. Node points were indicated on all images and target lines drawn on the first image in each view were warped for subsequent views. The automated processing and operator correction procedures described previously were then applied. Three-dimensional reconstructions and orientation-corrected densitometric measurements were obtained for all points in the cardiac cycle. The densitometric measurements were averaged on a point-by-point basis over all 3D tree reconstructions. An attempt to display this dynamic 3D information is

190

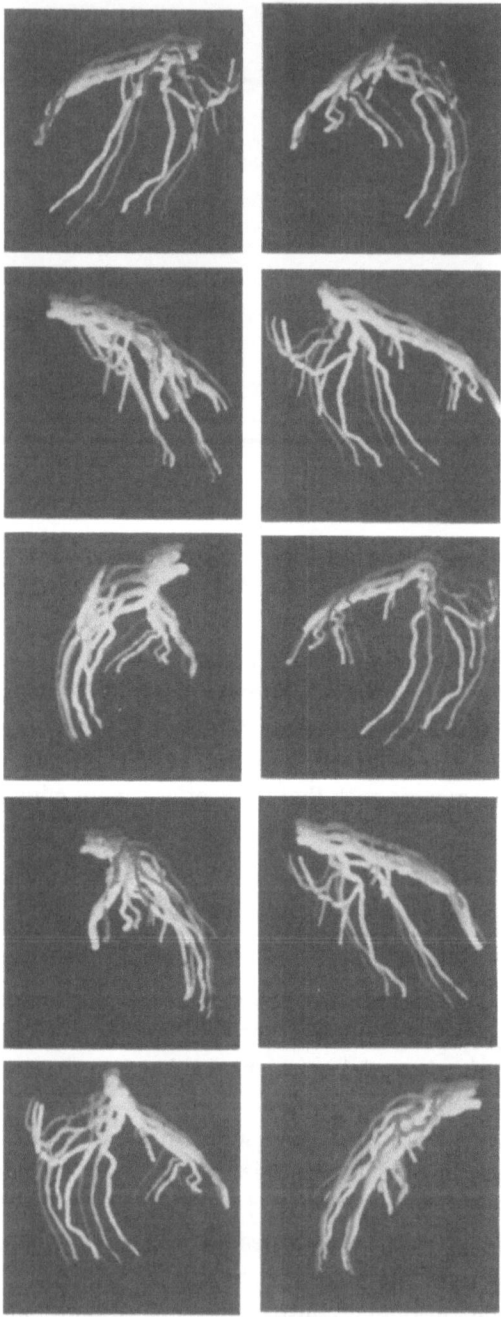

Fig. 7. Shaded surface reconstructions of human left coronary artery obtained from two sets of ECG-correlated views. To illustrate motion, reconstructions at the beginning, middle and end of systole are shown.

given in Fig. 7. In this figure, the arterial bed is displayed at the beginning, middle and end of systole. The changing brightness is used to separate the 3 representations and may be considered to portray motion with the brightest representation as the most recent. In some of the images, a lesion in the circumflex between the two marginals is clearly evident. Further studies are anticipated.

Summary

A system for three-dimensional reconstruction of moving arterial beds has been developed. This paper reports on initial results obtained with this system including preliminary evaluations of the accuracy of centerline position and vessel cross-section.

References

1. Brown BG, Bolson E, Frimer M, Dodge HT: Quantitative coronary arteriography estimation of dimensions, hemodynamic resistance, and atheroma mass of coronary artery lesions using the arteriogram and digital computation. Circulation 1977; 55: 329–337.
2. Sandor T, Spears JR, Paulin S: Densitometric determination of changes in the dimensions of coronary arteries. SPIE 1981; 314: 263–272.
3. Spears JR, Sandor TS, Als AV, Malagold M, Markis JE, Grossman W, Serur JR, Paulin S: Computerized image analysis for quantitative measurement of vessel diameter from cine-angiograms. Circulation 198; 68: 453–461.
4. Doriot PA, Rasoamanambelo L, Honegger HP, Merier G, Bopp P, Rutishauser W: Measurement of the degree of coronary stenosis by digital densitometry. Comput Cardiol Sept 1981; 329–332.
5. Nichols AB, Gabrieli CFO, Fenoglio JJ, Esser PD: Quantification of relative coronary arterial stenosis by cinevideodensitometric analysis of coronary arteriograms. Circulation 1984; 69: 512–522.
6. Kruger RA: Estimation of the diameter of and iodine concentration within blood vessels using digital radiography devices. Med Phys 1981; 8(5): 652–658.
7. See, for example, papers 1043, 1044, 1810 and 1813 in the Proceedings, AHA, 1985.
8. Detre KM, Wright E, Murphy ML, Takaro T: Observer agreement in evaluating coronary angiograms. Circulation 1975; 52: 979.
9. Zir LM, Miller SW, Dinsmore RE, Gilbert JP, Harthorne JW: Interobserver variability in coronary arteriography. Circulation 1976; 53: 627.
10. DeRouen T, Murray JA, Owen W: Variability in the analysis of coronary arteriograms. Circulation 1977; 55: 324.
11. Vlodaver Z, Frech R, Van Tassel RA, Edwards JE: Correlation of the antemortem findings in patients with oronary artery disease and recent myocardial revascularization. Circulation 1973; 47: 162.
12. Grondin CM, Dyrda I, Pasternac A, Campeau L, Bourassa MG, Lesperance J: Discrepancies between cineangiographic and post-mortem findings in patients with coronary artery disease and recent myocardial revascularization. Circulation 1974; 49: 703.

13. Robbins SL, Rodriguez FL, Wragy AL, Fish SJ: Problems in the quantitation of coronary arteriosclerosis. Am J Cardiol 1966; 18: 153.
14. MacKay SA, Potel MJ, Rubin JM: Graphics methods for tracking three-dimensional heart wall motion. Comp Biomed Res 1982; 15: 455–473.
15. Potel MJ, MacKay SA, Rubin JM, Aisen AM, Sayre RE: Three-dimensional left ventricular wall motion in man, coordinate systems for representing wall movement direction. Inv Radiol 1984; 19: 499–509.
16. Kim HC, Min BG, Lee TS, Lee SJ, Lee CW, Park JH, Han MC: Three-dimensional digital subtraction angiography. IEEE Trans on Med. imaging 1982; MI-1(2): 152–158.
17. Reiber JHC et al: Three-dimensional reconstruction of coronary arterial segments from two projections. In: Heintzen PH, Brennecke R (eds) Digital imaging and cardiovascular radiology. International symposium, Kiel, 1982.
18. Mol CR, Burridge JM, Morffew AJ: Three-dimensional graphics display of X-ray angiographic data. Comp Biomed Res 1986; 19: 47–55.
19. Kruger's circular tomography device.
20. Mawko GM, Peters TM: Iterative 3-D reconstruction of vascular images from a few views: Phantom study results. SPIE 1986; 671: 19–24.
21. Parker DL, Ppe DL, White KS, Tarbox LR, Marshall HW: Three-dimensional reconstruction of vascular beds. In: Bacharach SL (ed) Information processing in medical imaging; pp 414–430. Martinus Nijhoff, Boston, 1986.
22. Parker DL, Pope DL, Bree RE van, Desai R: Three-dimensional reconstruction of vascular beds from digital angiographic projections. SPIE 1986; 671: 50–59.
23. Parker DL, Pope DL, Bree RE van, Marshall HW: Three-dimensional reconstruction of moving arterial beds from digital subtraction angiography. Comp Biomed Res 1987; 20: in press.
24. Schmueli K, Brody WR, Macovski A: Estimation of blood vessel boundaries in X-ray images. SPIE 1981; 314: 279–286.
25. Pope DL, Parker DL, Clayton PD, Gustafson DE: Left ventricular border determination using a dynamic search algorithm. Radiology 1985; 155: 513–518.
26. Pope DL, Parker DL: Automated tracking of the coronary artery tree. Presented at RSNA, 1985.
27. Pope DL, Parker DL, Gustafson DE, Clayton PD: Dynamic search algorithms in left ventricular border recognition and analysis of coronary arteries. Comput Cardiol Sept 1984.

18. Fast Automatic Recognition and 3D Reconstruction of the Coronary Tree from DSA-Projection Pairs

K. BARTH, R. KOCH & P. MARHOFF
Siemens AG, Erlangen, FRG

Introduction

For a reliable quantitative assessment of vascular lesions the three-dimensional orientations and connections have to be known accurately. This information can be extracted systematically from two DSA-projections using a digital image processing system. Automatic identification and calculation of three-dimensional coordinates of the vessel centrelines are possible at angles of 15–45° between the two projections. The knowledge of the three-dimensional coordinates allows the determination of the true length and corrected densitometric values of foreshortened vessel sections.

Methods for the 3D reconstruction of the coronary vascular tree have been reported previously in the literature [1–6]. Some of the methods rely on manual interaction for the identification of arterial bifurcations [1, 2]. This paper proposes a fully automatic analysis and reconstruction of the coronary tree based on automatic vessel tracing. The number of data points for the reconstruction far exceeds the number of points that are used in a method which is based on manual interaction. Branching points are recognized and labelled automatically and they are used for a structural description of the tree.

Preprocessing

The first task is the object-oriented segmentation of the images. Binary images are generated where the pixels within the vessels are distinguished from all other pixels. With DSA images the background is homogeneous, so that threshold segmentation should give good results. However, due to motion artifacts and extra-arterial iodine contrast this segmentation does not work perfectly even if the local histogram is taken for local adaptation. Therefore more specific filtering for the extraction of vascular structures has to be applied. Theoretically, optimal results can be achieved with a matched filter as

P.H. Heintzen and J.H. Bürsch (eds), Progress in Digital Angiocardiography. ISBN 978-94-010-7093-5

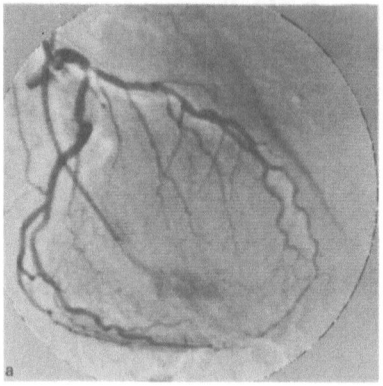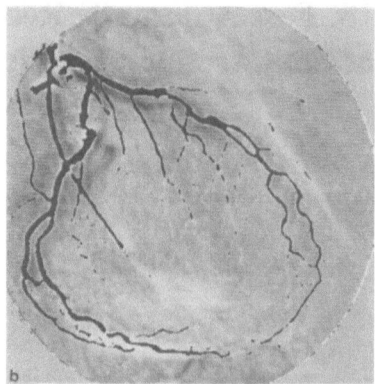

Fig. 1. Clinical image of the left coronary arteries. a. DSA image. b. Segmented binary image after application of the filter for vessel enhancement.

described in [3]. In this filter a template or convolution kernel is adapted to the vessel so that the squared differences (errors) between template and actual vessel densities are minimized. The correlation coefficient from the comparison between template and object data is the criterion used here. The template with the highest correlation coefficient (usually $r > 0.95$) is the optimal approximation to the actual vessel profile and also locates the vessel centreline.

Proceeding in this way, an 'iterative deconvolution' is realized. This means that a 'typical' vessel profile is assumed for the initial template, including the degradation by a realistic MTF. 'Typical' means e.g. a diameter of 4.0 mm for the left main coronary artery, circular cross section and homogeneous contrast filling. In the 'iterative' procedure the parameter for the vessel diameter and the pattern position are varied until the form of the template pattern optimally matches the local vessel profile.

This optimal filtering procedure requires a large computational effort. Therefore an abstraction of the convolution procedure has been implemented in the form of a filter which selectively enhances the vessels. Profile and template positions are not correlated contiguously but compared with bigger spacing, systematically covering the range of possible vessel diameters. In this way the complete correlation is approximated by the application of several three-point kernels. This involves difference operations symmetric to the vessel centre:

$$d_i = a\, f_{i-k} + b\, f_i + c\, f_{i+k},$$

where the f_i are samples from a profile across the vessel, and a, b and c are constants. This operation is numerically equivalent to correlating f_i and a template g_i, where $g_{-k} = a$, $g_o = b$, $g_k = c$ with typical values $a = -1$, $b = 2$, $c = -1$.

The operation range k >1 reduces the effect of local noise compared with difference operations on adjacent pixels. The output of the described filter is a transformed image with enhanced vessel contrast. This image is normalized globally and can be segmented by the application of a constant threshold. Remaining isolated noise structures are easily removed by rank order operations such as the median filter. Figure 1 shows an RAO view of the left coronary arteries with filtering and segmentation in Fig. 1b).

Vessel tracing

The tracing of the vascular trees is performed on the binary images from the preprocessing phase. Figure 2 shows one of the paired projection images of a left coronary vascular phantom. The tracing is started by marking the root of the tree with two points. The algorithm proceeds by looking for continuations in any direction similar to a radar scanner (Fig. 3). The fan-like geometry was found to follow curved vessel structures particularly well [3]. Stability is achieved by a small stepwidth compared with the fan radius. Vessel tracing is performed 'depth first', i.e. each path is traced down to a tip of the tree. Generally the main branch is processed first, but all alternatives at branching points are stored and processed later. If there is a vessel narrowing, a vessel may not be recognized as the main branch. This leads to a different processing order at the tracking stage, but does not affect correct projection matching in the 3D-synthesis.

In the top-down tracing process the backward 'parent' connections are registered. For the main path this is the relation to the preceding array cell. When a stored branch alternative is resumed, a link back to the coordinates of the parent node is entered in the tree(Fig. 5).

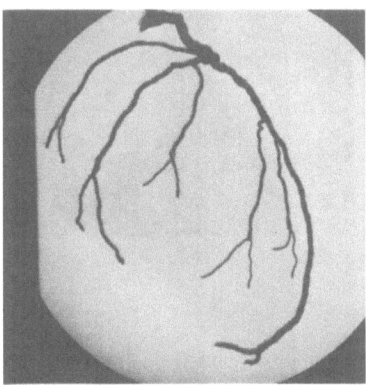

Fig. 2. Original image of the coronary phantom.

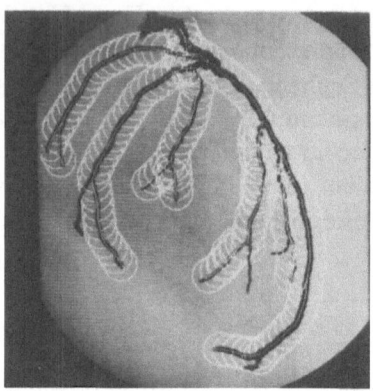

Fig. 3. Digital tracing scheme.

Structured tree processing

Once the tracing of all branches in the binary image has been completed (Fig. 4), the raw tree structure is checked, refined and segmented into subbranches. At this point, 'child' relations are established so that the tree can be traversed in all directions. As there may be several children nodes assigned to one parent node, a separate table for these connections is provided so that only one child-reference cell is needed in the long tree segment table (Fig. 6).

Begin and end markers are also entered in this table. They define the tree segments with the root segment between the start point (P_o) and the first branching. Leaf segments are the segments between the last branching point in a path and the peripheral tip of the artery. All the other segments lie between branching points.

The segments are stored in a segment table not shown in the figure, where

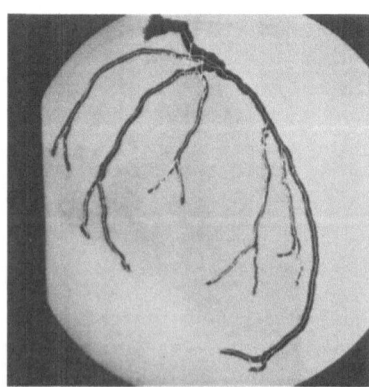

Fig. 4. Vascular skeleton obtained in the tracing process.

Data structures for the tree description (1)

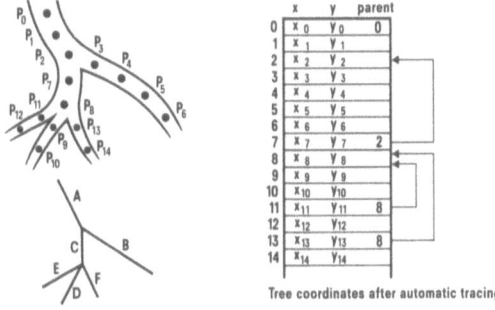

Tree coordinates after automatic tracing

Fig. 5. Data structure in the tracing stage.

the entry or segment A contains pointers 0 and 2 for the beginning and end, segment B points to 3 and 6, etc. While following the tree from the root down to any tip, a sequence of segments is traversed. For all such paths an entry in a path table is created, containing the names of the individual segments in the correct order. For the example in Figs 5 and 6 such paths are AB, ACD, ACE

Data structures for the tree description (2)

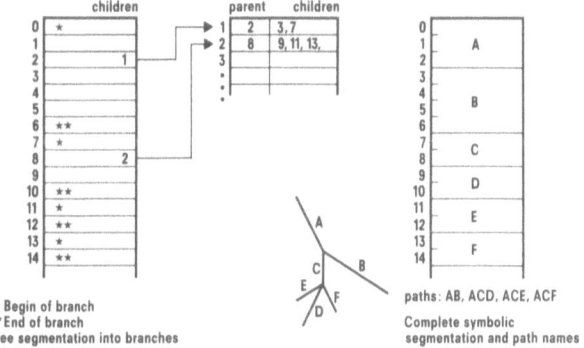

* Begin of branch
**End of branch
Tree segmentation into branches

paths: AB, ACD, ACE, ACF
Complete symbolic
segmentation and path names

Tree matching

– Stereo-like image pairs are compared automatically
– All paths from the root to any tip are associated pairwise

Procedure:

● Select one tree as the reference tree
● Check and mark it briefly
● Process the second tree

REPEAT the remaining steps for all paths in the reference tree:

● Select one path in the reference tree
● Compare this path with all »words« in the symbolic description of the other tree
● Select the optimal correspondence and calculate 3D-coordinates

Fig. 6. Data structures for the tree description (above) as the basis for tree matching (below).

and ACF. The tracing of a typical coronary tree yields several hundred points. For a complete matching of these points thousands of combinations would have to be considered. By the symbolic labelling of segments with letters and by the ordered path formation as 'words' the amount of computation is reduced to a small number of comparisons. Although only few segments are used for the 'syntactic' description, all the traced coordinates are accessible at any time. For the final three-dimensional reconstruction the complete set of original coordinates is used.

Tree matching and calculation of 3D-coordinates

For the 3D-synthesis one of the projections is taken as the reference tree to direct the matching process. The centre points from the top-down tracing are read in. Short side branches due to artifacts are deleted. For each path from the root of the reference tree to any leaf a corresponding path in the second projection is searched. All possibilities for corresponding paths in the path table are checked. The comparison for optimal correspondence is carried out by a pointwise cross correlation. Within each segment all individual coordinate pairs from the tracing stage are considered. When the X-ray imaging system is rotated about the y-axis, the x-coordinates are checked for similarity in the two projections. Usually there is no one-to-one correspondence of y-positions because the vessels are more or less inclined within the imaging planes of the two projections. Therefore an interpolation is carried out within each segment. At the segment transitions the correspondence is always defined by the branching points. When the point to point correspondences have been established along the complete path, the x_1-coordinate in the reference tree and the x_2-coordinate in the second image are associated for each y-coordinate from the reference tree. From these x_1- and x_2-pairs and the projection geometry, the depth coordinate z is calculated.

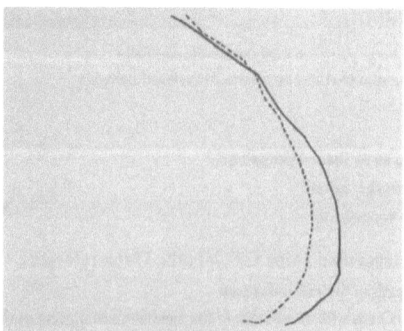

Fig. 7. Vessel pair matched from two projections.

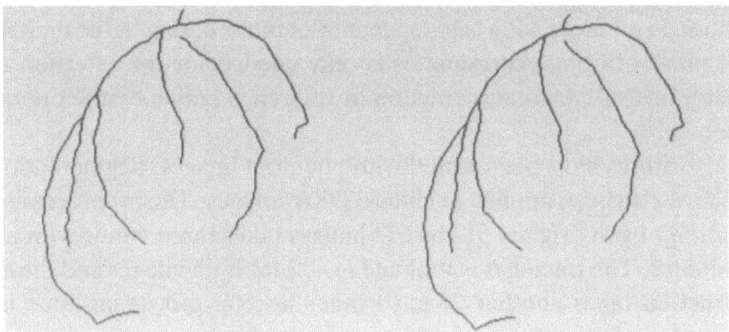

Fig. 8. Stereo pair of reconstructed tree skeletons.

Matching and 3D-calculation are carried out for all points down the reference tree similar to the path in Fig. 7. After matching all paths, the three-dimensional skeleton of the arterial tree is complete. It can be displayed immediately as a stereo pair from any selected viewing angle (Fig. 8).

It may also be used for the reconstruction of an animated display with original vessel densities, depth shading and hidden-point handling for continuous rotation of the vascular tree on the display. Fig. 9 shows a shaded stereo pair at 120° and 127° left posterior oblique. Clinically more important is the ability to access stenoses in any section of the vascular tree with 3D-data for the quantitative evaluation.

Performance and applications

A system for the comprehensive evaluation of the arterial tree in an automated procedure has been designed and implemented. Systematic tracing and three-dimensional processing of the coronary tree provide good positional accuracy, because the results are globally consistent. Errors by local matching problems

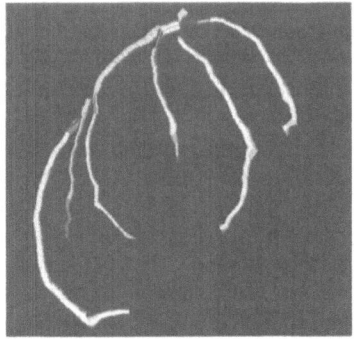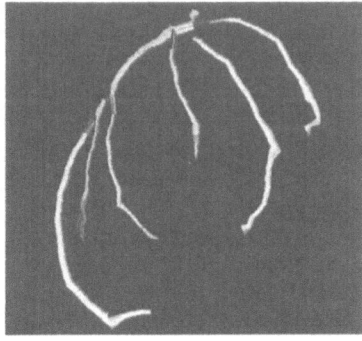

Fig. 9. Stereo pair of the 3D-vascular tree with grey-scale depth encoding.

are excluded and processing is independent of the ordering in the digital tree. Manual input of object coordinates is only needed for the selection of the processing field. A manual correction of reference points by the operator is possible.

The algorithms have been tested with phantom images. Segmentation and tracing have also been applied to clinical DSA-images. The preprocessing and binarization of two original 512 by 512 images takes three minutes on a VAX 750-computer. The tracing is completed in 40 s for both images and the spatial reconstruction takes another 20 s, so that the total processing time is four minutes. At this stage the program for preprocessing has been implemented as well on a modified DSA-system (Siemens DIGITRON I®) with a processing time of 20 s.

The fast generation of three-dimensional data provides the basis for quantitative arteriography. After 3D-processing a stenosis in any area of the major coronary arteries can be selected and analyzed in detail. As the complete arterial tree is available in structured graphical representation, a coronary score [7] can be obtained easily, which is a systematic way of combining the effects of distributed stenoses. The 3D-processing replaces the most tedious part of the evaluation in the case of multi-vessel disease, the determination of all the centrelines and orientations of various vessel segments in several projections.

When cardiac scenes are processed, pericardial motion can be inspected and a locally adaptive re-registration can be carried out. In clinical practice the three-dimensional reconstruction could provide planning assistance for bypass surgery, angioplasty and stereotactic operations.

References

1. Potel MJ, Rubin JM et al.: Methods for evaluating cardiac wall motion in three dimensions using bifurcation points of the coronary arterial tree. Invest Radiology 1983; 18: 47–57.
2. Parker DL, Pope DL et al.: Three dimensional reconstruction of vascular beds. In: Bacharach SL (ed) Information processing in medical imaging; pp 414–430. Martinus Nijhoff, Boston, 1986.
3. Barth K, Faust U et al.: A critical examination of angiographic stenosis quantitation by digital image processing. Proc IEEE ISMIII 1, Berlin 1982; 71–76.
4. Hoffmann KR, Doi K: Automatic tracking of the vascular tree in DSA images using a double-square-box region-of-search algorithm. Proc SPIE Medicine XIV, Newport Beach, 1986; 326–333.
5. Michel C, Barth K: Stenosebestimmung und dreidimensionale Rekonstruktion des Gefaessbaumes der Koronararterien aus digitalisierten Cineangiogrammen. Erg Bd Biomed Technik 1984; 29: 51–52.
6. Mawko GM, Peters TM: Iterative 3-D reconstruction of vascular images from few views. Proc AAPM Summer school, 1985.
7. Hamilton KK, Sanders WJ et al.: Computer reporting of coronary arteriograms using interactive graphics. Proc IEEE Comput Cardiol CH1462, 1979; 111–116.

19. Concepts for Coronary Flow and Myocardial Perfusion Measurements

J.H. BÜRSCH & P.H. HEINTZEN

Department of Pediatric Cardiology and Biomedical Engineering, University of Kiel, Kiel, FRG

Introduction and general comments

As a technique, coronary angiography provides an opportunity to evaluate not only morphologic but also functional information of the coronary circulation. Until recently, visual interpretation of the temporal course of vascular contrast flow was the only method to detect regional flow abnormalities. For example, delayed contrast opacification was considered a reflection of reduced blood flow. Obvious limitations in the visual assessment of abnormal vascular perfusion result from diagnostic uncertainties inherent in subjective evaluation. Consequently, several methods have been suggested that measure transit-times of the contrast bolus along vascular segments by roentgen densitometry [1, 2]. These studies were helpful both in testing specific applications and in understanding particular problems encountered in quantitative contrast dilution methods. However, limited practicality of this roentgen densitometric technique impeded its general acceptance for routine clinical use.

Digital image processing opens a new way to extract distinct qualities from angiographic image series and offers particular functional information that can be displayed in the angiographic image format [3–6]. Functional parameters can be obtained with adequate reproducibility that provide objective measurements of hemodynamic events.

Digital coronary angiography has been developed to extract temporal as well as density information to quantitate regional coronary blood flow [7–12]. These methods are intended to objectively study the severity of coronary vascular disease with particular reference to coronary flow reserve measurements as an index of vascular stenosis severity [13]. In this survey two concepts of digital processing will be described for assessment of coronary and myocardial perfusion. The first principle involves the analysis of temporal aspects of contrast flow. The second principle utilizes densitometric measurements of myocardial contrast accumulation as a relative measure of the magnitude of regional blood flow.

P.H. Heintzen and J.H. Bürsch (eds), Progress in Digital Angiocardiography. ISBN 978-94-010-7093-5

202

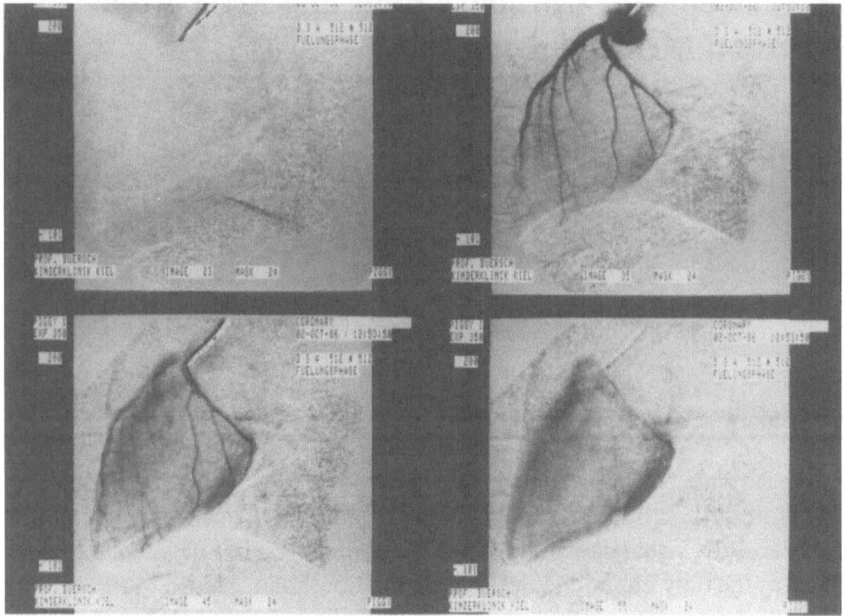

Fig. 1. Mask mode subtraction images of the left coronary artery branches in an animal study. Selective main coronary contrast injection was performed with a rate of 3 ml/s using a power syringe. End-diastolic images were selected from the pre-injection and contrast phase. The interval between subsequent subtraction images in this example corresponds to two cardiac cycles. *Top left:* subtraction of two pre-injection images indicating complete elimination of background densities. *Top right:* opacification of the main coronary artery vessels. *Bottom left:* washout of contrast medium from the coronary arteries with initial opacification of the myocardium. *Bottom right:* myocardial contrast image indicating mostly uniform distribution of radio-opaque indicator.

Great flexibility is a characteristic feature of computerized image processing that allows us to accomplish these tasks in various ways. The visual aspect of functional images may significantly vary depending on the specific algorithms and display modes being applied. Therefore, the interpretation of parametric images requires consideration of the respective image acquisition and processing modes, as well as a general understanding of indicator dilution theory. The display of functional images usually constitutes the first analytic step towards detailed quantitative analysis.

As stated above, the temporal course and the degree of regional contrast absorption are the physical determinants that form the basis for angiographic flow studies. An example of the so-called extraction of functional information from an image sequence is given by the rather simple modality of the combination of color-coded subtraction images. Figure 1 illustrates the temporal sequence of four coronary angiographic images in the mask subtraction mode.

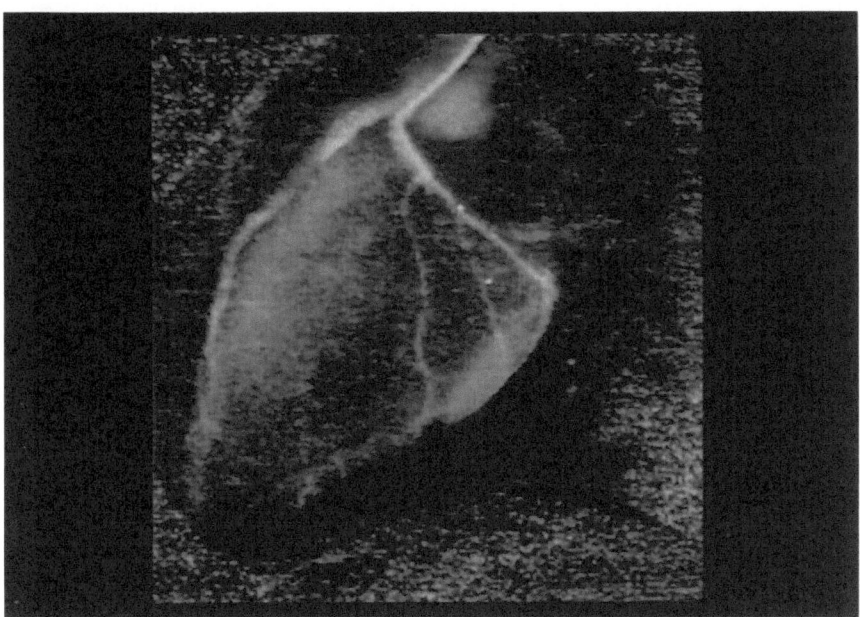

Fig. 2. Result of superimposition of the three subtraction images of Fig. 1 after color coding. The colors indicate the temporal sequence of contrast flow.

Elimination of non-specific background densities allows clear visualization of three phases of vascular opacification by the contrast bolus; the main coronary arteries, the early onset of myocardial opacification, and staining of the capillary bed in a normal animal. Conversion of gray intensities into colors and combination of colored images is used to superimpose contrast flow information in a single image (Fig. 2). The display of different colors in this image signifies the temporal sequence, while color intensities correspond to the degree of vascular opacification. Thus, the final, so-called functional image indicates the temporal course as well as the extent of regional contrast absorption.

Color coding has become a characteristic feature of parametric imaging and provides good separation of temporal events. In this particular case comparable degrees of capillary opacification, i.e. of the anterior and posterior left ventricular wall, is indicated by similar color tones and intensities of the two wall segments. Abnormalities of perfusion may be detected by non-uniform and non-homogeneous colors. This combination of images is the simplest processing mode, and yet has actually not been practiced frequently. Nevertheless, it illustrates the concept of displaying characteristic angiographic features such as temporal and contrast density information in a single image.

Coronary flow imaging and quantitative assessment

For the purpose of time parameter processing it is useful to consider temporal variations in roentgen density according to each picture element of the digital image matrix. The regional densograms can be analysed by applying the classical indicator dilution principle in order to define representative circulation-times of the contrast bolus for each picture element. In order to keep processing times reasonably low for the great number of densograms in each study (up to 65,000 densograms in a 256×256 matrix), the address of the pixel data must be internally arranged in the temporal domain. Otherwise, the conventional mode of data addressing in the spatial orientation of images is inefficient and may need more than one hour processing time depending on the number of serial images. An example of the recording of density variations is depicted in Fig. 3 for illustration of the primary densitometric process. Minute regions of interest were defined, for the detection of bolus travel along the two main left coronary arteries in an animal study. Each region of interest encompasses 4×8 picture elements. ECG-gated imaging was used to assure superimposition of the opacified vessels because of cardiac-vascular motion. This gated image acquisition mode, possibly combined with electrical pacing, has been most frequently used to minimize misregistration and motion artefacts. The concomitant discontinuity of data recording (time-interval of one cardiac length) definitely limits the accuracy with which time data are finally calculated. Nevertheless, interpolation between subsequent density values still allows application of most of the common indicator dilution algorithms. Limitation in temporal resolution must be regarded as one of several methodologic restraints that potentially degrade quantitative measurements of coronary blood flow. Therefore, it seems necessary to review the major sources of inadequate densitometric analysis and the resulting consequences.

Aside from low acquisition rates that may still be tolerable, the effect of parenchymal superposition with the coronary arteries may cause significant uncertainties due to alterations in the shape of densograms, particularly during the late contrast perfusion phase. Thus, it seems unlikely that accurate mean-transit time data as derived from the complete densogram will be obtained. Consequently, time parameters have been preferentially assigned to the initial section of the curve in order to exclude superposition phenomena during the late phase of densitometric recording. However, time values of the bolus front are compromised by dispersion phenomena of indicator in the streaming blood. A visual impression of these effects is obtained by comparing densograms from the proximal and distal vessel segments (Fig. 3) that show an increasing prolongation of the early curve section from the onset to maximum absorption of the contrast bolus. Many of these particular qualities in digital roentgen densitometry have been discussed in detail as limitations in the

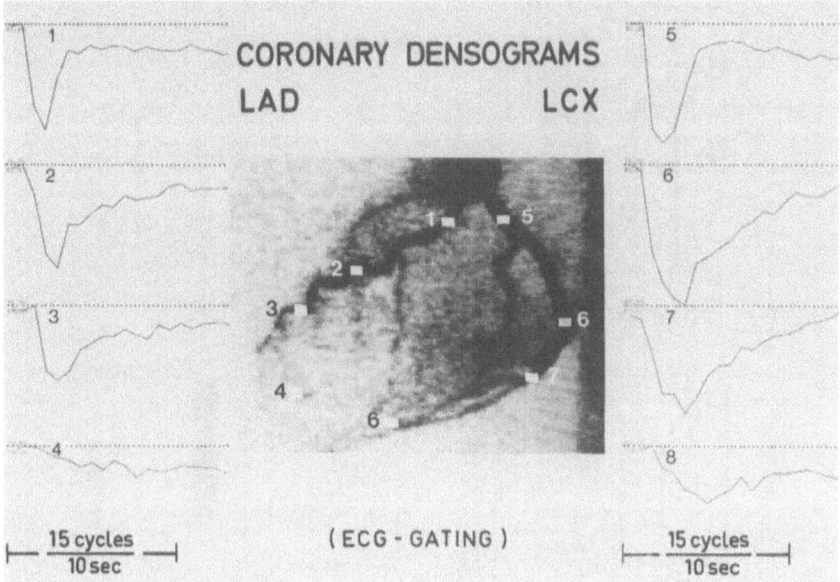

Fig. 3. Illustration of densograms from minute sampling areas assigned by the numbers 1 to 8. Density data were obtained for each densogram in intervals of one cardiac cycle length (ECG-gating). Densitometric curves were established by linear interpolation of the subsequently measured density values. Variations in shape of densograms with progression of the contrast bolus from the proximal to the distal vessel segments is mainly due to contrast dispersion as well as superimposition with the capillary perfusion phase.

interpretation of time parameters [14], and may give at best semi-quantitative information on regional contrast flow. Even though accurate measurements may not be expected, the diagnostic significance of parametric imaging seems relatively unaffected in some specific applications such as comparative studies of coronary blood flow, since many of the inherent methodologic deficiencies are canceled out. The fact that a variety of digital processing modes have been proposed for extraction of temporal information from image series results mainly from specific considerations of the various indicator effects, different algorithms, and the actual diagnostic goal. The latter has to account particularly for practical aspects and efficiency of the clinical examinations.

A simple version of ECG-gated image processing is depicted in Fig. 4. This schematic drawing illustrates that different colors are assigned to the sequence of serial contrast images. If one considers this set to be contrast images after mask subtraction, subsequent density values of each individual picture element reflect the densities of the contrast medium bolus at the respective site. A simple mathematical operator is applied to detect the one image that contains

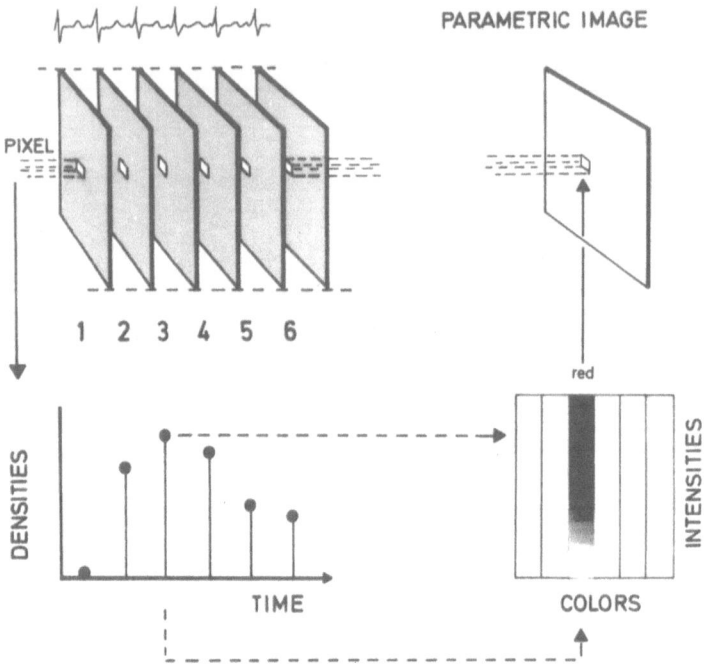

PARAMETRIC IMAGE

Fig. 4. Schematic illustration of time parameter extraction. Temporal variations in densities of a picture element (pixel) are depicted in the lower left panel. A computer program automatically detects the maximum density value, thus selecting the particular image and the corresponding time of maximal opacification, respectively. The fact that different colors are assigned to subsequent images allows conversion of temporal information into a color-coded parameter image. In addition, the degree of maximal contrast absorption may be used to vary the color intensities.

the maximal value of regional densities, thus selecting the appropriate color for each picture element in the parameter image. In addition, the degree of maximal absorption may be converted into color intensity for the final display. This method affords only short processing times and reveals time parameter images that indicate bolus progression in time intervals (different colors) of one ardiac cycle length. Similarly, other criteria than the maximum density can be used. Vogel and Le Free have used the elegant method of defining the time of the maximum change in contrast densities as a representative value [12, 15]. Figure 5 indicates that the so-called time-interval difference mode is applied for this purpose instead of the mask subtraction mode to calculate data of the time of the maximum derivative of density variations. Excellent presentation of the temporal aspects of the contrast bolus front was obtained yielding vascular perfusion segments of one cardiac cycle length.

We prefer a somewhat different approach by calculating the 'mean-rise

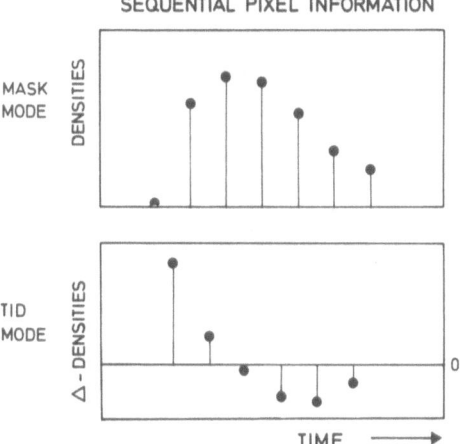

Fig. 5. Illustration of sequential density values for comparison of the mask subtraction mode (upper panel) and the time interval differences (TID) mode (lower panel). The latter derives from the difference of subsequent density values as depicted in the mask subtraction mode.

time' of the upslope of densitometric curves. This time value is defined as the front edge of a rectangle with the height of the maximum amplitude of the densogram and the area corresponding to the initial curve section. As the second processing step, the continuous increase in regional time values, according to bolus propagation, is converted into discrete increments. The time interval of these increments may be arbitrarily chosen, e.g. 250, 500, 750 msec. We believe that comparative studies will take advantage of this type of parameter processing, since the temporal aspect of regional flow is not dependent on variations in heart rates.

An early approach to estimate flow has been the calculation of myocardial appearance-times in different hemodynamic states of the circulation, e.g. by comparing the speed of flow in the control and hyperemic state [12]. However, interpretation of the temporal data as a reflection of coronary flow reserve was found to be inadequate unless intravascular volumes, in addition, were calculated. The three-dimensional coronary morphology, typically branching into multiple small diameter vessels, usually excludes relatively long vascular segments from dimensional measurements.

An alternative is the assessment of vascular volumes by regional density measurements within the confines of vascular segments. The fact, that selective coronary artery injection reveals mostly a homogeneous concentration of non-diluted contrast medium in the coronary arteries allows for the densitometric measurements from contrast images of the injection phase. Even though the accuracy has not yet been proven experimentally, it appears suitable for comparative studies of volume flow and the determination of flow ratios. Another method has been tested experimentally utilizing the density-time product (area under densograms) for estimation of relative volumes of vessel segments. The described methods are presently being tested to estimate hyperemic-to-baseline flow for the assessment of the hemodynamic significance of coronary stenosis.

Myocardial perfusion imaging and densitometric analysis

The alternative to time parameter extraction for relative flow measurements is to quantitate the amount of contrast medium that has entered the vascular bed according to regional artery supply [7, 16]. Basically, this approach requires minimal processing efforts since only digital subtraction is required prior to the densitometric analysis of a single image using large regions of interest (Fig. 6).

Selective coronary injection and myocardial contrast enhancement provides manual outlining of the region of interest for the integral density measurement of wall segments. It has been experimentally proven that summed densities from (large) regions of interest are linearly related to the amount of medium transradiated, if the exponential attenuation of roentgen absorption is adequately considered. Therefore, filtering of the incident roentgen radiation (0.1 mmCu) and logarithmic conversion of pixel data are the basic requirements needed for quantitative density measurements.

Myocardial densitometry includes the following steps:

1. Selective coronary angiography is performed preferably in an oblique view for adequate separation of the anterior and posterior myocardial wall. A contrast image is selected at the time of myocardial opacification before venous run-off occurs.

2. An optimal mask image is selected taking into account corresponding respiratory and cardiac phases. Suspended respiration is not mendatory since an optimal image mask may be alternatively selected out of a sequence of pre-injection images that have been acquired over at least one respiratory cycle length. Optimal matching of the contrast and the mask image is indicated by complete elimination of background densities, preferably visible at the cardiac wall circumference and the diaphragm.

3. Based on myocardial contrast enhancement the opacified wall contours are roughly delineated. This region of interest encompasses both the opacified myocardium and the superimposed coronary arteries.

4. Integration of densities within the region of interest produces a relative value of the amount of medium that has entered the vascular bed.

Calculation of coronary flow is primarily based on mass measurements of contrast medium from which volume data are derived. Volumes are easiest to

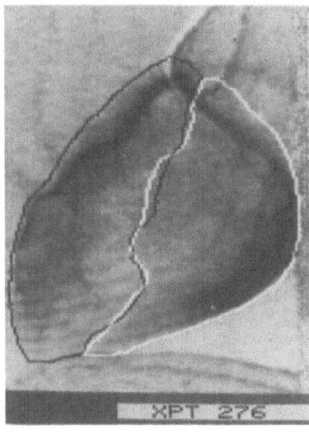

Fig. 6. Mask mode subtraction image at the termination of contrast injection from a digital coronary angiogram. The contours were manually outlined to define regions of interest for densitometric analysis of the anterior wall (black contour) and the posterior wall (white contour).

assess if the radio-opaque material is measured without any dilution effects and intravascular mixing with blood does not occur. Usually, this condition exists if selective injections are performed with rates higher than native coronary blood flow and retrograde flow of contrast medium into the aorta becomes visible. Thus, delivery of pure contrast medium during the time course of contrast injection is provided.

Assuming steady state circulatory conditions during the phase of injection a steady increase of amount of contrast medium in the coronary circulation can be theoretically expected. In fact, numerous experimental studies have demonstrated the feasibility of measuring linearly the increase in contrast opacification as indicated in the two densitometric recordings in Fig. 7.

The described technique is not substantially different from conventional coronary angiography. However, differences concern the injection mode, e.g. the use of a power syringe to provide contrast injection with a constant flow rate as well as the use of low viscous contrast medium in order to keep hemodynamic alterations low.

Relative flow can be assessed for each of the three main arterial vessels. A practical consideration is to avoid overlapping of myocardial regions that are perfused by the LAD and LCX coronary arteries. Since retrograde flow during injection is an essential methodologic condition a fractional amount of contrast medium may enter the other branch resulting in slight opacification of the opposite myocardial segment. In order to separate these two perfusion areas oblique projection is of particular importance.

We had the opportunity to test this technique in animal experiments for

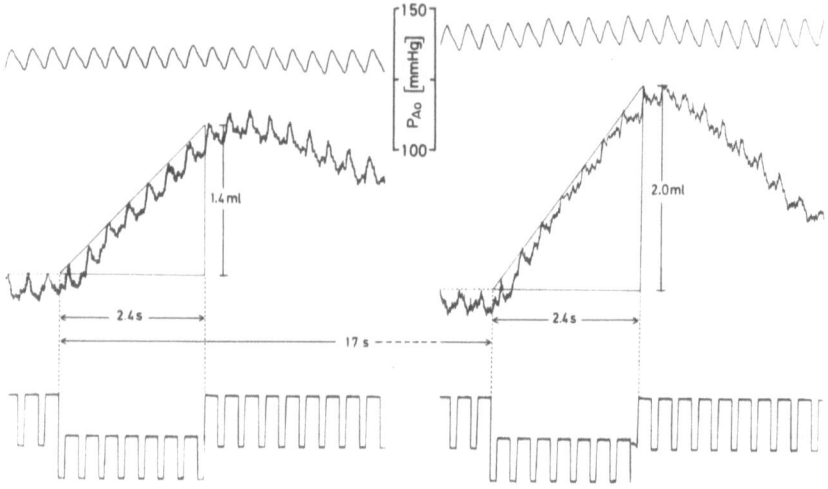

Fig. 7. Continuous densitometric recordings of summed densities from the anterior wall in an animal study. Two subsequent contrast injections were performed (3 ml Solutrast) into the left anterior descending coronary artery. The second injection was delayed by 17 seconds after the initial one indicating hyperemic response by increased contrast flow into the vasculature (right). It is noteworthy that there is a steady increase in contrast absorption during the phase of continuous contrast infusion reflecting a mostly linear recording system.

comparative flow studies in the hyperemic state and the control state for all three coronary arteries. In these studies duplicate contrast injections were performed using the first injection (control angiography) as the stimulus for hyperemic response. A second contrast injection was performed about 15 seconds after the initial one. The response of increased myocardial contrast flow is demonstrated in Fig. 8. Increased myocardial opacification was a regular finding in each of the hyperemic angiograms.

Comparative measurements in each set of angiograms revealed an increase in regional contrast amount by a factor of $1.8 \pm 20\%$ (mean, SD). It was even possible in these experiments to estimate myocardial contrast volume as a fraction of the delivered total injection volume. Thus the absolute volume flow of contrast medium that had entered the coronary arteries was calculated (Fig. 9). From our limited experience with these experimental studies we conclude that this particular method of myocardial densitometry can be easily practiced and seems to be adequate for clinical applications.

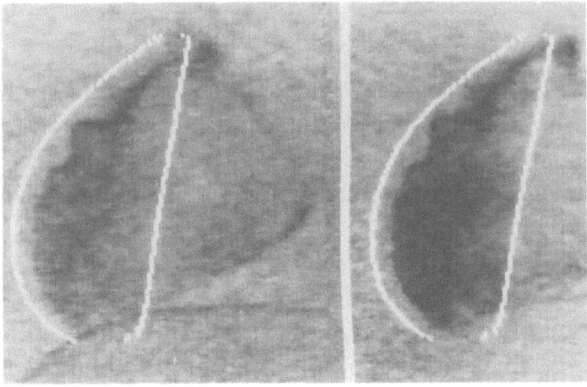

Fig. 8. Aspect of the contrast induced hyperemic response in an animal study using duplicate selective LAD contrast injections. These two mask subtraction images were processed according to the termination of injection applying identical contrast volumes and injection flow rates. Increased myocardial opacification in the right image is indicative for increased coronary flow and flow reserve, respectively. The contours were outlined to define regions of interest for summed densitometric measurements.

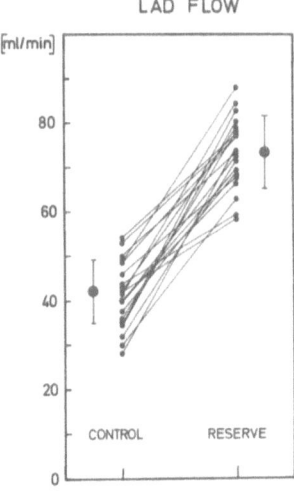

Fig. 9. Diagrammatic presentation of the left anterior descending (LAD) artery flow reserve in experimental pigs (20 kg body weight). Hyperemic response was induced by the initial angiographic contrast medium injection (Solutrast).

Summary

Advances in digital angiography and roentgen densitometry have focused attention on the potential benefits of parameter extraction for functional studies of the coronary circulation. Two approaches have been preferably applied to the challenge of coronary flow distribution and hyperemic flow reserve measurements:

1. The time parameter approach facilitates imaging of the sequential progression of the contrast bolus by different colors that indicate the time dependent perfusion of coronary artery segments. This information is extracted from ECG-gated images of the entire angiographic scene. Additional densitometric analysis is necessary to derive relative data of vascular volume flow. Practical limitations result from possible misregistration of this particular vasculature, as well as indicator dispersion and superimposition phenomena.

2. The alternative approach is myocardial densitometry applying large regions of interest for summed density measurement of myocardial contrast amounts in wall segments that are supplied by the main coronary artery branches. Only simple mask-mode subtraction is required (one subtraction image) for enhancement of myocardial opacification and subsequent digital densitometry. Comparative data of regional flow are established if selective coronary injections are performed with standardized flow rates that assure retrograde contrast flow into the aorta. A practical advantage of the latter technique is that it is rather little affected by motion and superimposition artefacts.

References

1. Heintzen PH, Bürsch JH (eds): Roentgen video techniques for dynamic studies of structure and function of the heart and circulation. Thieme Stuttgart, 1978.
2. Rutishauser W, Bussmann WD, Noseda G, Meier W, Wellauer J: Blood flow measurement through single coronary arteries by roentgen densitometry. Part I. A comparison of flow measured by a radiologic technique applicable in the intact organism and by electromagnetic flowmeter. Am J Roengenol 1970; 109: 12.
3. Brennecke R, Bürsch JH: Functional analysis of angiograms by digital image processing techniques. In: Nalcioglu O, Chow ZH (eds) Selected topics in image science: Applications to medical diagnosis and physical sciences; pp 182–220. Springer, Berlin/Heidelber/New York, 1984.
4. Brennecke R, Bürsch JH, Heintzen PH: Functional analysis of angiograms: basic physics and technology. In: Felix R, Frommhold W, Lissner J, Meaney TH, Niendorf HP, Zeitler E (eds) Contrast media in digital radiography; pp 37–50. Excerpta Medica, Amsterdam, 1983.
5. Heintzen PH, Brennecke R (eds): Digital imaging in cardiovascular radiology. Thieme, Stuttgart, 1983.

6. Heintzen PH, Bürsch JH, Hahne HJ, Brennecke R, Budach W, Lange PE: Assessment of cardiovascular function by digital angiocardiography. JACC 1985; 5 (I): 150–157.

7. Bürsch JH, Hahne HJ, Beyer C, Seemann S, Meissner L, Brennecke R, Heintzen PH: Myocardial perfusion studies by digital angiography. Comp Cardiol 1983: 343–346.

8. Ratib O, Chappuis F, Rutishauser W: Digital angiographic technique for the quantitative assessment of myocardial perfusion. Ann Radiol 1985; 28: 193–197.

9. Reiber JHC, Serruys PW (eds): State of the art in quantitative coronary arteriography. Martinus Nijhoff, Dordrecht/Boston/Lancaster, 1986.

10. Vogel RA: The radiographic assessment of coronary blood flow parameters. Circulation 1985; 72: 460–465.

11. Spiller P, Jehle J, Pölitz B, Schmiel FK: A digital image processing system for measurement of phasic blood flow in coronary arteries. Comp Cardiol 1982; 223–26.

12. Vogel RA, Le Free M, Bates E, O'Neill W, Forster R, Kirlin P, Smith DN, Pitt B: Application of digital techniques to selective coronary arteriography: Use of myocardial contrast appearence time to measure coronary flow reserve. Am Heart J 1984; 107: 153–164.

13. Gould KL, Lipscomb K, Hamilton GW: Physiologic basis for assessing critical coronary stenosis. Instantaneous flow response and regional distribution during coronary hyperemia as measures of coronary flow reserve. Am J Cardiol 1974; 33: 87–93.

14. Bürsch JH, Heintzen PH: Parametric imaging. Radiol Clin North Am 1985; 23 (2): 321–333.

15. Le Free MT, Vogel RA, O'Neill WW,Bates ER, Smith N, Pitt B: A digital radiographic technique for visualization and quantitation of regional myocardial perfusion. Comp Cardiol 1982; 153–156.

16. Bürsch JH: Densitometric studies in digital subtraction angiography: Assessment of pulmonary and myocardial perfusion. Herz 1985; 10: 208–214.

20. Blood Flow Measurements in Digital Cardiac Angiography using 3D Coronary Artery Reconstructions

DENNIS L. PARKER, DAVID L. POPE, RUDY E. VAN BREE &
HIRAM MARSHALL
Department of Medical Informatics, LDS Hospital/University of Utah, Salt Lake City, UT, USA

Introduction

Impaired blood flow, which can result in ischemia and death to tissues of critical organs, is a byproduct of several disease states. Examples of angiographic techniques which study blood flow include those

1. which measure uptake and washout of contrast media,
2. which measure the contrast dilution as an indicator, and
3. transit time measurements which measure the time it takes for the fluid to traverse a known volume.

This last technique provides the ability to measure absolute blood flow within individual segments and is the subject of this paper.

The importance of flow measurements in the coronary arteries has received significant attention recently with the demonstration of the clinical significance of coronary flow reserve [1–4]. Measurement of flow in the coronary arteries is difficult because of the motion of the arterial bed. This motion problem is compounded in angiographic imaging where the injection of contrast media can induce changes in the contraction pattern of the heart. For this reason, most techniques that study flow in the coronary arteries require pacing of the heart.

Several techniques for transit time measurements of blood flow through arterial segments have been presented [5–7]. Bateman and Kruger [5] developed a technique based on densitometric measurements of the contrast profile along and orthogonal to the vessel segment. The technique is valid for segments which do not change dimensions and are parallel to the imaging plane. In order to avoid problems associated with pulsatile blood flow, Colchester et al. [7] proposed using 3D reconstruction of arterial beds in order to measure the contrast profile along a vessel at one instant in time rather than finding the profile by temporal sampling at one location. Although this technique also works nicely when the vessel does not change dimensions, the theory as yet developed does not conveniently handle arbitrary branching vessel networks.

P.H. Heintzen and J.H. Bürsch (eds), Progress in Digital Angiocardiography. ISBN 978-94-010-7093-5
© 1988, Kluwer Academic Publishers, Dordrecht

In this paper we review the principles of transit time flow measurements and demonstrate how absolute flow can be measured in branches of an arterial bed for which the three-dimensional structure is known. Some initial phantom studies and a clinical example are presented.

Transit time flow measurements; theory

Transit time flow measurements are based upon the rate of passage of a contrast bolus down the known dimensions of an artery segment. The artery cross-section must be known or directly inferred from the measurement technique. Flow (Q) is then simply defined as the ratio of the volume traversed to the time of transit:

$$Q = \Delta V / \Delta t. \tag{1}$$

It is assumed that the bolus profile has some shape as a function of distance along the vessel. If the vessel changes dimensions, the vessel profile will also change shape as a function of distance along the vessel. In the absence of turbulence it is convenient to assume that the profile (iodine concentration) is a stationary function of volume along the artery:

$$\varrho_I(s,t) = \varrho_I[V(s) - V_f(s,t)], \tag{2}$$

where $V(s)$ is simply a measure of volume from some initial position to the point s on the vessel:

$$V(s) = \sum_{i=0}^{n(s)} A(s_i) \, \Delta s_i \,, \tag{3}$$

and V_f is the volume of flow through that position (s) from time 0 to time t:

$$V_f(s,t) = \int_0^t Q(s,t') \, dt'. \tag{4}$$

The digital density value of the profile is proportional to iodine density:

$$d_j(s_i) = g \, \mu_I \, \varrho_I(s_i) \, x_j(s_i) / \cos\beta_i, \tag{5}$$

where i and j are the indices parallel with and orthogonal to the vessel respectively, g is the sytem gain, μ_I is the iodine attenuation coefficient, x is the vessel thickness and β is the angle of inclination of the vessel relative to the imaging plane. The density at the position, s, at the center of the profile can be found as:

$$\varrho_I(s_i) = \frac{d_{max}(s_i)}{g \, \mu_I \, D(s_i)} \cos\beta_i. \tag{6}$$

Using equation (6) it is possible to determine the density profile along the artery segment, with correction for change in cross-section.

Measurement of the iodine bolus profile as a function of volume along the length of the artery segment can then be used to determine the location of the profile. For simplicity in this study we have chosen to use a point of specified density on the leading edge of the bolus. Use of the profile requires corrections for branching where flow rates differ between branches. Such corrections may prove unnecessary if simple point detection methods prove adequate.

Methods

Experimental flow determinations were obtained using a phantom consisting of 3.35 m diameter plastic tubing attached to the vertices of a plastic pyramid. Continuous flow of controlled rate was obtained using a Medrad Mark IV power injector. The phantom was immersed in a water bucket for imaging. The phantom was imaged using a Siemens Angioskop D interfaced to a Digitron II. Images were acquired in 512×512 digital format. For three-dimensional reconstruction, two views of the phantom separated by 57/ were obtained. Images were acquired at 6 frames/sec for flow rates of 1 and 2 ml/sec and 15 frames/sec for flow rates of 6, 8, 10, 12 and 16 ml/sec. Images were then transferred to a VAX 11/750 computer for 3D reconstruction and flow measurements.

Preliminary results

Three-dimensional reconstruction was performed as outlined previously and the accuracy of the reconstruction was determined [8]. A measure proportional to contrast bolus density was obtained using equation (6). Bolus endpoints were determined with no operator intervention as the first point along the vessel at which the bolus density dropped to 30% of the final density. Some examples of determined endpoints are shown in Fig. 1. Endpoints were determined for all images of all flow rates and the results are plotted in Fig. 2. Least squares fits of lines through the points are included in the Figure. Flow is defined simply as the slope of the lines. These flow computations, along with an estimate of the standard error, are plotted in Fig. 3.

Some initial results of flow measurements on the clinical study [8] are also presented. Bolus endpoints are again obtained as the point of 30% of the final, maximum, density as obtained from equation (6). Examples of the determined endpoints are shown in Fig. 4. Transit volumes and flow through the left main, left anterior descending (LAD) and circumflex branches are given in Fig. 5. The phasic nature of blood flow [9] is evident from the figure. In this case the

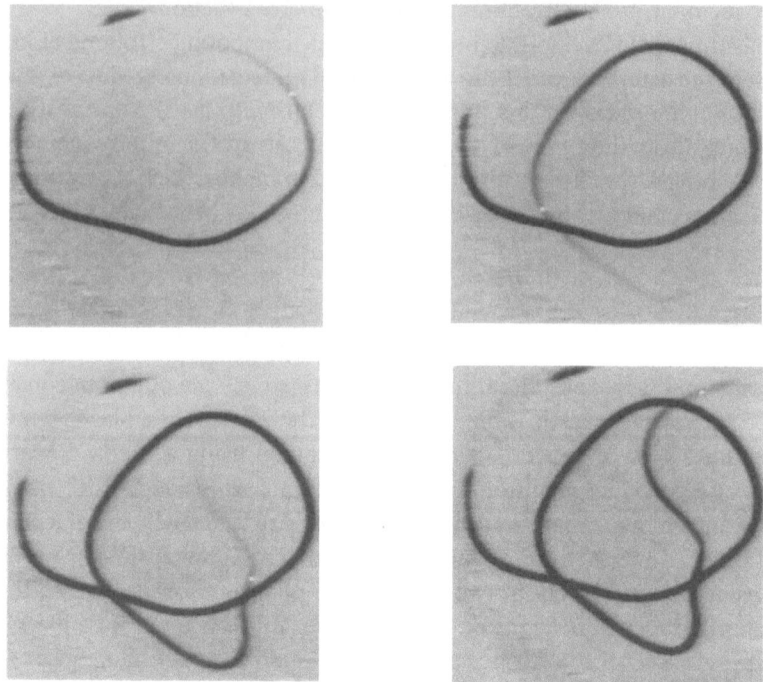

Fig. 1. Images showing contrast entering the flow phantom. Bolus endpoints have been determined using equation (6) (see text) as the point where the iodine density drops to 30% of the final density.

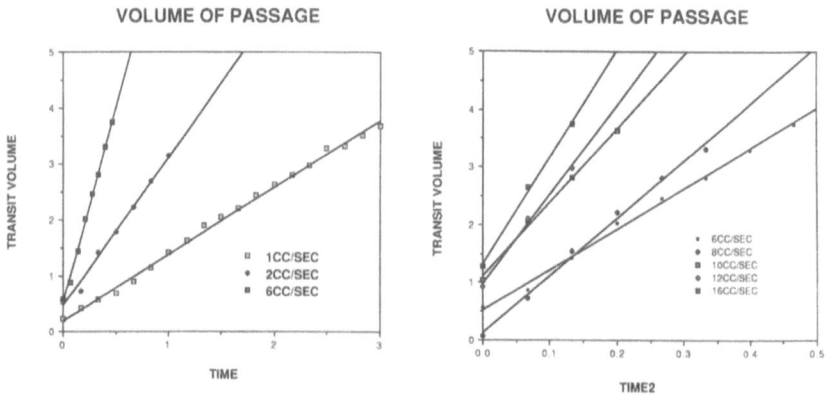

Fig. 2. Plot of the volume of passage through the flow phantom determined from the bolus endpoint locations. The lines are least squares fits through the points. Measured flow is defined simply as the slope of the lines.

FLOW MEASUREMENTS

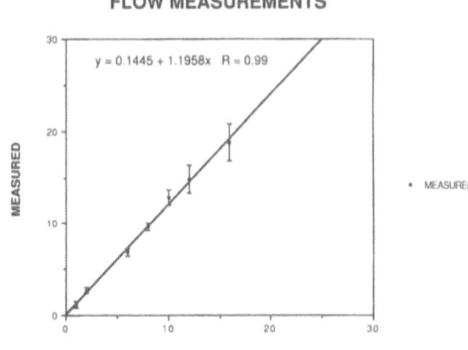

Fig. 3. Flow measurements obtained from the line slopes of Fig. 2. The error bars are estimates based upon the scatter in the volume of passage measurements.

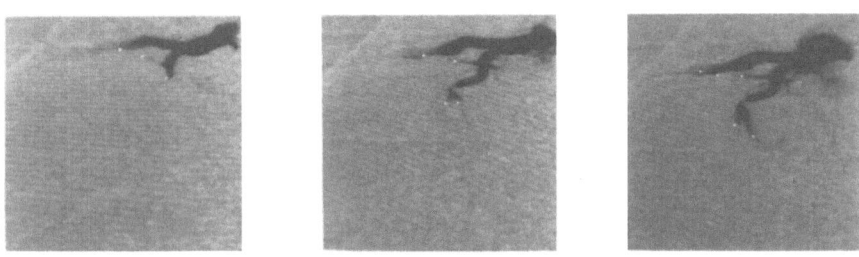

Fig. 4. Examples of bolus endpoints determined on an RAO view of the left main coronary artery.

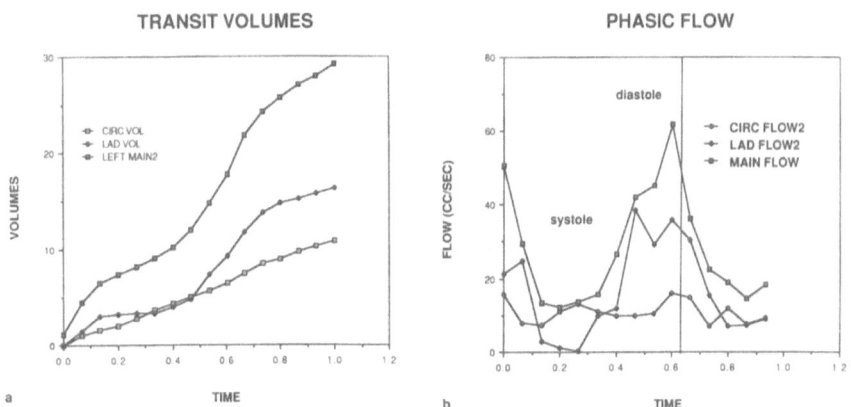

Fig. 5. a. Plots of volume passing through the left main, left anterior descending (LAD) and circumflex arteries. b. Flow measurements determined from the bolus endpoints for the entire left main artery and the LAD and circumflex branches. The vertical line represents the time at which the contrast media begins to appear outside of the computer-determined vascular tree structure.

flow through the LAD branch nearly stops during systole while the flow through the circumflex which feds the atrium continues.

Conclusions

Preliminary results indicate that three-dimensional reconstruction of vessel centerlines and cross-sectional area can be used in conjunction with bolus position determination to obtain transit time flow measurements. Both the phantom and clinical results are very encouraging. Further validation studies are ongoing.

Summary

A technique for measuring blood flow in the coronary arteries is presented. This technique relies upon tracking a bolus of iodine down the known dimensions of the three-dimensional reconstruction of the arterial bed. Results obtained fom a simple flow phantom are presented.

References

1. Gould KL Quantification of coronary artery stenosis in vivo. Circ Res 1985; 57: 341–353.
2. White CW, Wright CB, Doty DB, Hiratza LF, Eastham CL, Harrison DG, Marcus ML: Does visual interpretation of the coronary arteriogram predict the physiologic importance of a coronary stenosis: New Engl J Med 1984; 310: 819–824.
3. Vogel R, LeFree M, Bates E, O'Neill W, Foster R, Kirlin P, Smith D, Pitt B: Application of digital techniques for selective coronary arteriography: use of myocardial contrast appearance time to measure coronary flow curve. Am Heart J 1984; 107–153.
4. Koiwa Y, Bahn RC, Ritman EL: Regional myocardial volume perfused by the coronary artery branch: estimation in vivo. Circulation 1986; 74: 157–163.
5. Bateman WA, Kruger RA: Blood flow measurement using digital angiography and parametric imaging. Med Phys 1984; 11: 153–157.
6. Barrett W, Hines H, Scheibe P, Arnold B, Eisenberg H: Digital angiographic determination of relative blood flow from a single injection. Comp Cardiol Sept 1983; 335–338.
7. Colchester ACF, Hawkes DJ, Brunt JNH, Du Boulay G, Wallis A: Pulsatile blood flow measurements with the aid of 3-D reconstruction from dynamic angiographic recordings. In: Bacharach S (ed) Information processing in medical imaging; pp 247–265. Martinus Nijhoff, Boston, 1986.
8. Parker DL, Pope DL, Bree van RE, Marshall HW: Three-dimensional reconstruction and cross-secion measurements of coronary arteries using ECG-correlated digital coronary arteriography. In this volume, pp. 181–192.
9. Guyton AC: Textbook of medical physiology, 4th ed; p 359. WB Saunders, Philadelphia, 1971.

21. Coronary Blood Flow and Myocardial Perfusion Studied by Digitized Coronary Angiograms

W. RUTISHAUSER, O. RATIB, F. CHAPPUIS, P.-A. DORIOT & B. MEIER
Center of Cardiology, University Hospital, Geneva, Switzerland

Coronary angiography is since many years the key examination for the evaluation of coronary artery disease in man. While it is widely used to visualize coronary anatomy, it has until recently only sporadically been used to measure coronary blood flow. Early attempts for assessment of blood flow through single coronary arteries applied roentgendensitometric techniques [1, 2]. The principle is based on measurement of a vascular volume between two branching points and the mean transit time in order to get absolute coronary flow. It is obviously limited to major coronary vessel segments, which must be more or less perpendicular to the X-ray beam, if single plane angiograms are used.

Digital coronary artery imaging is not a simple technique, since one is trying to image structures of 3 mm down to fractions of a mm which may move with a speed of up to more than 10 cm/s. With this goal in mind a small focal spot, progressive video scanning and a matrix of 1024^2 with high frame rate should be available.

If one does not attempt to quantitate coronary artery flow but is satisfied with a regional index of perfusion, the progression of contrast medium through the coronary circulation can be visualized by parametric imaging with a coarser matrix and one frame per heart cycle.

Two sets of enhanced images can be generated:
1. a set where image enhancement is accomplished by serially subtracting the selected image obtained before injection (mask image) from the following frames obtained in phase with each QRS-complex;
2. a second set can be obtained by a so-called ECG-gated time interval difference, where each frame is subtracted from the frame in phase with the QRS-complex of the next cardiac beat.

Vogel and Mancini [3] have described a new approach for the assessment of the arterial, myocardial and venous phases of contrast medium transit and the visualization of the spatial distribution and timing of contrast flow obtained from standard cinearteriograms. The results are displayed in a color-coded functional image, where intensity and color modulation are used to respectively depict the magnitude and timing of the appearance of contrast medium

P.H. Heintzen and J.H. Bürsch (eds), Progress in Digital Angiocardiography. ISBN 978-94-010-7093-5

in each picture element. Such a method is based on the hypothesis that the visualization of the time of passage of the contrast through the myocardial circulation would be less sensitive to veiling glare and scatter than integrating time-videodensity curves, and would still provide an index of regional flow [4–6].

In the Geneva University Hospital similar approaches were developed and tested [7–9]. Four different temporal parameters of the progression of the contrast medium through the heart are calculated and displayed in corresponding color-coded functional images. This type of image analysis was applied to measure differences in perfusion between myocardial segments supplied by normal or by stenosed coronary vessels. Earlier, it was shown that the mean transit time of a bolus of tracer through the circulation is inversely related to the quantity of blood flowing through it [10]. However, it was also demonstrated that at resting state there is no change in flow between normal coronary vessels and vessels with mild or moderate stenosis ($< 70\%$ reduction in diameter) [11]. Interventions are therefore needed to better visualize the differences in the capacity to increase the blood flow between normal and abnormal vessels. The hyperemic response to vasodilation is indeed reduced downstream in a stenosed vessel. The coronary flow reserve defined as the ratio of hyperemic to resting blood flow is an excellent indicator of the physiologic significance of a coronary lesion in the perfusion of non-infarcted myocardium [12]. Intracoronary administered ionic contrast medium or intravenous injection of dipyridamole or intracoronary papaverine can be used to create hyperemic states. Since ionic contrast medium and intracoronary papaverine lead to acute changes in flow, which vary according to the dose [13], we have confined our investigations to the intravenous application of 0.5 mg/kg dipyridamole which is a reliable coronary vasodilator. Subsequent quantitative evaluation of changes in perfusion from baseline to hyperemic state provide useful information about the functional significance of coronary stenosis. Non-ionic contrast medium (4 ml Iopamidol 370 mgI/ml) is injected starting in early diastole. Selective injection of contrast medium 60/ LAO projection is well suited to separate the territories of the two main branches of the left coronary artery.

Six successive end-diastolic frames are selected starting one cycle before injection of contrast medium, digitized in 256×256 matrix, and stored on disk; subsequent pixel-by-pixel analysis is then performed, where the progression of contrast medium through the myocardium is displayed on four color-coded parametric images:

1. *Mask mode image,* obtained by giving each of the five successive frames after mask subtraction a predefined color in the sequence of the rainbow, and by combining all the colored frames in one by adding the different color intensities of each pixel in each frame.

2. The *time interval difference* image also referred to as the image of contrast medium 'appearance' time [14] obtained from a set of five gated time interval images by determining the maximum magnitude (pixel value) and timing (frame number), i.e. the maximum increase of each pixel. This corresponds to the fastest change of intensity (maximal rate of opacification), and is coded into 256 intensity levels and the corresponding timing coded into five predefined colors used as the colored time scale representative of five successive cardiac cycles.

3. The *time of maximum intensity* image is obtained by displaying the maximum opacification magnitude into a 256 intensity scale and the time of maximum opacification into the five colors time scale.

4. The *time of center of gravity* image is obtained by computing the center of gravity of the surface below the time intensity curve of each pixel. Because this does not involve the whole curve, the term may be misleading. The resulting value is color-coded similar to the three other images using a five-colors time scale modulated in 256 intensity levels representing the magnitude of the center of gravity.

In each of these images the independent parameters of magnitude and timing of the progression of the contrast medium through the heart are simultaneously depicted, and regional differences in each of these parameters are clearly visualized.

For further quantification of the progression of contrast medium through the heart, the operator outlines regions of interest using a joystick cursor. Several parameters are then calculated and averaged in each region of interest. The comparison between areas perfused by normal or stenosed coronary vessels rarely shows differences already at baseline but after maximal hyperemia by dipyridamole, the progression of contrast medium downstream from significant stenoses is delayed. That is immediately visible on the parametric image.

The methods presented here, based on a pixel-by-pixel analysis of the progression of contrast medium through the total heart, allows the visualization of contrast medium within its myocardial phase. Although it has been demonstrated that the time of arrival of the contrast material to a certain region of the myocardium is inversely related to the regional blood flow, the parameter which best reflects the timing of the progression of the contrast medium needs still to be determined.

Our current clinical applications include the evaluation of the significance of coronary artery stenosis by comparing regional differences in myocardial contrast appearance time and time of maximum intensity between resting and hyperemic state after intravenous dipyridamole infusion. Our results tend to confirm data recently published by Vogel et al. [3, 14] on the evaluation of coronary reserve from digitized cinearteriograms. These results suggest that

224

such computerized analysis can provide useful clinical informations on relative regional coronary blood flow.

In a recent study [15], digitized coronary angiograms were analyzed at rest and during dipyridamole-induced hyperemia in 28 patients, 18 with coronary heart disease and 10 normals. Using a biharmonic Fourier fit, densograms were constructed in each pixel and the times of maximum upslope and of maximum density determined with a high temporal resolution. Regions of interest were manually selected over the left anterior descending and circumflex areas and defined as abnormal if they contained a > 70% stenotic artery. Means and standard errors of the times of maximum upslope and of maximum density were computed in each region of interest. The means and standard errors were used as indices of the synchrony of transit times within a region of interest. At rest, there were no differences between normal and abnormal regions of interest. During hyperemia the mean times of maximum upslope and of maximum density occurred significantly later in abnormal than in normal regions of interest; also, the means and standard errors were higher in abnormal than in normal regions of interest (times of maximum upslope means and standard errors: 0.78 ± 0.22 cycles versus 0.63 ± 0.24, $p < 0.05$; times of maximum density means and standard errors: 0.91 ± 0.33 versus 0.66 ± 0.26, $p < 0.005$), reflecting the inhomogeneity of contrast medium progression. This was visualized on color-coded parametric images. Thus, Fourier analysis of digitized coronary angiograms accurately assesses the delay and asynchrony of contrast medium progression within regions of interest containing > 70% stenoses, and thus may be useful for clinical determination of their hemodynamic significance.

Acknowledgments

This work was supported by a grant of the Swiss National Foundation for scientific research. The authors are grateful to Drs P. Chatelain, J.-P. Melchior and A. Righetti for their contributions, and M.M. J.-J. Adatte, J.-P. Bodenmann and J.-P. Killisch for their technical assistance. We thank Ms M. Turrian for her excellent secretarial performance.

References

1. Rutishauser W, Bussmann W, Noseda G, Meier W: Blood flow measurement through single coronary arteries by roentgen densitometry. I. A comparison of flow measured by a radiologic technic applicable in the intact organism and by electromagnetic flowmeter. Am J Roentgenol 1970; 109: 12–20.
2. Rutishauser W, Noseda G,Bussmann W, Preter B: Blood flow measurement through single

coronary arteries by roentgen densitometry. II. Right coronary artery flow in conscious man. Am J Roentgenol 1970; 109: 21–24.

3. Vogel RA, Mancini GBJ: Cardiac applications of digital radiography. Cardiol Clin 1985; 3: 3–17.

4. Haude M, Jehle J, Löss B, Pölitz B, Schmiel FK, Spiller P: Beurteilung der Myokard-perfusion anhand der mittels digitaler Subtraktionsangiokardiographie gemessenen Kontrastmittel-Einstromzeiten. Z Kardiol 1985; 74: 692–699.

5. Nissen SE, Elion JL, Booth DC, Evans J, DeMaria AN: Value and limitations of computer analysis of digital subtraction angiography in the assessment of coronary flow reserve. Circulation 1986; 73: 562–571.

6. Whiting JS, Drury JK, Pfaff JM, Chang BL, Eigler NL, Meerbaum S, Corday E, Nivatpumin T, Forrester JS, Swan HJC: Digital angiographic measurement of radiographic contrast material kinetics for estimation of myocardial perfusion. Circulation 1986; 73: 789–798.

7. Chappuis F, Ratib O, Meier B, Righetti A, Rutishauser W: Assessment of coronary flow reserve by digitized coronary angiograms at rest and after dipyridamol infusion (Abstract). J Am Coll Cardiol 1985; 5: 475.

8. Chappuis F, Ratib O, Meier B, Righetti A, Rutishauser W: Mesure de la perfusion myocardique régionale par analyse computérisée de coronarographies digitalisées. Schweiz Med Wschr 1985; 115: 1618–1621.

9. Ratib O, Chappuis F, Rutishauser W: Digital angiographic technique for the quantitative assessment of myocardial perfusion. Ann Radiol 1985; 28: 193–197.

10. Rutishauser W, Simon H, Stucky JP, Schaad N, Noseda G, Wellauer J: Evaluation of roentgen densitometry for flow measurement in models and in the intact circulation. Circulation 1967; 36: 951–963.

11. Widmann T, Moret P, Ritschard J, Donath A: Perfusion myocardique régionale dans les sténoses coronaires de divers degrés. Schweiz Med Wschr 1980; 110: 1666–1669.

12. Hoffmann JIE: Maximal coronary flow and the concept of coronary vascular reserve. Circulation 1984; 70: 153–159.

13. Bussmann W, Rutishauser W, Noseda G, Meier W, Preter B: Influence of a new contrast medium (metrizoate) on coronary blood flow. In: Heintzen PH (ed) Roentgen-, cine- and videodensitometrie. Proc 1st Int Conf on Roentgen-, cine- and videodensitometry; p 133. Thieme, Stuttgart, 1971.

14. Vogel R, LeFree M, Bates E: Application of digital techniques to selective coronary arteriography: Use of myocardial appearance time to measure coronary flow reserve. Am Heart J 1984; 107: 153–164.

15. Chappuis FP, Ratib O, Chatelain P, Meier B, Rutishauser W: Fourier analysis of digitized coronary angiograms: a new way to evaluate regional myocardial perfusion (Abstract). Circulation 1986; 74: II–486.

22. Comparison of Time Parameters Derived from Myocardial Time-Density Curves in Patients before and after Percutaneous Transluminal Coronary Angioplasty

T. VAN DER WERF[1], R.M. HEETHAAR[2], H. STEGEHUIS[2], N.H.J. PIJLS[1] & F.L. MEIJLER[2]

[1] Department of Cadiology, Catholic University, Nijmegen, The Netherlands, and [2] Departments of Cardiology and Medical Physics, State University, Utrecht, The Netherlands

Introduction

Much uncertainty exists about the pathophysiological significance of narrowings in the coronary arteries, especially those of moderate degree, as well as about the importance of diffuse coronary artery disease. Analysis of the contrast dynamics in the myocardium may provide pathophysiological information with which these problems can be solved or at least approached in a quantitative manner.

In a previous study [1] we demonstrated that digital coronary subtraction angiography can produce images of myocardial filling of high quality provided the correct triggering method has been applied. This method, called apparent cardiac arrest, comprises two special measures. First, heart rate is kept strictly regular by stimulating the right atrium with an external pacemaker via an electrode catheter. Secondly, heart rate is made synchronous with the X-ray frequency, which is effected by triggering the stimulator at its external input with the appropriately divided main's signal. These precautions are necessary to obviate mismatching of the mask image and the subsequent contrast images. Previously, we demonstrated that a mismatch of only 20 or 40 milliseconds may produce white areas in the subtracted images, caused by shifting, although no contrast had been injected in between [1].

The time-density curves obtained over the myocardium after injection of contrast material into a coronary artery resemble dye dilution curves. Until now these myocardial time-density curves can, however, not be treated like dye dilution curves to calculate absolute flow, because of uncertainty about
1. the injected quantity of contrast, caused by the backflow into the aorta,
2. the distribution of the injected quantity over normal and pathological areas, and
3. the volume of the vascular fraction of the myocardium.
On the other hand, time parameters can be calculated rather accurately.

P.H. Heintzen and J.H. Bürsch (eds), Progress in Digital Angiocardiography. ISBN 978-94-010-7093-5

Therefore, they form potential measures for relative myocardial perfusion in comparison to other areas or to other circumstances such as before and after a therapeutic procedure like percutaneous transluminal coronary angioplasty (PTCA).

A variety of time parameters has been suggested, as described in more detail in the Methods section. We applied five of these parameters to forty-four curves obtained over the myocardium in eleven patients before and after PTCA in order to evaluate their feasibility and discriminating power.

Methods and patients

Practical realization of the concept of apparent cardiac arrest

A strictly regular heart rate was obtained by stimulating the heart at a frequency slightly above sinus rhythm by means of an externally triggered stimulator connected with a pacing catheter positioned against the right atrial wall. The X-ray equipment produced 25 cine frames/s in synchrony with the frequency of the electric main alternating current (50 cycles/s in Europe). To achieve synchrony between X-ray film frames and heart rate, the stimulator is also triggered by the alternating electric current. Therefore, the main current's signal is fed into an electronic circuit that delivers a short pulse each time the main voltage exceeds a certain value, resulting in a sequence with 20 ms between subsequent pulses. Adequate selection (by division) of these pulses results in a pulse train that is fed into the external input of the stimulator leading to intervals that are multiples of 40 ms. Optical insulation units prevent the occurrence of leakage currents in accordance with international safety standards.

Patients

Ten patients, scheduled for left-sided percutaneous transluminal coronary angioplasty (PTCA), were studied, all but one having a single stenosis in the left anterior descending artery and a normal circumflex artery. One patient had two stenoses, one in the left anterior descending artery and one in a large diagonal branch; this patient was counted twice. In the first four patients the contrast medium was injected manually into the left main stem through a size 9 guiding catheter for PTCA. Thereafter, this protocol was changed in two ways. Contrast was injected with a power injector with a flow rate of 4 ml/s and a volume of 8 ml in order to standardize the injection technique. Furthermore, an especially for this purpose introduced size 8 Judkins catheter was used; it had been observed that a size 9 catheter could occlude the left main stem as was seen in two patients (not included in this paper) impeding contrast run-off. Sodium meglumine ioxaglate (Hexabrix^R) was used as contrast medium.

Catheterization procedure

The cineangiographic investigations were performed before as well as after the PTCA procedure. In most patients the same stimulation rate could be maintained in the cine-runs before and after the PTCA procedure. In four patients the rate after the PTCA procedure had to be set slightly higher. At the start of the dilation procedure, nifedipine (Adalat^R) was routinely administered sublingually. In some patients intracoronary nitroglycerine was given in case of a difficult crossing of the narrowing with the dilation catheter. The cine-run after the PTCA procedure was always performed after at least 10 minutes following the last contrast administration, obviating the vascular dilating effect of the contrast medium.

In all but one case the left anterior oblique projection (usually 50–60°) was chosen with a slight cranial angulation (about 20°). In one case a 30° right anterior oblique projection was chosen. The angiographic projections before and after PTCA were always identical. The angiographic investigations were performed with Siemens X-ray equipment using a focal spot size of 0.6 mm at about 70 KVp and a tube current of about 100 mA. The automatic brightness control was turned off. During the cine-run the ECG and the cine-puls signal were recorded. The Kodak film (2496 RAR) was developed with a gradient of about 1.65. All data used for this study were obtained during routine procedures with informed consent of the patient.

Subtraction procedure

In the laboratory, the film was analyzed in an off-line mode. It was placed on a spooler, equipped with a microprocessor-controlled motordrive. Following identification of the first frame, the desired frame number was touched in and the film automatically advanced to this particular frame. The video signals, obtained with a Vidicon high resolution camera with locked automatic light compensation, were connected to an image analysis system (VICOM). After analog-to-digital conversion, comparable non-contrast and contrast images were stored into memories I and II, respectively, with a spatial resolution of 512×512 pixels and 256 gray levels. Subtraction was performed and the results stored in memory III. For better visual inspection, the gray levels of the resulting images were amplified by a factor 4 or 8. After digital-to-analog conversion, the results could be displayed on a video monitor and stored on a video disk. Regions of interest were placed in subtracted images in which the mean pixel grayness was computed. For this study only end-diastolic frames were analyzed. The regions of interest were positioned over the left main stem, over a myocardial area of about 12×16 pixels in the region supplied by the narrowed and subsequently dilated vessel, the so-called ischemic area, and over an area supplied by the normal circumflex artery, the control area.

Analysis of the time-density curves

Time-density curves were obtained over the left main stem, the ischemic area and the control area in all patients before and after the PTCA procedure. The following time intervals were measured:

1. appearance time = the time from the start of the injection to the moment the curve reaches 5% of its top amount;
2. t_{max} = the maximum concentration time = the time from the start of the contrast injection to the moment the curve reaches the top amount;
3. t_{bu} = the build-up time = the difference between maximum concentration time and appearance time;
4. $\triangle t_{bu}$ = the difference in build-up times between the myocardial area of interest and the left main stem;
5. t_{mean} = the mean circulation time.

Estimation of coronary stenosis

The degree of coronary stenosis before and after PTCA was estimated by two experienced angiographers not belonging to our study group and unaware of the results of the calculations of the time parameters. The degree of stenosis was classified into the following categories:

1. less than 25% diameter narrowing;
2. 25–50% diameter narrowing;
3. 50–70% diameter narrowing;
4. 70–90% diameter narrowing;
5. subtotal stenosis.

These percentages thus refer to diameter narrowing as appreciated by inspecting the film on a Steenbeck professional viewer. We share the general scepticism about the accuracy of these estimates. Furthermore, it is highly improbable that stenoses of 90% or more of the diameter really do exist. Nevertheless, we performed this analysis to compare the results of the calculation of time parameters with customary clinical methods.

Statistical analysis

Statistical analysis was performed by calculating mean and standard deviation of the results obtained during certain conditions. It is questionable whether the observations in areas supplied by stenosed vessels may be considered as samples taken from a normally distributed population. Therefore, statistical analysis aimed at the comparison of certain conditions was performed with the Wilcoxon test for paired observations.

Results

The results for the different time parameters are summarized in Table 1 (mean ± SD). In Fig. 1 the results for the maximum concentration time are depicted also in a bar diagram. In case of the mean circulation time (t_{mean}) it appeared not to be possible to measure this parameter in all curves. In fact, it was only possible in about half the curves. This was caused by the fact that the curves remained on a high level or that they did not exhibit a semilogarithmic linear decay, because of which extrapolation of the first contrast passage was impossible.

Significant differences at the $p < 0.05$ and $p < 0.01$ level between the situation before and after PTCA were encountered only for the parameters t_{max} and $\triangle t_{bu}$.

Because for none of the time parameters, obtained over the control area, a significant difference between the pre- and post-PTCA value could be demonstrated, we also took these corresponding values for all patients together to establish a first approximation of 'normal values'.

In Fig. 2 the estimated degree of coronary diameter narrowing is compared to t_{max}. The points all the way to the left represent the maximum concentration

Table 1. Time parameters derived from myocardial time-density curves in 11 patients. Values in seconds (mean ± SD).

	Ischemic area		Control area		
	Before PTCA	After PTCA	Before PTCA	After PTCA	Before + after (n = 22)
t_{app}	1.1 ± 0.5	0.7 ± 0.5	0.7 ± 0.4	0.8 ± 0.5	0.8 ± 0.4
t_{max}	7.1 ± 1.8	4.4 ± 0.8[a]	4.6 ± 0.9	4.4 ± 0.8	4.5 ± 0.9
t_{bu}	6.0 ± 2.2	3.8 ± 0.7	3.9 ± 1.0	3.7 ± 0.9	3.8 ± 1.0
$\triangle t_{bu}$	3.9 ± 2.6	2.0 ± 1.1[b]	1.7 ± 1.2	2.0 ± 1.2	1.8 ± 1.2
t_{mean}	8.0 ± 0.9[c]	5.0 ± 1.3[c]	5.1 ± 0.8[d]	5.4 ± 1.1[c]	5.2 ± 0.9[e]

[a] $p < 0.01$
[b] $p < 0.05$
[c] only n = 5
[d] only n = 8
[e] only n = 13

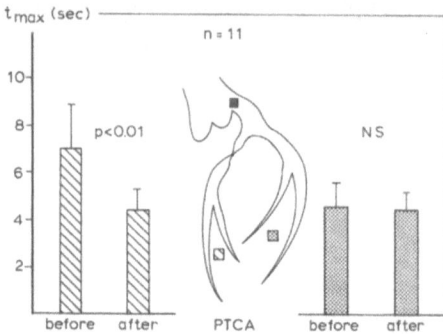

Fig. 1. t_{max} before and after PTCA in ischemic and control areas. The drawing of the coronary system indicates the position of the narrowing necessitating the PTCA procedure. Furthermore the position of the regions of interest are indicated. The bars to the left represent mean ± SD of t_{max} before and after the PTCA procedure in the ischemic area. The bars to the right indicate these respective values obtained over the control area. (NS = not significant.)

time in the control area from which results the normal range was assessed (mean ± 2 SD). The points between 0% diameter narrowing and subtotal stenosis are pooled data from pre- and post-PTCA results. Up till stenoses not exceeding 70% diameter narrowing the maximum circulation times remain within the normal range. In the category 70–90% diameter narrowing all but one determinations are in the higher normal limits; one is prolonged. All but one values found over the myocardium distal from a subtotal stenosis, on the

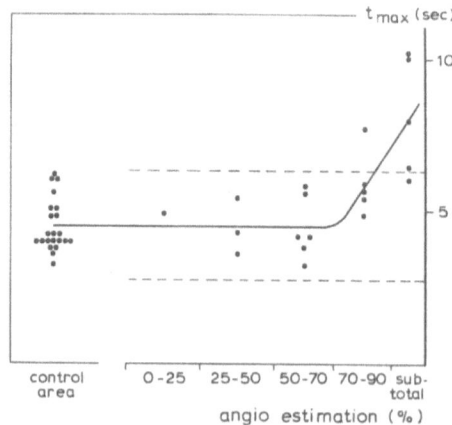

Fig. 2. t_{max} and estimated degree of stenosis. Maximum concentration time (t_{max}) of time-density curves over a myocardial region of interest as a function of percentage diameter narrowing of the coronary artery supplying that region. The values to the left belong to 'normal' coronary arteries (see discussion). The dotted lines represent mean ± two times SD of these normal values. The solid line connects the mean values per category stenosis.

contrary, are prolonged. The mutual differences in this category are, however, strikingly large.

Discussion

In our opinion it is necessary to take precautions for exact matching of mask and contrast images. Simply selecting images near to the QRS-complex is insufficient because heart rate is never strictly regular and because of the asynchrony between heart rate and exposure rate. Each variance in RR-interval affects myocardial contractility and therefore the similarity of myocardial images [2]. To obviate these problems we developed the concept of apparent cardiac arrest resulting in subtracted images with a very high signal-to-noise ratio.

In this way we could obtain time-density curves over the myocardium, in many instances resembling dye dilution curves. Before these time-density curves can be treated in a quantitative manner as usual for dye dilution a number of fundamental problems have, however, to be solved.

The theory of dye dilution technique presupposes constancy of flow during the period from injection till the end of sampling. In case of injection of X-ray contrast material into a coronary artery flow increases considerably (after an initial decrease). Furthermore, important differences between reactions of normal parts of the coronary tree and parts distal of tight stenoses may be expected.

A second fundamental problem is the impossibility to calibrate the vertical axis of the curves. Supposing the law of Lambert-Beer to be applicable, the vertical axis shows a quantity of iodine. This quantity is the product of concentration and the vascular volume studied, supposing that the contrast does remain intravascularly as in a one-compartment model. As mentioned in our results only about half of the curves had a descending limb that showed the characteristic behaviour of a linear relation between time and the logarithm of the iodine quantity. Therefore, our research is now oriented towards finding a contrast agent that does not produce a hyperemic response and towards calibration of the density axis.

Being aware of the problem in considering time-density curves as dye dilution curves, the question remains which time parameters are most suitable to derive the desired information from these curves. A variety of time parameters has been suggested. Vogel [3] measured the 'appearance' time, which is the time from the start of the injection to the moment at which the curve reaches 10% of the peak value. Note that in dye dilution appearance time means the time at which the first amount of dye appears at the measuring site. This value of 10% was used by the authors because of baseline noise. Spiller et

234

al. [4] measured the time from injection to halfway the top of the curve. They called this parameter $T_{1/2}$ (see below). Rutishauser [5] measured the time from injection to the moment of the steepest slope of the ascending limb. The use of the maximum concentration time is inherited from dye dilution techniques. The build-up time is the time from appearance to the maximum of the curve. Bürsch [6] calculated the difference in build-up time over a vascular bed. The difference in mean transit time between two measuring areas over a non-branching vascular segment, like in dye dilution, was used by Rutishauser et al. [7] and Smith et al. [8]. Ikeda et al. [9] introduced recently the contrast disappearance half-life time, also abbreviated as $T_{1/2}$. With this measure they mean the time from the start of the injection to the moment the downward slope of the curve reaches a level, half the maximum amount.

Of the time parameters, calculated here, only the maximum concentration time and the difference in build-up times over the vascular bed under study showed significant differences between the situation before and after the successful PTCA procedure. Significance was also expected for the mean circulation time but this parameter could not be evaluated in a sufficient number of patients.

A note must be made to the right most column of Table 1 and to the horizontal broken lines in Fig. 2. These numbers and lines suggest 'normal' values. These measurements were, however, performed over the myocardium, supplied by so-called normal vessels in patients with signs of coronary atherosclerosis. It is questionable whether these 'normal' vessels are indeed normal.

The relation between the estimated degree of narrowing of the coronary arteries before and after PTCA and the maximum concentration time is at least not in contradiction with established pathophysiologic data [10]. Only very severe narrowings produce delayed circulation times. Poisseuille's law, however, predicts that the human eye (and brain) must be unable to make a further differentiation in the domain of very severe narrowings.

Our results suggest that the study of time-density curves might produce the possibility to make further pathophysiologic differentiations in case of severe narrowings.

In the opening of this article it was stated that uncertainty exists about the pathophysiological importance of narrowings in the coronary arteries, especially those of moderate degree. Our results indicate that in order to disclose the impact of stenoses of *moderate degree* an intervention procedure necessarily must be applied.

Summary

Computer-aided densitometry was applied to subtraction images of digitized coronary arteriograms. Heart rate was in synchrony with cine frequency by main's triggered right atrial stimulation. Eleven candidates for PTCA were studied after injection of 8 ml Ioxaglate in 2 s into the left main stem (LMS). Mean grayness was determined in regions of interest over the LMS, the myocardium supplied by the stenosed vessel (ischemic area) and the normal vessel (control area) in end-diastolic frames, acquired during 15 s before and after the PTCA procedure. From the time-density curves obtained in this way the maximum concentration time (t_{max}) and the differences in build-up time between the myocardium and the LMS ($\triangle t_{bu}$) were calculated. Both parameters showed the expected improvement of myocardial perfusion by PTCA to values similar to those obtained over control areas. Computerized densitometry of subtraction images of digitized coronary arteriograms makes quantitative analysis of parameters related to myocardial perfusion possible.

Acknowledgments

The authors wish to thank P.W. Westerhof, M.D., and B.T.J. Meursing, M.D., for estimating the stenoses and Miss Tanja van den Heuvel for the preparation of the manuscript.

References

1. Werf T van der, Heethaar RM, Stegehuis H, Meijler FL: The concept of apparent cardiac arrest as a prerequisite for coronary digital subtraction angiography. JACC 1984; 4: 239–244.
2. Meijler FL, Kuyer PJP, Dam-Koopman I van, Heethaar RM, Werf T van der: The clinical relevance of postextrasystolic potentation. Mayo Clinic Proc 1982; 57(Suppl): 34–40.
3. Vogel RA: The radiographic assessment of coronary blood flow parameters. Circulation 1985; 72: 460–465.
4. Spiller P, Schmiel FK, Pölitz B, Block M, Fermon U et al.: Measurements of systolic and diastolic flow rates in the coronary artery system by X-ray densitometry. Circulation 1983; 68: 337–347.
5. Rutishauser W, Ratib O, Chappuis F, Doriot P-A, Meier B: Coronary blood flow and myocardial perfusion studied by digitized coronary angiograms. In this volume.
6. Bürsch JH: Use of digitized functional angiography to evaluate arterial blood flow. Cardiovasc Intervent Radiol 1983; 6: 303–310.
7. Rutishauser W, Noseda G, Bussman WD, Preter B: Blood flow measurement through single coronary arteries by Röntgen densitometry. Am J Roentgenol 1970; 109: 21–24.
8. Smith HC, Sturm RE, Wood EH: Videodensitometric system for measurement of vessel blood flow, particularly in the coronary arteries in man. Am J Cardiol 1973; 32: 144–150.
9. Ikeda H, Koga Y, Utsu F, Toshima H: Quantitative evaluation of regional myocardial blood

flow by videodensitometric analysis of digital subtraction coronary arteriography in humans. JACC 1986; 8: 809–816.

10. Gould KL, Lipscomb K, Hamilton GW: Physiologic basis for assessing critical coronary stenosis. Instantaneous flow response and regional distribution during coronary hyperemia as measures of coronary flow reserve. Am J Cardiol 1974; 33: 87–94.

23. Methods for Calculation of Coronary Flow Reserve by Computer Processing of Digital Angiograms

STEVEN E. NISSEN, JONATHAN L. ELION &
ANTHONY N. DEMARIA
Division of Cardiology, Department of Medicine, University of Kentucky College of Medicine, Lexington, KY, USA

Coronary arteriography is widely utilized to assess the severity of coronary artery disease (CAD) and to guide therapy in patients with coronary obstructions. However, the accuracy of conventional arteriography in accurately depicting the severity of CAD has been seriously questioned [1]. There is significant intra- and interobserver variability in the interpretation of coronary angiograms and several pathological studies have demonstrated that angiographic estimates of coronary obstruction do not necessarily correspond to subsequent pathological examination [2, 3].

Traditionally, the severity of a stenosis is reported as per cent reduction in luminal area. However, this measure is significantly influenced by overlapping of vessels, collateral blood flow, and angle of view [4, 5]. Furthermore, many patients with coronary artery disease have diffuse vessel involvement with focal stenoses superimposed upon a generalized narrowing. In this setting, per cent luminal area reduction cannot accurately reflect the severity of the disease [1].

Even when conventional coronary arteriography is accurate in classifying the severity of stenoses, arteriography provides no data regarding functional consequences of stenoses. Furthermore, there is a non-linear relationship between per cent luminal reduction and functional impairment which further complicates accurate visual interpretations of films [6].

In contrast to the limitations inherent in arteriography, coronary flow reserve has been shown to be an excellent descriptor of functional impairment secondary to epicardial coronary obstructive lesions [6, 7]. Coronary flow reserve has traditionally been measured by determination of coronary reactive hyperemia defined as the increase in blood flow produced following temporary coronary occlusion. Such methods require operative coronary exposure and are thus not suitable for application in man except during cardiac surgery. Therefore, other methods of evaluating coronary reserve have been sought.

Several groups have recently attempted to measure coronary flow or flow reserve by computer processing of contrast coronary angiograms. The ob-

P.H. Heintzen and J.H. Bürsch (eds), Progress in Digital Angiocardiography. ISBN 978-94-010-7093-5

jective of these efforts has been to develop a reliable method whereby the physiological consequences of coronary lesions could be determined in man. Three distinct approaches to coronary flow analysis have been presented in the literature to date. These approaches have been based upon

1. the measurement of coronary transit-time,
2. the calculation of myocardial contrast washout,
3. the application of indicator dilution principles to intracoronary contrast injection.

Each of these three approaches has inherent methodological assumptions and individual limitations. We have evaluated these methods in an animal model of CAD with the intention of evaluating the strengths and limitations of the various approaches. Specifically, we have sought to validate the accuracy of digital angiographic methods to detect and quantify reductions in coronary flow reserve secondary to artificial stenoses of varying magnitude produced in open-chest dogs.

Concept of coronary flow reserve

Because of the limitations of conventional angiography in accurately identifying physiologically insignificant coronary stenoses, digital angiographic methods have focused on measurement of coronary flow reserve. It is well established that coronary reactive hyperemia – that is the increase in blood flow following a vasodilator stimulus – is significantly blunted in the presence of epicardial CAD [6]. Thus, reactive hyperemic flow is diminished from $4 - 7 : 1$ under control conditions to $1 : 1$ in the presence of a critical stenosis. Measurement of resting coronary flow is not a sensitive indicator of the severity of stenoses since only very severe lesions ($> 90\%$) will reduce resting flow.

For investigative and clinical purposes, reactive hyperemia can be induced not only by temporary coronary occlusion but also by administration of vasodilator drugs, including papaverine, dipyridamole or iodinated contrast. Computer methods for assessing coronary flow reserve from coronary angiography have attempted to measure reactive hyperemia from images obtained before and after one of these interventions.

Physiological basis for computer methods

Coronary transit-time

Techniques based upon the measurement of coronary transit-time were the first methods proposed for assessment of coronary flow or flow reserve by

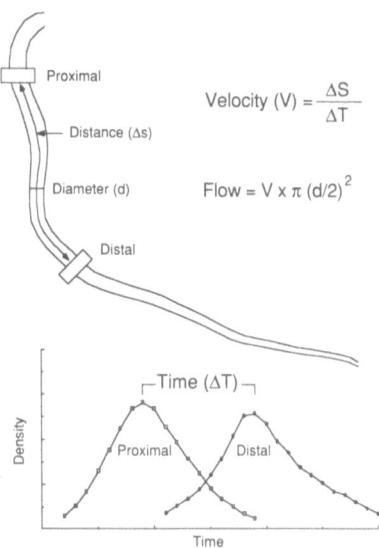

Velocity $(V) = \dfrac{\Delta S}{\Delta T}$

Flow $= V \times \pi \, (d/2)^2$

Fig. 1. Schematic illustration of the scientific basis for calculation of coronary flow from the transit time. The time Δ T for passage of a contrast bolus from a proximal to a distal coronary region of interest is measured. The velocity (V) and flow (F) can be calculated from the distance Δ S between the regions of interest and the diameter of the coronary.

angiography. Rutishauser et al. in Switzerland and Wood et al. in Rochester, Minnesota, demonstrated that simultaneous measurement of contrast intensity curves at two sites in the coronary circulation could be utilized to measure transit-time [8–14]. If the distance between two sites is known then mean coronary flow velocity can be calculated as distance divided by transit-time. If mean cross-sectional area of the coronary is also measured, then a mean coronary flow can be calculated as the product of mean velocity and mean cross-sectional area. This method has been shown to correlate closely with electromagnetic measurement of coronary blood flow in both an animal model and in man [8–14]. The scientific basis for the transit-time method is schematically illustrated in Fig. 1.

Recently, Vogel et al. have re-introduced the transit-time approach [15–16]. However, the approach of Vogel and co-workers differs fundamentally in many respects from the earlier attempts at transit-time analysis. Using digital angiography, rather than film, they measure the 'myocardial contrast appearance time', which is defined as the time from contrast injection until opacification of myocardium. Contrast administration and image acquisition are ECG-triggered so that appearance time is measured in units of cardiac cycles. The method has been further refined by its proponents to calculate an index of coronary flow based upon two factors, the appearance time of contrast and the

240

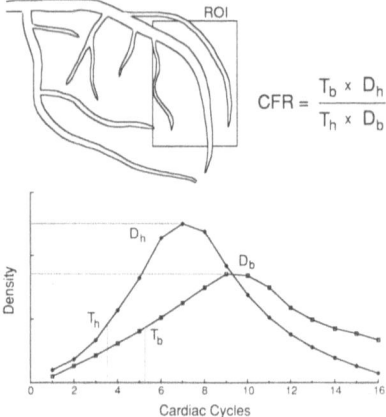

$$CFR = \frac{T_b \times D_h}{T_h \times D_b}$$

Fig. 2. Calculation of myocardial contrast appearance time. The time intensity values for a large region of interest are measured and the coronary flow reserve calculated as shown. CFR = coronary flow reserve, T_b = time from injection until 10% of peak density under basal conditions, T_h = time to 10% maximal for hyperemic conditions. D_h and D_b represent maximal density under hyperemic and basal conditions respectively.

peak opacification achieved in the myocardium. This contrast appearance time index thus reflects both transit-time and volume of distribution of contrast. A schematic illustration of the contrast appearance method is shown in Fig. 2.

Unlike the earlier transit-time approach, the myocardial appearance time method seeks to calculate not total coronary blood flow but rather coronary flow reserve. This calculation is accomplished by comparing the contrast appearance time under two conditions, the basal state and following induction of coronary reactive hyperemia with contrast dye or intracoronary papaverine. In experimental animals, the index of myocardial contrast appearance has been shown to correlate with coronary flow reserve measured by electromagnetic flow probe. The method has also been extensively investigated in man.

Myocardial contrast washout

A second method proposed for calculation of coronary flow reserve is based upon the measurement of contrast washout. This method is possible using digital subtraction angiography because the subtraction process enhances visualization of the myocardial phase of contrast dye clearance. Several groups have proposed that the disappearance rate of myocardial contrast following digital coronary arteriography could be utilized to calculate coronary flow reserve [17–19]. This method generally assumes that contrast dye behaves as a

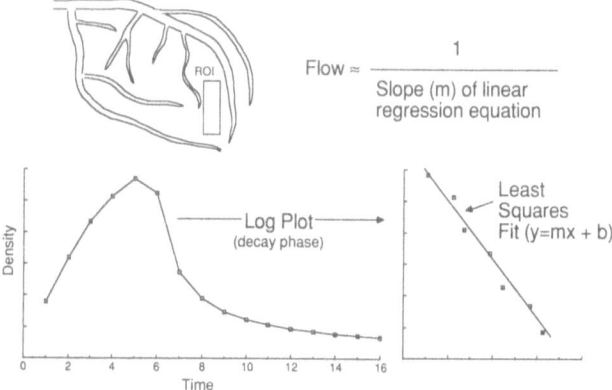

$$\text{Flow} \approx \frac{1}{\text{Slope (m) of linear regression equation}}$$

Fig. 3. Measurement of coronary flow from the washout phase of myocardial contrast. The decay phase is assumed to be mono-exponential and is plotted on a logarithmic scale. A linear regression least squares fit is determined for the decay phase. Flow is proportional to the inverse of the slope (m) of the regression equation.

typical tracer substance with a mono-exponential decay function representing its disappearance phase from the myocardium. The method of analysis assumes that the disappearance rate of contrast from the myocardium will be increased under conditions of hyperemia. Presumably this increase in contrast washout rate under hyperemic conditions would be attenuated in the presence of physiologically significant stenosis. The scientific basis for this method of analysis is schematically illustrated in Fig. 3.

Indicator-dilution analysis

Another method for analysis of coronary reserve from digital angiograms is based upon the principles of indicator-dilution techniques. In this case, the indicator is radiographic contrast medium. Indicator-dilution theory utilizes the equations of Stewart and Hamilton which have been widely applied to other indicators (such as indocyanine green) or iced saline in thermodilution cardiac output determination. Indicator-dilution theory predicts that the area under a contrast time curve will be directly proportional to the quantity of contrast injected and inversely proportional to the flow. If the same quantity of contrast is administered under basal and hyperemic states and if the region of interest analyzed is unchanged, then the inverse ratio of the area under the two time-intensity curves will reflect coronary flow reserve. This method is schematically illustrated in Fig. 4. The indicator-dilution method was applied by Forester et al. [20] and has been subsequently evaluated by our group in an animal model of coronary artery disease [21].

242

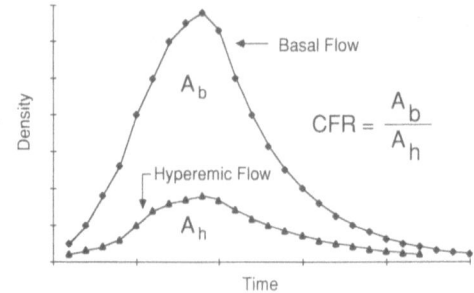

Fig. 4. Calculation of coronary flow reserve from indicator-dilution curves. Coronary flow reserve is equal to the ratio of the area under a time density curve for a coronary region of interest obtained under basal conditions (A_b) divided by the area of the curve of an identical region of interest obtained under hyperemic flow conditions (A_h). CFR = coronary flow reserve.

Study design

Experimental protocol

To determine the value and limitations of each of the three proposed methods for assessment of coronary hyperemia, we investigated each method in an animal model of coronary artery disease. Nine dogs were instrumented with an electromagnetic flow probe and two pneumatic occluders placed on the circumflex coronary artery. One occluder was used to create a variable stenosis and the other to produce temporary coronary occlusion as a stimulus for reactive hyperemia. The animal was paced via an epicardial needle electrode at 10 beats/minute greater than the resting heart rate. A 5 French catheter was subselectively placed in the circumflex coronary artery from the right carotid artery. The coronary electromagnetic flow signal, arterial pressure, and electrocardiogram were continuously monitored on a multichannel physiological recorder.

Imaging procedure

Digital subtraction fluoroscopy was performed following ECG-gated power injection of radiographic contrast. The quantity of contrast injected was adjusted until the maximum dose was determined that did not result of reflux of contrast into the left anterior descending coronary artery. This was typically from 2–3 ml over 2 seconds. Fluoroscopic images underwent real-time analog-to-digital conversion into a 256 × 256 pixel matrix with 256 shades of gray (8 bits). Each image underwent logarithmic transformation prior to mask mode subtraction. Although 30 frames/second were acquired, only the end-diastolic

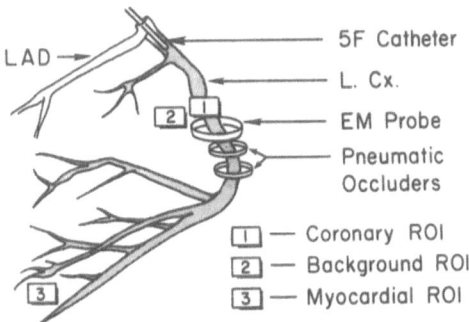

Fig. 5. Location of instrumentation and regions of interest curves in the animal model of coronary disease. ROI = region of interest, LAD = left anterior descending coronary artery, EM = electromagnetic. L. Cx. = left circumflex.

images were analyzed in a dedicated image analysis computer (Kontron Electronik, Munich, FRG).

ECG-triggered power injection was performed under basal conditions and following induction of hyperemia by total obstruction of coronary flow for 15 seconds. Subsequently, partial coronary stenoses were produced by inflating the second pneumatic occluder positioned on the circumflex. For each level of stenosis, hyperemia was produced by total obstruction of the coronary for 15 seconds and imaging sequence performed under both the basal and hyperemic state.

Image analysis

Analysis of digital coronary angiograms was performed with a computer program that allowed the operator to select regions of interest, rectangular in shape, that could be varied in size. For each region of interest, summated pixel values for each end-diastolic frame were measured so as to generate a time-intensity curve. Three regions of interest (ROI) were analyzed with ROI-1 positioned over the proximal left circumflex coronary artery, ROI-2 outside the vessel just adjacent to ROI-1, and ROI-3 over the myocardium perfused by the left circumflex coronary artery (Fig. 5).

Two families of time-intensity curves for these regions of interest were produced by plotting summated intensity vs. time. In one set of curves, the summated intensity values were plotted for the proximal coronary region of interest (ROI-1) minus the summated gray values for the background (ROI-2). The subtraction of values for ROI-2 served as a method to correct for the contribution of myocardial opacification to the summated gray values in the coronary region of interest. A second family of curves was generated from the single myocardial region of interest (ROI-3). These curves represented the summated pixel values for ROI-3 minus the value obtained from the first end-diastolic frame of each injection for this same region. Thus, these latter curves reflect the incremental changes in intensity for the myocardial region of interest referable to the first cardiac cycle.

Data analysis

For each pair of injections, the mean electromagnetic coronary blood flow under hyperemic conditions were divided by the mean flow under basal conditions to obtain an index of coronary reserve capacity. A similar index of coronary reserve was calculated for each of the three computer methods described previously. Thus, for the myocardial region of interest, the ratio of time-to-peak myocardial opacification was compared under basal and hyperemic conditions and similarly, myocardial contrast disappearance rate was determined under both basal and hyperemic flow states. For the background-corrected proximal coronary region of interest, an index of coronary reserve was obtained by dividing the area of the basal time-intensity curve by the area under the curve during hyperemic flow conditions. The coronary flow reserve ratios calculated from electromagnetic flow were compared by linear regression analysis to values obtained by computer analysis of the digital images.

Results

In the nine dogs, 76 coronary injections were performed for 38 separate stenoses. The ratio of hyperemic-to-basal coronary flow by EMF for these injections ranged from $0.8:1$ to $4.2:1$.

Appearance time

For the myocardial region of interest, hyperemic-to-basal flow ratios derived from the time-to-peak myocardial opacification exhibited a smaller range than ratios derived from EMF, varying from a low of $0.95:1$ to a high of $1.8:1$ (Fig. 6). When linear regression analysis was performed, the ratio of measurements of resting and hyperemic flow derived from the time-to-peak myocardial opacification correlated moderately well with EMF flow ratios ($r = 0.68$), but with a slope much less than unity ($y = 0.16x + 0.97$).

RESERVE RATIO: TIME TO PEAK CONTRAST

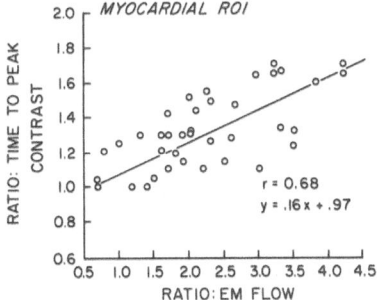

Fig. 6. Results of linear regression analysis comparing coronary flow reserve determined by electromagnetic probe with flow reserve calculated from the time-to-peak opacification of a myocardial region of interest.

Contrast washout

Comparison of EMF to coronary flow reserve ratios calculated from myocardial contrast washout is shown in Fig. 7. The correlation between resting hyperemic flow ratios derived from contrast decay rate compared to those obtained by EMF was poor ($r = 0.34$). Thus, the change in the disappearance rate of contrast for a myocardial region of interest was not closely related to the extent of hyperemia recorded by EMF in this animal model of coronary artery disease.

RESERVE RATIO: CONTRAST WASHOUT RATE

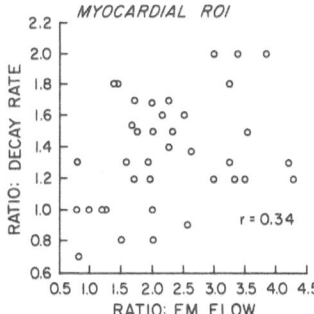

Fig. 7. Results of linear regression analysis comparing coronary flow reserve obtained by the electromagnetic probe with coronary reserve calculated from the contrast decay rate for a myocardial region of interest.

246

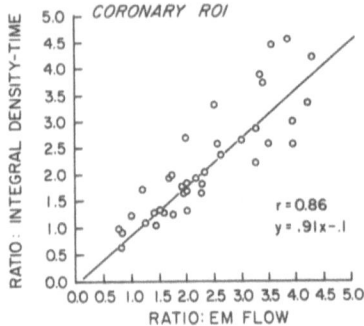

RESERVE RATIO: DENSITY-TIME INTEGRAL

Fig. 8. Linear regression analysis comparing coronary flow reserve determined from an electromagnetic probe with flow reserve calculated from the integral of the density-time curve for a coronary region of interest.

Indicator-dilution analysis

For the coronary region of interest, the flow ratios calculated from the area under the time-intensity curves derived from digital angiography yielded values that varied from 0.9 : 1 to 4.5 : 1. Thus, the ratios of area measurements derived from background-corrected proximal coronary curves (ROI-1 minus ROI-2) were similar in magnitude to those obtained by EMF. Further, linear regression analysis revealed a close relationship between indices of coronary reserve calculated by this method and those obtained by electromagnetic flow probe measurements, with a correlation coefficient of r = 0.86.

Discussion

Conventional assessment of luminal narrowing from film-based angiography has major limitations in assessing the severity of coronary stenoses and provides virtually no information regarding the physiological consequences of coronary lesions. However, coronary reactive hyperemia is an excellent physiological descriptor of coronary reserve capacity. Computer analysis of digital angiography offers the potential to calculate coronary flow reserve from angiographic coronary images, and thereby to accurately evaluate coronary reserve capacity in the setting of coronary obstructive disease.

The three major approaches to assessing coronary reserve from angiography have consisted of:
1. coronary transit-time measurement,

2. myocardial contrast washout decay rate,

3. indicator-dilution analysis.

Each of the methods has a physiologic basis, relies upon inherent scientific assumptions, and has characteristic limitations.

Transit-time measurements such as those introduced by Rutishauser, Wood, and colleagues were the first methods utilized to measure coronary flow by angiography. This method is based upon measurement of the time for a contrast bolus to progress between two points in the coronary separated by a distance, $\triangle$ S. (Fig. 1). However, because of the serpiginous nature of the coronary circulation with many curves in three dimensions, the distance between sampling points cannot be easily determined even with biplane angiography. This uncertainty has limited application of the transit-time technique for coronary vessels. A further limitation is the need for a very high temporal resolution, since the transit of contrast dye in the coronaries can take place within a single cardiac cycle, particularly during induced hyperemia. Ideally, 90 or more frames/second would be optimal for transit-time measurement. Furthermore, coronary arteries differ from a straight wall pipe in that the cross-sectional area is constantly changing from proximal to distal vessel. Side branches represent another confounding variable in transit-time analysis which are frequently encountered in the coronary circulation.

Because of these inherent limitations, Vogel et al. introduced a simpler method for transit-time calculation. This method, termed 'myocardial contrast appearance time', measures the transit-time from contrast injection until myocardial opacification. Typically, myocardial opacification is defined as the time at which 10% of maximal myocardial summated pixel gray value is achieved. In studies done in our laboratory, this simple index of contrast appearance correlated moderately with flow reserve ratios calculated by the electromagnetic flow method. The contrast appearance time analysis assumes that coronary cross-sectional area is constant under both basal and hyperemic conditions and therefore that appearance time is proportional to both velocity and volumetric flow. It is likely that this assumption is not completely accurate, since the induction of hyperemia should be expected to augment the cross-sectional area of coronary resistance vessels.

To overcome this limitation, the proponents of the contrast appearance time method have recently modified the technique so that the myocardial contrast appearance time is divided by the maximal myocardial pixel gray value to obtain a new index of coronary flow reserve. This approach is schematically illustrated in Fig. 2. Utilizing the corrected appearance time, Vogel [22] has reported close correlation between electromagnetic flow reserve and the computer method.

Several assumptions and limitations are also inherent in the contrast appearance method. The technique relies upon total replacement of coronary blood with contrast medium. Thus, very large and rapid injections are required which must be performed with a power injector. At the high levels of flow required, the potential for coronary injury is enhanced. Furthermore, complete replacement of coronary blood with contrast medium may not be possible under maximal hyperemic conditions. Maximal contrast flow rates may augment the hemodynamic consequences of contrast injection, including bradycardia and hypotension. In addition, the method is quite sensitive to misregistration artifact. Well-registered mask-mode subtraction, a requisite condition for accurate appearance time calculation, can be performed only if the patient does not breathe or move.

The spatial distribution of flow reserve represents another confounding variable to appearance time analysis. The contrast appearance method utilizes large regions of interest encompassing both segments of myocardium and epicardial vessels. It is not always clear from myocardial images which areas are supplied by the circumflex and which areas are supplied by the left anterior descending coronary. Collateral vessels may further confuse the observer since they represent flow that is often out of phase with normal antegrade flow.

The disappearance rate of contrast from the myocardial region of interest has not correlated closely with EMF flow reserve in our experimental studies ($r = 0.34$). Several requisite assumptions which result in major limitations in this method are apparent. Radiographic contrast is not inert but is capable of inducing an intense hyperemic response. Thus, attempts to measure contrast disappearance rate are strongly influenced by the presence of contrast medium which augments its own decay rate even in the absence of other stimuli for hyperemia. Furthermore, the washout phase for myocardial contrast is quite prolonged, with a half-life as long as 10 seconds. Thus, patients would be required to hold their breath for 20 to 30 seconds during the imaging procedure in order to maintain good registration. This may be realistic in only a small fraction of patients.

The shape of the decay curve for myocardial contrast does not appear to be mono-exponential. This likely represents the non-steady state nature of coronary flow during the washout phase secondary to the influence of contrast-induced hyperemia. Finally, there may be some tissue iodine accumulation in the myocardium which represents an additional confounding variable since it is unaccounted for by traditional tracer theory. This latter situation is supported by the fact that myocardial contrast effect is present even after all of the dye should have cleared the capillary circulation.

In the animal experimental model, analysis of digital angiograms based upon the principles of indicator-dilution techniques was the most successful technique for assessing coronary reserve which we encountered. There are several assumptions inherent in the application of indicator-dilution analysis to contrast angiography. First, the brightness of an individual pixel must be proportional to the quantity of contrast presence. Since X-ray attenuation is exponential, a logarithmic transformation is necessary. A second requirement for using radiographic contrast in dye dilution analysis is that all the contrast medium must pass through the vessel to be analyzed. This requires careful adjustment of dosing and injection. Another requirement is that complete mixing of the contrast agent with blood takes place proximal to the region of interest.

A further methodological problem was presented by the assumption that contrast injected in the coronary vessel was the sole source of opacification within the region of interest during the period of analysis. Because injection of contrast in the epicardial vessel ultimately results in myocardial opacification, it was necessary to subtract the contrast density for an adjacent myocardial region of interest from the coronary region of interest values.

Despite these limitations, when carefully applied in the animal model, indices of coronary reserve derived by the indicator-dilution method correlated closely with those obtained by the electromagnetic flow probe ($r = 0.86$). There are several significant advantages to estimation of coronary reserve by analysis of area under a time-density curve derived from a coronary region of interest. Since the transit-time is short, an imaging sequence of only 6–8 seconds rather than 15 seconds is required for analysis of myocardial contrast appearance and disappearance. Thus, if applied in a clinical setting a shorter duration of motion-free imaging would be required with shorter periods of breath holding. Furthermore, since the curves are derived from multiple measurements, the effect of artifact in a single frame is minimized. Thus the area under a time-intensity curve can be accurately described even with low tempral resolution during image acquisition.

Several practical problems require consideration with regard to their clinical application of each of the three angiographic methods, for the assessment of coronary flow reserve in man. Digital subtraction requires precise registration of images over many cardiac cycles and therefore would be unsuitable in patients with atrial fibrillation or other arrhythmias. In addition, misregistration artifact secondary to respiratory motion represents a major limitation. For each of the three methods, power injection of dye in the coronaries is probably necessary to prevent variability secondary to the rate and volume of contrast injected by hand. It is likely that some clinical practitioners would consider power injections unacceptable.

Despite the limitations noted for each of the three methods, digital angiography holds great promise in the calculation of coronary flow reserve in man. Given the inherent limitations of anatomic coronary imaging in the assessment of the severity of coronary stenoses, it is likely that computer-based DSA methods will be increasingly utilized in the future.

References

1. White CW, Wright CB, Doty DB, Hiratzka LF, Eastham CL, Harrison DG, Marcus ML: Does visual interpretation of the coronary angiograms predict the physiologic importance of a coronary stenosis? N Engl J Med 1984; 310: 819.

2. Lesperance J: Discrepancies between cineangiographic and post-mortem findings in patients with coronary artery disease and recent myocardial revascularization. Circulation 1974; 49: 703.

3. Gray CR, Hoffman HA, Hammond WS, Miller KL, Oseashon RO: Correlation of arteriographic and pathologic findings in the coronary arteries in man. Circulation 1962; 26: 497.

4. Levin DC, Baltaxe HA, Sos TA: Potential sources of error in coronary arteriography. II. Interpretation of the study. Am J Roentgenol 1975; 124: 386.

5. Zir LM, Miller SW, Dinsmore RE, Gilbert JP, Hawthorne JW: Interobserver variability in coronary angiography. Circulation 1976; 53: 627.

6. Gould KL, Lipscomb K: Effects of coronary stenoses on coronary flow reserve and resistance. Am J Cardiol 1974; 34: 48.

7. Gould KL, Lipscomb K, Hamilton GW: Physiologic basis for assessing critical coronary stenosis, instantaneous flow response and regional distribution during coronary hyperemia as measures of coronary flow reserve. Am J Cardiol 1974; 33: 87.

8. Rutishauser W, Bussmann WD, Noseda G, Meier W, Wellauer J: Blood flow measurement through single coronary arteries by roentgen densitometry. I. A comparison of flow measured by a radiologic technique applicable in the intact organism and by electromagnetic flow meter. Am J Roentgenol 1970; 109: 12.

9 Rutishauser W, Noseda G, Bussmann WD, Preter B: Blood flow measurement through single coronary arteries by Roentgen densitometry. II. Right coronary artery flow in conscious man. Am J Roentgenol 1970; 109: 21.

10. Rutishauser W: Application of roentgendensitometry to blood flow measurement in models, animals and in intact conscious man. In: Heintzen PH (ed) Roentgen-, cine- and videodensitometry; pp 108–118. Georg Thieme, Stuttgart, 1971.

11. Smith HC, Frye RL, Donald DE, Davis GD, Pluth JR, Sturm RE, Wood EH: Roentgen videodensitometric measure of coronary blood flow: determination from simultaneous indicator-dilution curve at selected sites in the coronary circulation and in coronary artery-saphenous vein grafts. Mayo Clinic Proc 1971; 46: 800.

12. Smith HC, Sturm RE, Wood EF: Videodensitometric system for measurement of vessel blood flow, particularly in the coronary arteries in man. Am J Cardiol 1973; 32: 144.

13. Smith HC, Frye RL, Davis GD, Pluth JR, Sturm RE, Wood EF: Simultaneous indicator dilution curves at selected sites in the coronary circulation and determination of blood flow in coronary artery-saphenous vein graft by roentgen videodensitometry. In: Heintzen PH (ed Roentgen-, cine- and videodensitometry; pp 152–157. Georg Thieme, Stuttgart, 1971.

14. Rutishauser W, Simon HJ, Stucky JP, Schd N, Noseda G, Wellauer J: Evaluation of roentgen cinedensitometry for flow measurement in models and in the intact circulation. Circulation 1967; 36: 951.

15. Vogel R, LeFree M, Bates E, O'Neill W, Foster R, Kirlin P, Smith D, Pitt B: Application of digital techniques to selective coronary arteriography: use of myocardial contrast appearance time to measure coronary flow reserve. Am Heart J 1984; 107: 153.

16. Hodgson , LeGrand V, Bates E, Mancini J, Aueron M, O'Neill WW, Simon SB, Beauman GJ, LeFree MT, Vogel RA: Validation in dogs of a rapid digital aniographic technique to measure relative coronary blood flow during routine cardiac catheteization. Am J Cardiol 1985; 55: 189.

17. Johnson RA, Wasserman AG, Katz RJ, Leiboff RH, Bren GB, Tannenbaum ES, Ross AM:

Correlation of coronary anatomy and function using contrast density decay curves by on-line subtracted digital fluoroscopy. Circulation 1984; 70(suppl II): II–32.

18. Nissen SE, Elion JL, Booth DC, Evans J, DeMaria AN: Digital angiographic measurement of radiographic contrast material kinetics for estimation of myocardial perfusion. Circulation 1986 73: 789–798.

19. Detrano R, Yiannikas J, Simpfendorfer C, Hobbs RE, Salcedo EE: Quantitative assessments of regional myocardial perfusion by digital subtraction angiography. J Cardiogr 1985; 15: 603–612.

20. Foerster JM, Link DP, Lantz BM, Lee G, Holcroft JW, Mason DT: Measurement of coronary reactive hyperemia during clinical angiography by video dilution technique. Acta Radiol 1981; 22: 209.

21. Nissen SE, Elion JL, Booth DC, Evans J, DeMaria AN: Value and limitations of computer analysis of digital subtraction angiography in the assessment of coronary flow reserve. Circulation 1986; 73.

22. Vogel RA: The radiographic assessment of coronay blood flow parameters. Circulation 1985; 72: 460–465.

24. Parametric Encoding of Coronary Arteriograms for the Evaluation of Hyperemic Reserve

JONATHAN L. ELION & STEVEN E. NISSEN
Division of Cardiology, Department of Medicine, University of Kentucky College of Medicine, Lexington, KY, USA

Introduction

There is a growing body of evidence to suggest that traditional assessments of the severity of coronary stenosis (visual grading of the coronary arteriogram) correlate poorly with the actual anatomy [1], and fail to predict the actual physiologic significance of the lesion [2, 3]. Reactive hyperemia has long been recognized as a sensitive index of the severity of the physiologic impairment, as the presence of a significant stenosis limits the ability of the coronary bed to increase its flow in response to a hyperemic stimulus [4–6].

Research in our laboratory has previously demonstrated the feasibility of determining the extent of coronary flow reserve of an arterial bed using radiographic methods [7]. This approach requires extensive operator interaction, leading to the introduction of inter- and intraobserver variability, and providing results as a single numerical value. We therefore undertook a project to develop a method which would be more directly applicable to clinical catheterization practices, combining physiologic measurements with the actual anatomic display, eliminating the need for operator interaction, and displaying the results in a format familiar to clinicians.

Methods

The experimental preparation used has been described previously [7]. Briefly, an open-chest canine model of coronary stenosis was used. The left circumflex coronary artery of mongrel dogs was instrumented with an electromagnetic flow probe and two pneumatic occluders. The proximal occluder was used to produce variable degrees of coronary stenosis, while the distal one was used to produce brief complete coronary occlusions to stimulate hyperemia. Digital angiograms were recorded using an acquisition system which was gated to the electrocardiogram, providing a sequence of end-diastolic images. Small bolus-

P.H. Heintzen and J.H. Bürsch (eds), Progress in Digital Angiocardiography. ISBN 978-94-010-7093-5
© 1988, Kluwer Academic Publishers, Dordrecht

es of radiographic contrast were injected subselectively into the circumflex artery using an ECG-gated power injector ensuring that no dye refluxed out of the artery. Image sequences were taken first under basal conditions, then repeated following the production of hyperemia by a 15 second total coronary occlusion.This paired acquisition was repeated under several different levels of coronary stenosis.

All images were processed on a commercial medical image processing system, which allowed for the control of the radiographic acquisition of the images, ECG-gating, and triggering of the power injector on an R-wave. To allow the analysis of the change of a pixel's variance in the time domain, it was necessary to achieve optimal registration of the images, with each end-diastolic frame registered with the preceding and following frames, and with the basal sequence aligned with the hyperemic sequence. This was achieved by using a cross-correlation approach to calculate the optimal spatial translations necessary to align the images [8, 9].

It was recognized early on that it was necessary to correct the measurements made in a coronary artery for those of the subadjacent myocardium. Since X-rays are a silhouette technique, any measurement of intensity within a coronary artery is actually the sum of the intensity within the artery itself and that within the underlying myocardium. The first attempts at correcting the background were based on the same methods used by Nissen et al. for the pure numerical approach [7], namely the selection of a single background region of interest in the proximal artery. Measurements taken in this region of interest were then applied as a correction factor for all pixels within the entire coronary bed by subtracting the area under the background curve from the area under the coronary curve. A representative image using this simplified background correction scheme is shown in Fig. 1. The area under the time-intensity curve for all pixels within the boundaries of the coronary arteries were corrected using the area under the time-intensity curve of a single region of interest in the proximal myocardial bed. Corrected areas under the curve were computed under basal and hyperemic conditions, and the resulting area ratio (basal divided by hyperemic) used to assign the color of each pixel (described in greater detail below). Indicator dilution principles state that the flows measured should be related to flow at the site of the injection, not at the site of the reading, so a uniform flow ratio can be expected to be obtained throughout the entire arterial bed. As can be seen in Fig. 1, however, such a uniform result was not obtained. There is a clear predominance of the correct encoding proximally (representing a greater than 4 : 1 flow reserve, as was known to be present in this experiment), but as one moves distally in the artery, the values change considerably. Review of the myocardial contribution to the image data illustrates the basis for this nonuniformity (Fig. 2). This figure shows the results of adding together all of the end-diastolic frames with the resulting intensity of

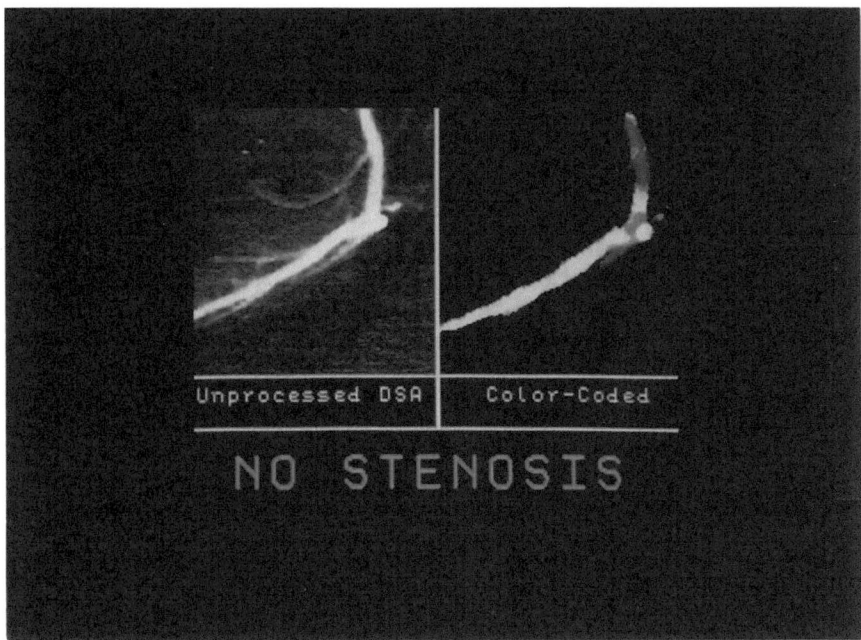

Fig. 1. An early attempt at producing a parametric representation of flow reserve. A frame from the original angiographic sequence is shown on the left following digital subtraction of the background and shows a subselective injection of a canine circumflex coronary artery. The parametrically encoded image on the right used a single background correction factor derived from the proximal artery, resulting in improper correction of the distal artery and a nonuniformity in parametric encoding.

each pixel being proportional to the area under its time-intensity curve. The measurement for myocardial correction was taken at the proximal artery immediately adjacent to the flow probe artifact and indicated by the (1) in the figure. In fact, there is very little myocardial contribution to the signals at this location. The distal myocardial indicated by the (2) in the figure demonstrates a bright myocardial blush. Because of the spatial nonuniformity of these myocardial intensities, it is not possible to apply a measurement from single location as a correction factor for the entire coronary bed. Instead, for each pixel within a coronary artery, it is necessary to search for the immediately adjacent myocardial pixel, and use the value obtained there for local corrections. In order to accomplish this without extensive operator interaction and tedious identification of large numbers of myocardial regions, a method for automatically segregating coronary from myocardial pixels was necessary.

The basis for this classification can be seen in Fig. 3 which shows typical time-intensity curves for a region of interest within a coronary artery and for

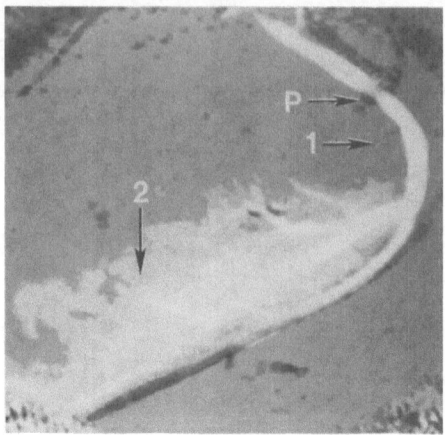

Fig. 2. The result of adding together all end-diastolic frames in an image sequence. The intensity of each pixel is proportional to the area under its time-intensity curve. The nonuniformity of the myocardial intensities is readily apparent.

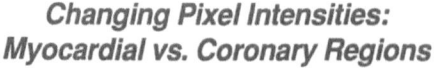

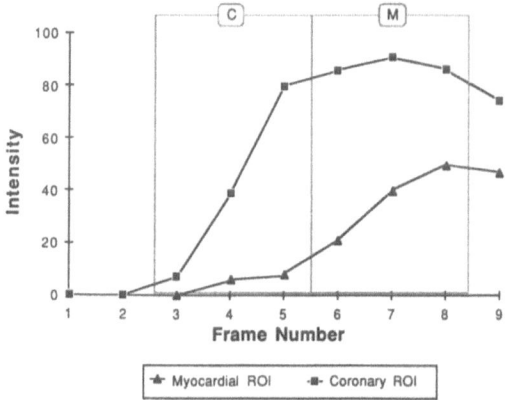

Fig. 3. Representation of typical time-intensity curves for two adjacent regions of interest; one within the borders of the mid-portion of the coronary artery (closed squares), and one within the adjacent myocardium (closed triangles). The coronary region of interest shows an early rise in intensity (during the time period labeled 'C'), while the myocardial region shows a later change (time period labeled 'M').

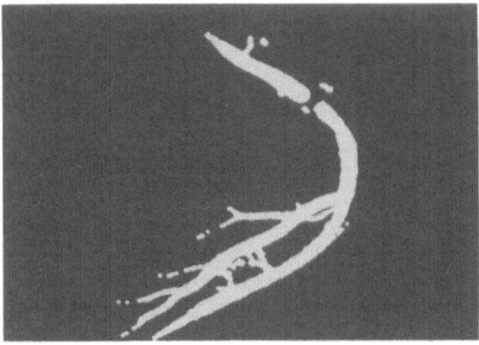

Fig. 4. A classification image, derived by comparing the statistical variance of the pixels early in the image sequence against a predetermined threshold. Pixels classified as belonging to coronary structures are represented as white, while all other pixels are black.

one in the immediately adjacent myocardium. Note that the intensity within the coronary region of interest rises very abruptly and early during the image sequence, while the intensity in the myocardial region of interest shows changes which are much slower and later in the sequence. This difference makes it possible to identify pixels within the coronary arteries by simple statistical variance; those pixels which demonstrate a variance of intensity early on in the cardiac cycle (the time period labeled 'C' in Fig. 3) would be classified as belonging to a coronary artery, while those demonstrating a change later in the sequence (time period 'M') would be classified as myocardial. Those pixels demonstrating no change of intensity (either remaining bright or remaining dark) would, by definition, belong to background structures.

Using this statistical approach, it is possible to arrive at a classification image which demonstrates those pixels which the computer feels on statistical grounds belong within the boundaries of a coronary artery [10]. Such an image is shown in Fig. 4. Pixels which are white have a variance which exceeds a predetermined threshold early in the image sequence, while the remaining pixels are noncoronary either myocardial or background.

Armed with this ability to identify and classify coronary pixels automatically, it is then possible to devise a scheme to apply background corrections to coronary pixels using values from immediately neighbouring myocardial pixels The processing is done on entire image frames at a time, rather than rising time-consuming 'loops' in the computer programs for pixel-by-pixel computations. This allows optimal use of the specialized hardware and software capabilities of the image processing computer. The steps used to derive the final images are shown schematically in Figs 5 and 6 and include:

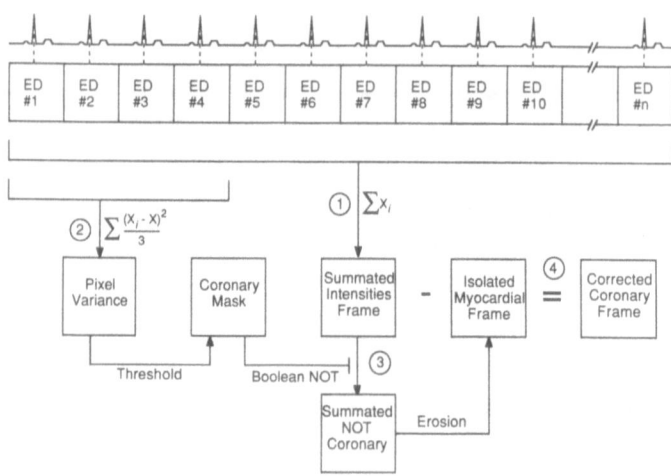

Fig. 5. Computation of an image frame which represents the corrected area under the coronary time-intensity curve (see text).

1. A summated frame is computed by adding together all of the end-diastolic frames in the sequence (Fig. 2). Pixels within such a summated image are therefore proportional to the area under the time-intensity curve, but lack a factor for the sampling interval the time between images). The time factor is not necessary to compute, as it will cancel out mathematically during a subsequent division step.

2. A classification image is created by computing the statistical variance of pixels early in the image sequence (the first four end-diastolic frames are used in this example). The variance information is used to produce a binary mask using discrimination against a predetermined threshold. Pixels whose variance exceeds the threshold are assigned to Boolean TRUE (white), and all others assigned to Boolean FALSE (black).

3. A frame containing only the myocardial background information is created using the classification image of the coronaries to mask out all of the coronary intensities. The holes left in the image by the masking procedure can be filled using classic image processing erosion methods. The resulting frame therefore represents pure myocardial information with the coronary contribution removed.

4. By subtracting the myocardial image (obtained in Step 3) from the summated image (from Step 1), a complete frame of corrected coronary information results. Corrected coronary frames are computed for both the basal and hyperemic sequences.

5. The ratio of the areas under time-intensity curves under basal and hyperemic conditions can be computed by simply dividing the corrected coronary

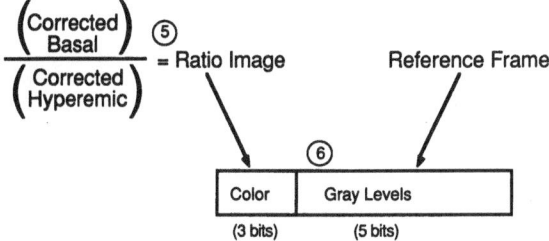

Fig. 6. The ratio of basal to hyperemic areas is computed by simple frame division. The ratio is represented in the upper three bits of each final pixel, while the gray level information, taken from the basal sequence, is contained in the lower five bits.

frame obtained under basal conditions by that obtained during hyperemia.

6. The resulting ratio image is then used to describe the color overlay (upper three bits of each pixel) which is added to the data from the representative frame of the sequence (placed into the lower five bits of each pixel).

Results

Representative images from one experimental preparation are shown in Figs 7 and 8. The color scale which was used for the representation of the flow reserve assigns flow ratios of 4:1 or greater to the blue end of the color spectrum, while blunted flow reserve (in the range of 1:1, signifying an absent flow reserve) are represented by the red end of the color spectrum. In Fig. 7, there is no coronary stenosis present, and the measured flow reserve (by the electromagnetic flow probe) is greater than 4:1. Note that the majority of the coronary pixels have been coded blue, indicating that the computations reflect a greater than 4:1 flow reserve by the area method. The few pixels which have been coded yellow or orange are caused by misregistration artifact resulting in the inability of the computer to accurately derive time intensity curves for the very small distal vessels. In the same experimental preparation, a coronary stenosis was produced by partial inflation of the distal pneumatic occluder (Fig. 8), and the experiment repeated. In this case, the actual flow reserve ratio was 1.2:1 and the color encoding shows a corresponding shift to the red end of the color spectrum.

We evaluated the ability of clinicians to meaningfully interpret these images. Clinical angiographers were given a brief training session concerning the significance of coronary flow reserve as a measure of the physiologic impact of a coronary stenosis. A random sequence of images, including both the original black-and-white frames and color-encoded computer images, were presented

260

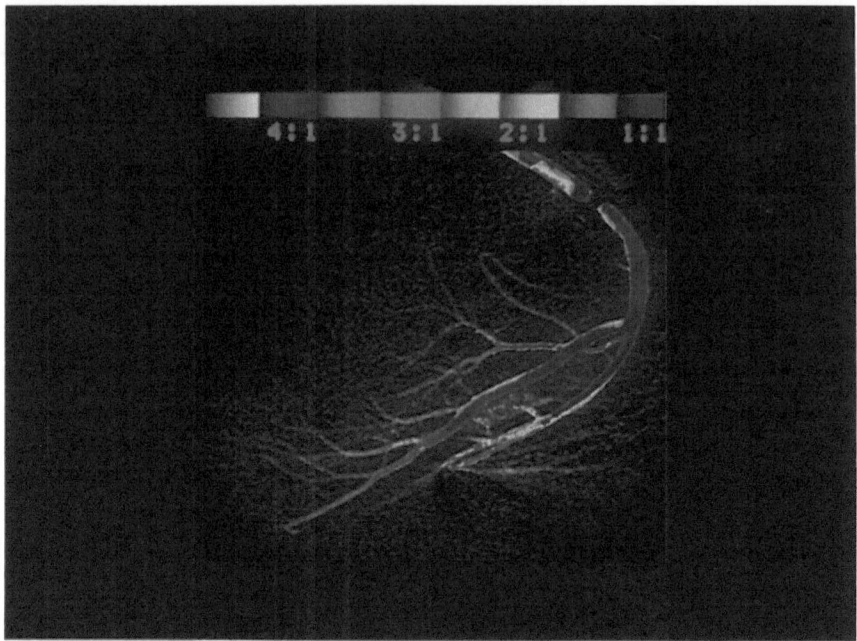

Fig. 7. Parametric image of normal flow reserve (canine model). Blue is used to represent basal-to-hyperemic flow ratios greater than 4 : 1, which in this example is the value obtained by direct electromagnetic flow probe determinations. The apparent stenosis seen proximally in the artery is in fact an artifact produced by the radio-opaque electromagnetic flow probe.

to the evaluators. They were asked to grade the suspected level of physiologic impairment associated with the lesions on a scale of one (severely impaired) to four (normal physiology). The correlation between their grades for the un-coded black-and-white images and the actual electromagnetic flow probe determinations of the true flow reserve ratios was poor (r = 0.57). When they used the color-encoded images to make their evaluations, however, the ability to estimate true impairment was improved markedly, with an excellent correlation between their grades and the actual measured flow determinations (r = 0.97).

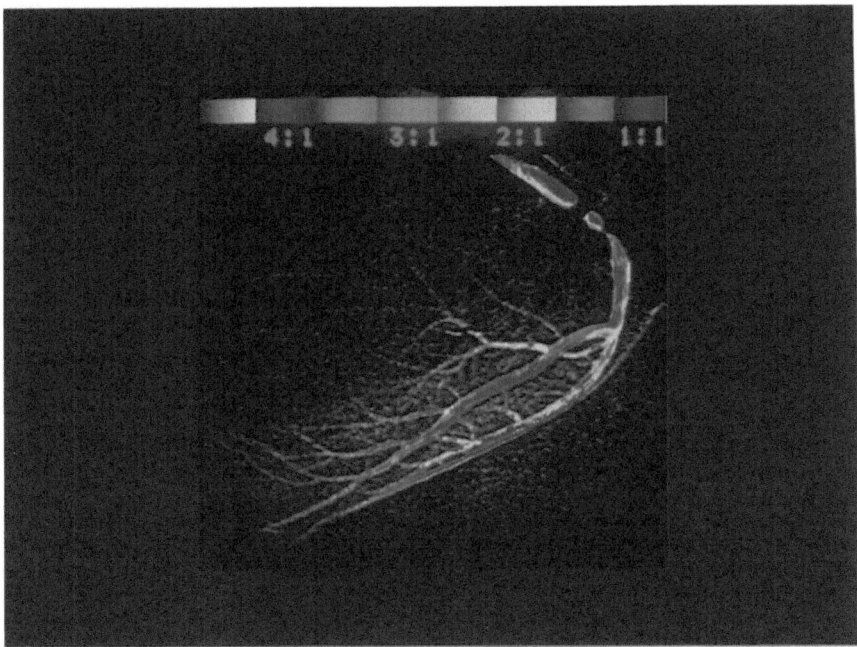

Fig. 8. Parametric image of impaired flow reserve. A stenosis has been introduced in the same experimental preparation shown in Fig. 7 (seen here just distal to the flow probe artifact). The measured flow reserve was 1.2 : 1 and results in a shift in the color coding to the red end of the color spectrum.

Discussion

We have therefore shown that images can be derived by the computer which accurately reflect both anatomy and the physiology of coronary lesions in a single frame. The method allows rapid computer processing which is free from the need for operator interaction. The images can be accurately interpreted by clinicians to derive a meaningful index of the physiologic impairment associated with a given coronary stenosis.

There are several limitations which remain for the method before it can see widespread clinical application. The nature of the hyperemic response itself is such that it can be expected to be altered in several disease and clinical states, including the presence of cardiac hypertrophy, previous myocardial infarction, vasoactive drugs, and recent coronary ischemia. The indicator-dilution principles which are used mandate that the radiographic contrast dye must be injected subselectively in the artery to be evaluated, and therefore requires the use of special catheterization methods for subselective injection (such as would be used during coronary angioplasty). Finally, the method requires exquisite registration of all of the end-diastolic images, and is very sensitive to even minor motion either during image acquisition, or between the basal and hyperemic image sequences. New methods for reregistration of images which have been degraded by complex motion artifact should be a great help in reducing this limitation.

Summary

A method has been developed for encoding a single frame of a coronary arteriogram with colors which represent the hyperemic flow reserve of the coronary arterial bed. The methods are based on the application of indicator dilution principles using a radiographic approach which has been previously validated and shown to correlate closely with flow ratios measured by electromagnetic flow probes. Following injection of contrast dye, coronary flow is proportional to the area under the radiographic time-intensity curve, with ratios of the areas under basal and hyperemic conditions computed for every pixel within the boundaries of a coronary artery. This ratio is used to assign the color overlay to the pixel, with blue shades used to represent a normal hyperemic reserve (flow ratio of greater than $4:1$), and red shades used to represent a blunted hyperemic response (ratio of $1:1$). Evaluations have shown that clinical angiographers can be easily trained to accurately interpret these images, thereby providing valuable insight into the physiologic consequences of a stenosis not otherwise possible with traditional image displays.

References

1. Marcus ML, Armstrong ML, Heistad DD, Eastham CL, Mark AL: Comparison of three methods of evaluating coronary obstructive lesions: postmortem arteriography, pathologic examination and measurement of regional myocardial perfusion during maximal vasodilation. Am J Cardiol 1982; 49: 1699.
2. White CW, Wright CB, Doty DB, Hiratzka LF, Eastham CL, Harrison DG, Marcus ML: Does visual interpretation of the coronary arteriogram predict the physiologic importance of a coronary stenosis? N Engl J Med 1984; 310: 819.
3. Harrison DG, White CW, Hiratzka LF, Doty DB, Barnes DH, Eastham CL, Marcus ML: The value of lesion cross-sectional area determined by quantitative coronary angiography in assessing the physiologic significance of proximal left anterior descending coronary arterial stenoses. Circulation 1984; 69: 1111.
4. Gould KL, Lipscomb K, Hamilton GW: Physiologic basis for assessing critical coronary stenosis: instantaneous flow response and regional distribution during coronary hyperemia as measures of coronary flow reserve. Am J Cardiol 1974; 33: 87–94.

5. Gould KL, Kelley KO: Physiologic significance of coronary flow velocity and changing stenosis geometry during coronary vasodilation in awake dogs. Circ Res 1982; 50: 695.
6. Hillis WS, Friesinger GC: Reactive hyperemia: an index of the significance of coronary stenoses. Am Heart J 1976; 92: 737.
7. Nissen SE, Elion JL, Booth DC, Evans J, DeMaria AN: Value and limitations of computer analysis of digital subtraction angiography in the assessment of coronary flow reserve. Circulation 1986; 73: 562.
8. Pratt WK: Correlation techniques of image registration. IEEE Transactions on aerospace and electronic systems, May 1974.
9. Barnea DI, Silverman HF: A class of algorithms for fast digital image regitration. IEEE Transactions on computers 1982; C-21: 179–186.
10. Elion JL, Nissen SE, DeMaria AN: Classification of cardiac structures in digital angiograms by the analysis of pixel variance. Comp Cardiol Oct 1986.

25. Digital Angiographic Transfer Function Analysis of Regional Myocardial Perfusion: Measurement System and Coronary Contrast Transit Linearity

NEAL L. EIGLER, J.MARTIN PFAFF, JAMES S. WHITING,
ANDREAS ZEIHER, JAMES S. FORRESTER & H.J.C. SWAN
Division of Cardiology, Cedars-Sinai Medical Center, Los Angeles, CA, USA, and the School of Medicine, University of California, Los Angeles, CA, USA

Introduction

Digital angiography produces high resolution images of contrast material transit through the coronary microcirculation from which quantification of the regional density of contrast material as a function of time can be derived. Analysis of these time-density curves with descriptive parameters such as time of arrival, time to peak, washout rate, etc. [1–5] has not produced reliable absolute flow measurements because of four unsolved problems: lack of a validated physiologic model, uncorrected systematic errors in densitometry, dependence on contrast agent injection technique, and the transient or variable effects of contrast material itself or other hyperemic stimuli on flow.

The purpose of this study was to overcome these problems by using linear systems theory to model the transit of contrast material through the coronary circulation. Our goals were: first, to study the linearity of digital coronary angiographic imaging in a phantom model; and second, to determine the linearity of regional coronary contrast transit in vivo by evaluating the sensitivity of perfusion parameters to injection technique and hyperemic stimuli.

Methods

System description

A linear system can be represented by the system transfer function which is totally defined by its input and output signals [6, 7]. For this study, the upstream time-density function acquired over a proximal coronary artery segment served as input, while the downstream time-density function over a region of myocardium supplied by this artery is the output. The system consists of the multiple pathways interconnecting the input and output which disperse, mix, and wash-out contrast material according to the system's blood flow and

P.H. Heintzen and J.H. Bürsch (eds), Progress in Digital Angiocardiography. ISBN 978-94-010-7093-5
© 1988, Kluwer Academic Publishers, Dordrecht

contrast material distribution volume characteristics.

A system is linear if it meets two criteria:

1. The output function in response to a combination of simultaneous inputs equals the sum of the outputs in response to the inputs applied separately; this is the principle of superposition.
2. The system's parameters must remain constant during measurement; this is the principle of stationarity.

If these criteria are fulfilled, the transfer function predicts the output of the system to any input.

Transfer function algorithm

The transfer function algorithm first generates a lagged-normal density function to model coronary contrast transit [8, 9]. This is a two-compartment model (Fig. 1): the first compartment (a Gaussian or normal density curve) simulates the temporal dispersion of indicator flowing through a conduit which we postulate occurs, for the most part, at the tip of the injecting catheter and in the large coronary arteries:

$$h'_1(t) = (1/\sigma/\sqrt{2\pi}) \cdot \exp(-0.5(t-T_c/\sigma)^2) \qquad \text{for } t > 0,$$

where $h'_1(t)$ represents a symmetric random distribution of transit times about a central time, T_c, with standard deviation σ. The second compartment, a monoexponential decay function, represents mixing in a branched network which may correspond, for the most part, to the myocardial microcirculation:

$$h'_2(t) = (1/\tau) \cdot \exp(-t/\tau) \qquad \text{for } t > 0,$$

where τ is the mean transit time. The mathematical convolution of these two functions yields a lagged-normal density curve:

$$h'(t) = h'_1 * h'_2.$$

Hereafter, $h'(t)$ is referred to as the model which closely resembles transfer functions derived from indocyanine green dye indicator dilution curves observed in the central circulation. The transfer function was obtained by iterative convolution as previously described [10, 11]. In brief, the lagged-normal density model was convolved with the input and the parameters were serially adjusted until the result of the convolution converges on the observed output. The system mean transit time, T_{sys}, is the sum of the individual compartment transit times and the inverse of each mean transit time is equal to the flow in that compartment divided by its volume:

$$T_{sys}^{-1} = \text{flow/volume.}$$

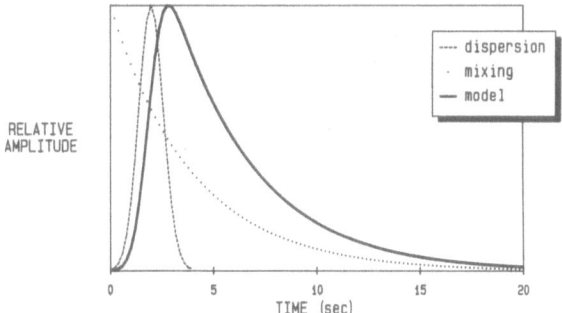

Fig. 1. The lagged-normal density function is a two-compartment model. The normal density curve and the monoexponential curve model dispersive and mixing processes respectively. The convolution of these two curves yields a lagged-normal density curve which is the model for the system transfer function.

Densitometric corrections

Transfer function analysis requires linear densitometry; both the input and output signal must be proportional to contrast concentration. This was achieved by acquiring time-intensity curves over a region of interest (ROI) and over an adjacent lead blocker which quantifies X-ray scatter and image intensifier veiling glare (SVG), and subtracting the SVG curve frame-by-frame from the ROI. The resultant curve was logarithmically transformed to correct for the Lambert-Beers effect, inverted and background subtracted. High frequency variations due to cardiac motion were reduced by temporal smoothing (4).

Phantom model

To determine the linearity, potential accuracy, and sources of error of the digital angiography system, we developed a linear X-ray phantom model of the coronary circulation (Fig. 2). This phantom consisted of 3.0 mm inner diameter polyethylene tubing which served as inflow and outflow conduits for a cylindrical mixing chamber (length 48 mm, diameter 20 mm). A baffle was placed near the chamber inflow to create turbulence for enhanced mixing and the remaining volume was filled with 2.0 mm diameter spherical glass beads to provide multiple interconnected path lengths to simulate a branched vascular network.

The phantom was perfused with saline by constant volume syringe pumps which were precalibrated and reproducibly delivered fluid at rates from 10 to 450 ml/min ± 1.0%. Contrast material (sodium meglumine diatrizoate, Re-

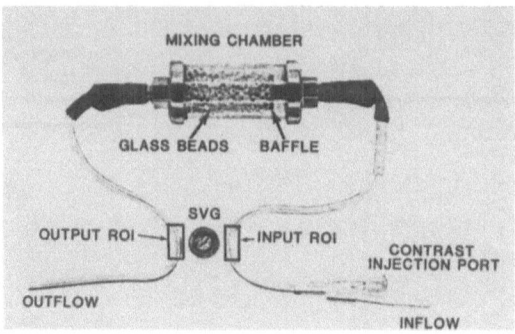

Fig. 2. Dynamic coronary X-ray phantom for determining linearity of digital angiographic measurement system.

nografin-76 370 mgI/ml, R-76) was delivered by a power injector connected to the inflow tubing (total 46 injections). To evaluate superposition, contrast injection rate (1–3 ml/sec), volume (2–8 ml), and bolus shape (single and dual peaks) were varied. The phantom was immersed in 20 cm of water to simulate tissue scattering and was imaged by digital angiography using a 512^2 pixel by 256 gray level format at 10 frames/sec. Rectangular 200 pixel ROIs were placed over the inflow and outflow tubing to acquire the input and output time-density functions.

Animal model

Six anesthetized open-chest dogs were fitted with an electromagnetic flow probe on the left circumflex coronary artery. A snare occluder was positioned immediately proximal to the flow probe to create variable degrees of stenosis. Hand-injected selective digital left coronary angiograms (n = 102) were performed in the left lateral position and recorded at 6 frames/sec during four coronary flow states: normal arteries under resting flow conditions (31 injections), stenotic arteries at resting flow (31 injections), normal arteries with hyperemic flow (23 injections), and stenotic arteries during hyperemia (17 injections).

To evaluate superposition and stationarity, several types of injection techniques and hyperemic stimuli were used. Normal and stenotic resting arteries were hand-injected with a single 4 ml bolus of undiluted R-76, a double bolus of R-76 (2 ml twice separated by approximately 1 sec), or a single 4 ml bolus of the nonionic contrast agent Iohexol (Omnipaque 350 mgI/ml,). Hyperemia was induced by four methods: dipyridamole infusion (0.56–1.02 mg IV over 5–10 min), dipyridamole plus norepinephrine infusion (titrated to raise mean blood pressure to 100–150 mm Hg), 20 second coronary occlusion, or following intracoronary contrast injection with 4 ml of R-76.

Flowmeter perfusion was defined as the immediate 3 sec pre-injection mean flow in ml/min /100 gm of left circumflex myocardium. At the conclusion of each study, total occlusion of the left circumflex artery was created and 50 ml of Monastral blue was injected into the left ventricle, immediately followed by KCl (50 meq) to produce cardiac standstill. The heart was excised, cut into 1 cm thick short axis sections, weighed and photographed. The mass of the left circumflex-supplied myocardium was calculated from the sum of the mass of each section multiplied by the percent unstained myocardium.

Time density curves were obtained by placing a 400 pixel ROI over the left main coronary artery just distal to the tip of the catheter for the input. A large > 9,000 pixel irregular ROI drawn over the projected left circumflex supplied myocardium for output.

Results

Phantom studies

Fig. 3 compares angiographically derived T_{sys}^{-1} with calibrated phantom flow/ volume ratios for each category of contrast material injection, over the full range of phantom flow rates (15–450 ml/min). Although contrast injection volume ranged from 2–8 ml and injection rate varied from 1–3 ml/sec, including double-peaked bolus injections, transfer function analysis accurately and reproducibly predicted phantom flow/volume (r = 0.99, SEE = 1.6) with the regression equation not significantly different from the line of identity.

Animal studies

Fig. 4 illustrates the derivation of the transfer function by iterative convolution in a dog. A trial lagged-normal density model was convolved with the input curve to yield a simulation of the output curve and the model parameters were serially adjusted and iteratively convolved until a best fit with the output curve was obtained. The final model is the system transfer function.

Fig. 5 compares T_{sys}^{-1} with flowmeter perfusion for each of the flow states. There was a close linear correlation between T_{sys}^{-1} and flowmeter perfusion (n = 102, r = 0.90, SEE = 3.6) over a wide range – from 0 to 514 ml/ min/100 gm myocardium. Moreover, when injections under normal resting conditions were excluded from analysis, an even stronger correlation was seen (n = 71, r = 0,94, SEE = 3.2). This occurred because T_{sys}^{-1} was significantly higher for normal arteries at rest compared to subcritically stenotic vessels where resting flow was not compromised (10.6 ± 1.3 vs 6.5 ± 1.9 min^{-1} respectively; p < 0.001).

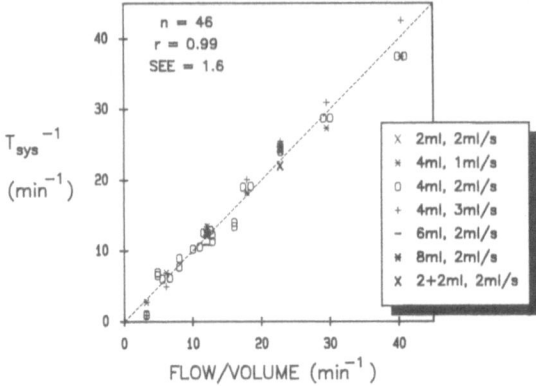

Fig. 3. Phantom study comparing the inverse of the system mean transit time, T_{sys}^{-1}, obtained by digital angiography with calibrated flow/volume ratios. Each symbol represents a different combination of contrast volume, injection rate and bolus shape.

Fig. 6 demonstrates the effects of injection shape and type of contrast agent on T_{sys}^{-1} for normal arteries in the absence of pre-existing hyperemia. A single peaked injection of R-76 in normal arteries produced a $400 \pm 60\%$ transient increase in flow, while Iohexol injection resulted in a transient rise of only $220 \pm 35\%$ ($p < 0.001$). The data show that the complexity of the bolus shape and the type of contrast material have no effect on T_{sys}^{-1}.

Fig. 7 compares T_{sys}^{-1} with flowmeter perfusion for the four different

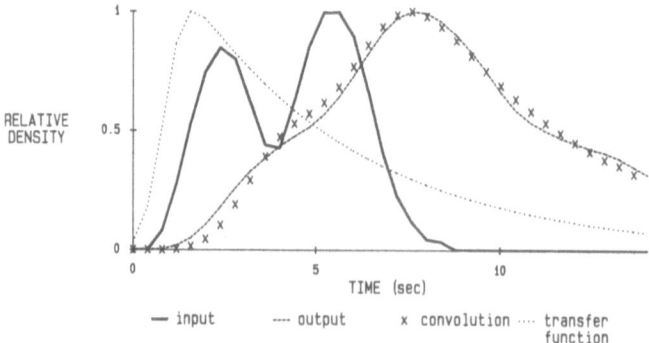

Fig. 4. Derivation of the system transfer function by iterative convolution. The input time-density function over the left main coronary artery has a complex double-peaked bolus shape which is reflected in the output function acquired over the left circumflex-supplied microcirculation. A lagged-normal density model was iteratively convolved with the input curve and its parameters serially adjusted until the result of the convolution converged on the observed output function. The final model is the system transfer function.

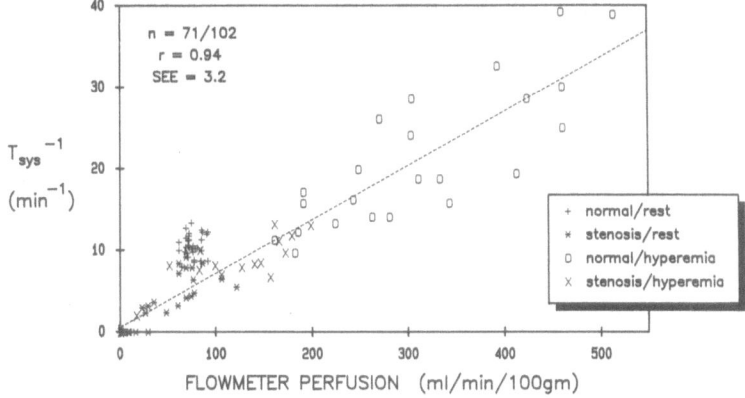

Fig. 5. Animal study comparing angiographic T_{sys}^{-1} with flowmeter perfusion for all injections during four flow states. A bimodal relationship is evident with normal/rest values of T_{sys}^{-1} greater than stenosis/rest for the same flow. The regression line has been plotted for all states except normal/rest.

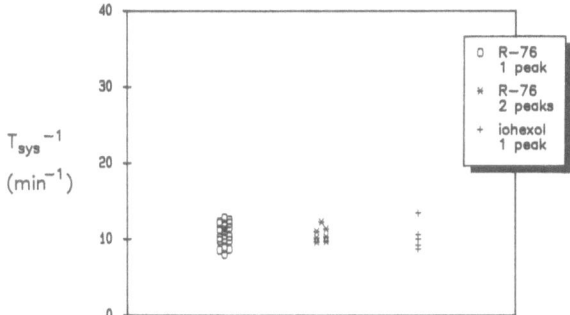

Fig. 6. Effect of bolus shape and type of contrast material on T_{sys}^{-1} in normal arteries at resting flow.

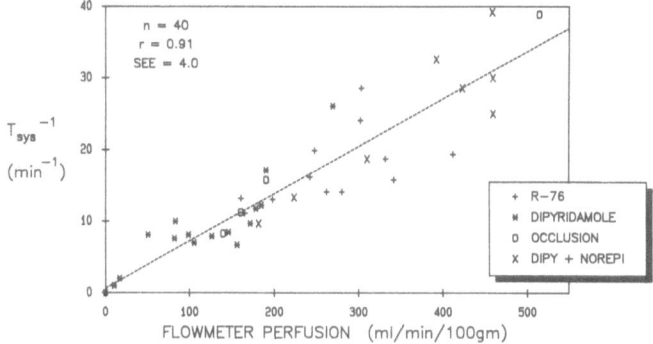

Fig. 7. Effect of type of hyperemic stimulus on T_{sys}^{-1}.

hyperemic stimuli. Whether coronary blood flow was augmented by dipyrida-mole, dipyridamole + norepinephrine, 20 second coronary occlusion, or R-76, the linear relationship was maintained. Variability was greater at the highest flows and when hyperemia was induced by R-76 or 20 second occlusion/release.

Discussion

Our goal was to study if both digital angiography and the coronary circulation contrast transit behave as linear systems. This was accomplished by using a linear mathematical model of the coronary circulation to calculate the system transfer function from time-density curves recorded over the left main coronary artery and the left circumflex territory myocardial contrast perfusion blush. The inverse of the mean transit time of the transfer function, T_{sys}^{-1} was the single parameter studied which we compared to directly measured flow/volume ratios in a phantom and to flow per mass of myocardium under varying conditions of stenosis, hyperemia and contrast injection technique in the dog. The potential advantages of this method are:
1. minimal sensitivity to signal noise because all the data points from both the input and output curves are used in an integrative process with the model serving as a smooth template for the transfer function;
2. ability to obtain the transfer function when the output signals have not returned to baseline by the end of acquisition; and
3. individual compartment transit time may have anatomical or physiologic correlates (beyond the scope of this study).

Digital angiographic system linearity

Linear analysis requires that both the system being measured and the measurement system be linear. We tested the linearity of our digital angiographic measurement system by imaging a dynamic X-ray phantom which simulated the flow, volume, contrast concentration and scatter conditions expected in vivo. Previous studies in our laboratory have documented the necessity for accurate densitometry by using fixed X-ray technique, and correcting for scatter, veiling glare, video camera and A/D converter non-linearities.

We tested linearity by applying the superposition principle; contrast injection rate, volume and bolus shape were widely varied while stationarity of system flow and volume were maintained. Linearity was demonstrated by showing that the mean transit time of the transfer function was independent of the shape of the recorded time-density curves; the most critical test being the dual peaked injections [10]. Furthermore, the measurement system was shown to be highly accurate and reproducible for determining phantom flow/volume ratios over a wide range of flow rates, from 15–450 ml/min.

Coronary circulation system linearity

Our studies show a strong linear correlation between angiographic T_{sys}^{-1} and regional myocardial perfusion in the dog over the wide range of flow rates produced by various combinations of stenosis and hyperemic stimuli. An interesting finding was the difference in T_{sys}^{-1} between normal and sub-critically stenotic arteries at rest where flow was the same. We speculate that this difference reflects increased contrast distribution volume due to stenosis-induced vasodilitation of the microcirculation

Our data show that the complexity of the input bolus shape and the type of contrast agent used, ionic vs nonionic, have no effect on T_{sys}^{-1} in normal arteries at resting flow rates. The former is a test of the superposition principle while the latter suggests system stationarity despite wide differences in the hyperemic response to each contrast agent. We hypothesize that this apparent stationarity occurs because:

1. the hyperemic phase occurs sufficiently after the peak of the output function;
2. hyperemic flow may be accompanied by nearly proportional increases in contrast distribution volume and therefore, transit time will be minimally affected.

Furthermore, for non-resting flow conditions, our data show that the mean transit time is independent of the type of hyperemic stimulus.

In conclusion, both digital coronary angiography and coronary contrast transit, appear to behave as linear systems, thus legitimizing transfer function analysis. Secondly, transfer function analysis accurately and reproducibly predicts regional coronary blood flow in dogs. Finally, transfer function analysis eliminates the need for standardized intracoronary contrast injections and can be used with a variety of hyperemic stimuli. These data suggest that transfer function analysis may replace traditional indicator dilution curve parameters for assessing regional myocardial perfusion.

Acknowledgments

This work was supported in part by NIH SCOR-IHD grant HL 17651. Dr Eigler is the recipient of NHLBI Clinical Investigator Award IK08HL 01578-01(MR). Dr Zeiher is the recipient of a research grant from the Deutsche Forschungsgemeinschaft.

274

References

1. Vogel RA, Lefree M, Bates E, et al.: Application of digital techniques to selective coronary arteriography: use of myocardial contrast appearance time to measure coronary flow reserve. Am Heart J 1984; 107: 153–164.
2. Hodgson JM, LeGrand V, Bates ER, et al.: Validation in dogs of a rapid digital angiographic technique to measure relative coronary blood flow during routine cardiac catheterization. Am J Cardiol 985; 55: 188–193.
3. Whiting JS, Drury JK, Pfaff JM, Chang BL, Eigler NL, Meerbaum S, Corday E, Nivatpumin T, Forrester JS, Swan HJC: Digital angiographic measurement of radiographic contrast material kinetics for estimation of myocardial perfusion. Circulation 1986; 73: 789–798.
4. Ratib O, Chappuis F, Rutishauser W: Digital angiographic technique for the quantitative assessment of myocardial perfusion. Ann Radiol (Paris) 1985; 28: 193–197.
5. Ikeda H, Yoshinori K, Utsu F, et al.: Quantitative evaluation of regional myocardial blood flow by videodensitometric analysis of digital subtraction coronary arteriography in humans. J Am Coll Cardiol 1986; 8: 809–816.
6. Bassingthwaighte JB: Physiology and theory of tracer washout techniques for the estimation of myocardial blood flow: flow estimation from tracer washout. Prog Cardiovasc Dis 1977; 20: 165–189.
7. Bassingthwaighte B: Blood flow and diffusion through mammalian organs. Science 1970; 167: 1347–1353.
8. Bassingthwaighte JB, Warner HR, Wood EH: A mathematical description of the dispersion in blood traversing an artery. Physiologist 1961; 4: 8.
9. Bassingthwaighte JB, Ackerman FH, Wood EH: Applications of the lagged normal density curve as a model for arterial dilution curves. Circ Res 1966; 18: 398–415.
10. Bassingthwaighte JB: Plasma indicator dispersion in arteries of the human leg. Circ Res 1966; 19: 332–346.
11. Hazelrig JB, Ackerman E, Rosevean JW: An iterative technique for conforming mathematical models to biomedical data. Proc 16th Ann Conf Eng Biol 1963; 5: 8–9.

26. Relation between Coronary Flow Reserve and Severity of Coronary Obstruction, Both Assessed from Coronary Cineangiogram

JOHAN H.C. REIBER, FELIX ZIJLSTRA, JAN VAN OMMEREN
& PATRICK W. SERRUYS
Erasmus University Rotterdam, Rotterdam, The Netherlands

Introduction

Coronary angiography is the only technique that allows the high resolution visualization of the coronary anatomy in man. In our and other laboratories quantitative techniques have been developed for the objective and reproducible assessment of the dimensions of coronary arterial segments from 35 mm cineframes [1–3]. In addition to assessing the accurate anatomic description of the severity of coronary obstructions, it is of great interest to obtain information about the functional significance of such obstruction, i.e. the question is posed: to what extent does the obstruction limit the flow through that artery?

During the last five years techniques have been developed at several institutes for the determination of time and flow parameters in digital angiography [4–9]. By means of these parameters the functional significance of anatomically defined coronary obstructions can be determined in terms of regional coronary flow reserve (CFR), defined by the ratio of maximal blood flow to resting flow. With the introduction of intracoronary papaverine, maximal coronary blood flow can be safely induced during routine cardiac catheterization [10, 11].

In this chapter the methodology and clinical application of a digital cineangiographic technique is described, which allows the quantitation of relative regional coronary blood flow on the basis of myocardial contrast perfusion measurements. This technique was introduced by R.A. Vogel et al. [5, 6]. Although this technique is usually applied to video images of the coronary arterial system acquired directly from the image intensifier of the X-ray system, we have implemented the technique for 35 mm cinefilm.

We were particularly interested in studying the relation between the quantitatively assessed coronary artery dimensions with the regional CFR in a group of 17 patients with single discrete proximal stenoses and in 12 angiographically normal individuals [12].

P.H. Heintzen and J.H. Bürsch (eds), Progress in Digital Angiocardiography. ISBN 978-94-010-7093-5
© 1988, Kluwer Academic Publishers, Dordrecht

Patients

Seventeen coronary arteries of patients with single vessel coronary artery disease (CAD) and 12 coronary arteries of patients with normal coronary arteries were studied. The 17 coronary artery lesions were all single discrete stenoses in the proximal parts of the vessels before any significant sidebranch occurred. Coronary angiography was performed for chest pain syndromes, with the Sones or Judkins technique. Informed consent was obtained for the additional investigation. All patients were studied without premedication, but their medical treatment (nitrates, calcium antagonists and β-blockers) was continued on the day of the investigation. None had systemic hypertension, cardiac hypertrophy, anemia, polycythemia, documented previous myocardial infarction, valvular heart disease or angiographic evidence of collateral circulation.

The procedures for the determination of the CFR and the quantitative assessment of coronary arterial dimensions from 35 mm cinefilm have been implemented on the computer-based Cardiovascular Angiography Analysis System (CAAS), which has been described extensively elsewhere [2, 13].

Methods CFR measurements

Angiographic procedure and induction of a maximal hyperemic response

The heart was atrially paced at a rate just above the spontaneous heart rhythm. Iopamidol at 37/C was injected into the coronary artery with an ECG-triggered Medrad Mark IV$^{(R)}$ infusion pump. This non-ionic contrast agent has a viscosity of 9.4 cP at 37/C, an osmolality of 0.796 osm.kg^{-1} and a iodium content of 370 mg/ml. For the left coronary artery 7 ml was injected at a flow rate of 4 ml/sec; the coronary angiogram was obtained in a left anterior oblique projection. For the right coronary artery 5 ml was injected at a flow rate of 3 ml/sec and the angiogram was taken in a left or right anterior oblique projection. The injection rate of the contrast medium was judged to be adequate when backflow of contrast medium into the aorta occurred. The angiogram was repeated 30 sec after a bolus injection of 10 mg papaverine into the coronary artery. The film speed for coronary cineangiograms was taken at 50 frames/sec.

Angiographic image analysis procedure

Cineframe digitization. For the quantitation of the relative coronary blood flow, five to eight end-diastolic (ED)-cineframes were selected for digitization

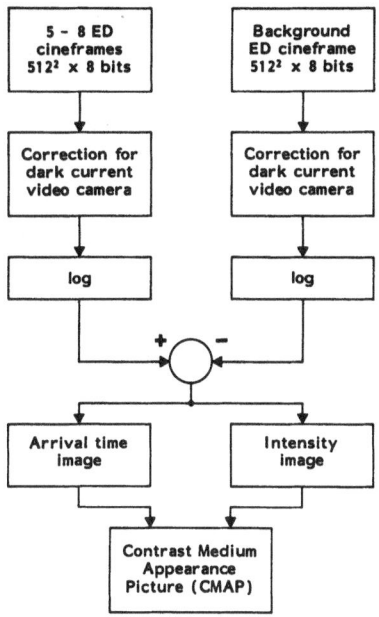

Fig. 1. Flow diagram for the digitizing and processing of the end-diastolic cineframes for the assessment of the CFR from 35 mm coronary cineangiograms.

from successive cardiac cycles. These cineframes were digitized with a high quality cinedigitizer at a resolution of 512×512 pixels and 256 gray levels (Fig. 1) [1–3]. The digitized images were corrected for the dark current of the video camera. Logarithmic mask-mode background subtraction was applied to the image subset to eliminate non-contrast medium densities. The last ED-cineframe prior to the contrast administration was chosen as the mask. The intensity level in the background-subtracted cineangiograms was found to be proportional to the irradiated amount of contrast material [14]. An example of a series of 6 consecutive background- subtracted ED-cineframes is shown in Fig. 2.

For the calculation of relative regional blood flow within a user-defined myocardial region-of-interest (ROI) two parameters are required, i.e. relative regional vascular volume and mean contrast appearance time. How these parameters can be determined will be explained in the following sections.

Time parameter extraction. From the sequence of background-subtracted cineframes a contrast medium appearance time picture was generated, using a fixed threshold (12%) in pixel brightness level. The individual pixels in this image were color-coded, based on the sequence number of the heart cycle in

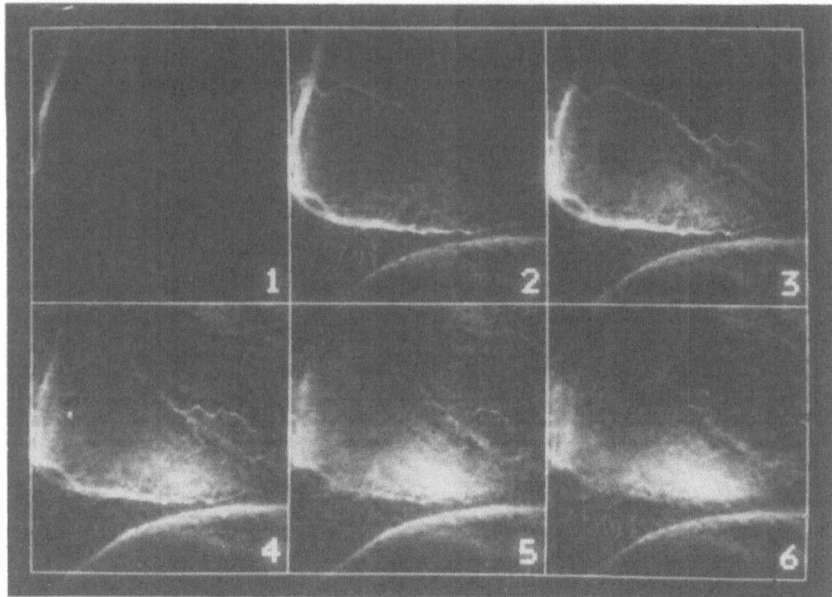

Fig. 2. End-diastolic cineframes, digitized in 512 × 512 eight-bit matrices from 6 consecutive heart beats following contrast injection. Stationary background structures were eliminated by means of logarithmic mask-mode background subtraction using the ED-cineframe acquired prior to contrast administration as a mask.

which the pixel intensity for the first time exceeded the threshold, starting from the beginning of the ECG-triggered contrast injection. Red was assigned to the pixels whose intensity surpassed the threshold during the first post-injection cycle, yellow for the second cycle, white for the third one, green for the fourth one, and so on.

Contrast medium appearance in the first post-injection cycle counts as 0.5 cycle, in the second as 1.5 cycle, and so on. The contrast medium appearance in consecutive heart cycles for the example of Fig. 2 is demonstrated in Fig. 3.

Regional vascular volume determination. The relative regional vascular volume, the second parameter required in the calculation of relative regional coronary blood flow, was calculated from a maximum intensity image, which is to be generated from the sequence of background-subtracted cineangiograms. Each picture element in this image represents the maximal pixel intensity level found within the series of background-subtracted cineframes. As a result, the maximum intensity image contains information on the maximum contrast medium concentration within the displayed vessels as it occurred during the acquisition period. The maximum intensity image generated from the image

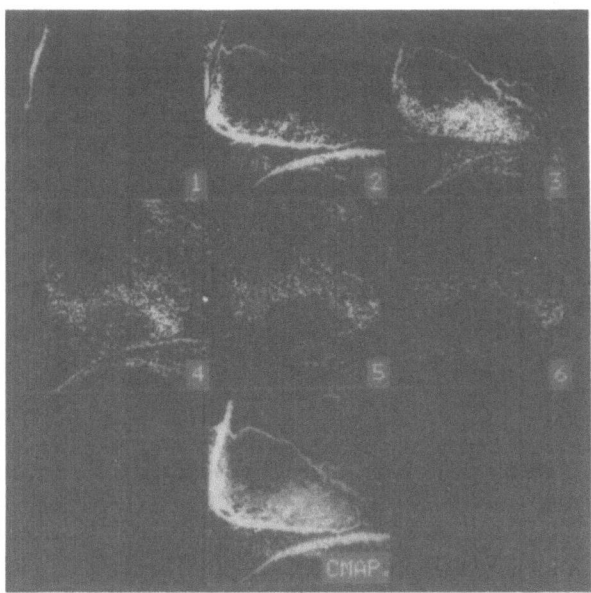

Fig. 3. Contrast medium appearance in 6 consecutive cardiac cycles from the example of Fig. 2. The first two cycles show the arterial phase, while the other cycles show the myocardial perfusion phase. The 6 individual cycles are finally combined into the last image (bottom center), being the color-coded contrast medium appearance picture (only shown in black/white).

series of Fig. 2 is demonstrated in Fig. 4. This maximum intensity image shows the distribution of contrast agent over the cardiovascular system. As stated before [14], the intensity value in background-subtracted cineangiograms is proportional to the transradiated amount of contrast material within the vessels. Under the assumption of homogeneous mixing of the contrast medium with the blood, the regional vascular volume V for a user-defined ROI is proportional to the mean radiographic intensity within that ROI:

$$V = k \int_{ROI} D(p)\ dp = k\overline{D},$$

where k is a radiographic constant, D(p) the radiographic intensity per pixel and $\overline{D}$ the mean radiographic intensity within the ROI.

Relative regional flow. Next, the color-coded time parameter image, shown as a grey-tone image in Fig. 3 (bottom, center), was combined with the maximum intensity image, resulting in a dual parameter image, which contains both time and density information. In this dual parameter image, the Contrast Medium Appearance Picture (CMAP), appearance time is color coded and contrast

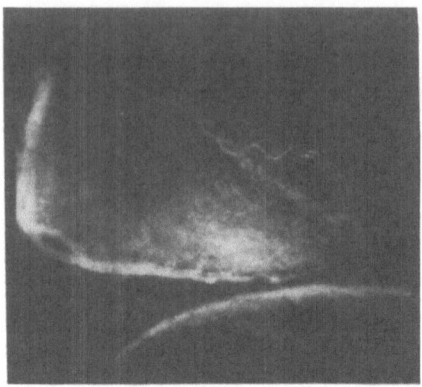

Fig. 4. Maximum intensity image, generated from the image series of Fig. 2. Each individual pixel intensity in this image represents the maximum intensity for that particular pixel as it occurred over the entire image series.

medium accumulation is represented by the individual pixel intensity values.

Regional flow values can then be determined quantitatively using the following videodensitometric principle:

$$Q = V/\overline{T},$$

where Q is the regional flow, V the regional vascular volume, and $\overline{T}$ the mean appearance time.

We are interested in the ratio of the coronary flow under normal (baseline) conditions and under maximal flow (hyperemic) conditions for the determination of the so-called coronary flow reserve factor. As flow *ratios* are determined, only relative and not absolute regional flow values for baseline and hyperemic conditions are required. Therefore, coronary flow reserve (CFR) is defined as the quotient of relative hyperemic and baseline flows Q_h and Q_b, respectively:

$$CFR = \frac{Q_h}{Q_b} = \frac{V_h \cdot \overline{T_b}}{\overline{T_h} \cdot V_b} = \frac{\overline{D_h} \cdot \overline{T_b}}{\overline{T_h} \cdot \overline{D_b}}.$$

Mean contrast intensity and appearance time were computed within the user-defined ROIs. Each ROI was chosen such that the large epicardial arteries, the aortic root and the coronary sinus were excluded from the analysis.

Quantitative coronary cineangiography

In the group of patients with single vessel coronary artery disease, the severity of the obstructions in terms of absolute and relative arterial dimensions was

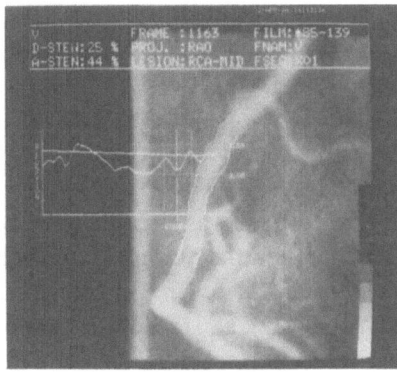 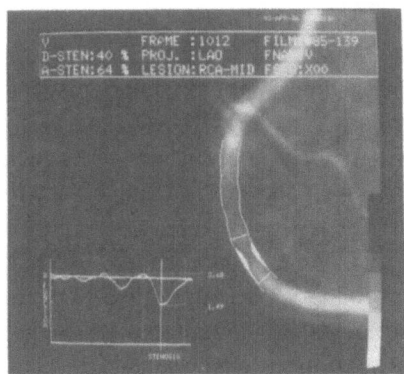

Fig. 5. Representative example of the assessment of the anatomic severity of a lesion in the mid-portion of the right coronary artery of the patient of Fig. 2. In the RAO-view (left) the interpolated percent diameter- and area stenosis were 25% and 44%, respectively, in the LAO-view 40% and 64%, respectively.

assessed with the CAAS [2, 13]. The percent diameter and area stenoses of an obstruction were calculated with the interpolated or computer-defined reference technique. Each lesion was analyzed in at least two, preferably orthogonal views, and mean values were used for the calculations. The results of the automated contour detection on the lesion in the mid-portion of the right coronary artery of the patient of Fig. 2 are demonstrated in Fig. 5. In the RAO-view the percentages diameter- and area-stenosis (assuming circular cross sections) were found to be 25% and 44%, respectively; in the LAO-view these numbers were 40% and 64%, respectively. Therefore, at the average the percentages diameter and area stenosis for this lesion were 32.5% and 54%, respectively.

From the measured arterial dimensions of the obstruction, including obsruction area, normal distal area and its length, the theoretical pressure gradient over the obstruction can be calculated at flows of 1, 2 and 3 ml/sec according to the well-known formulas described in the literature [15–18]. The coronary perfusion pressure distal of the stenosis is then equal to the mean aortic pressure minus the calculated pressure loss over the stenosis. From these data pressure-flow relations can be determined.

Statistical methods

The Student's t-test was used for the comparison between groups. Least-squares regression analyses were used to find the 'best fit' relationship between CFR and the quantitatively assessed coronary artery dimensions.

Results

The mean age of the 29 patients was 55 years (range 31–71); 4 patients were female, 25 male. All 17 patients with CAD had single vessel disease and all 23 patients had a normal left ventricular ejection fraction (> 55%).

A summary of the results from the quantitative analysis of the coronary arteries is shown in Table 1. The investigated vessel was the left anterior descending coronary artery in 16 of the patients (6 in the normal individuals and 10 in the patients with CAD), the right coronary artery in 7 patients (3 in the normal individuals and 4 in the patients with CAD), and the left circumflex coronary artery in the remaining 6 patients (3 in the normal individuals and 3 in the patients with CAD). An average of 2.3 angiographic projections was used for the quantitative morphologic analyses of the coronary angiogram. The 12 normal coronary arteries showed a mean cross-sectional area of $7.6 \, mm^2$ (s.d. $= 1.8 \, mm^2$), measured in the proximal parts before any branching occurred. The interpolated reference cross-sectional area of the vessels with coronary artery disease was $7.0 \, mm^2$ (s.d. $= 1.7 \, mm^2$). In the vessels with coronary artery disease the percent area stenosis (AS) ranged from 51% to 93% (mean 76%). The minimal luminal cross-sectional area (MLCA) ranged from 0.4 to $4.1 \, mm^2$ (mean $1.7 \, mm^2$), while the mean length of the obstructive lesions was $7.0 \, mm$ (range: 3.0 to $13.6 \, mm$).

The 12 normal coronary arteries had a mean CFR of 5.0 (s.d. $= 0.8$), while the CFR in vessels with coronary artery disease ranged from 0.5 to 3.9 (mean $= 1.6$); these CFR values differed significantly ($p < 10^{-5}$) from the CFR of normal coronary arteries. The relation between CFR and MLCA was best described by a quadratic equation:

Table 1. Summary of the results from quantitative analysis of the coronary arteries.

	Quantitative coronary cineangiography	
	Normals	CAD
Vessels		
RCA	3	4
LAD	6	10
LCX	3	3
Ref. area (mm^2)	7.6	7.0
AS (%)	–	76 (51–93)*
MLCA (mm^2)	–	1.7 (0.4–4.1)*
Length (mm)	–	7.0 (3.0–13.6)*

* mean (range)

Abbreviations: AS = percent area stenosis; MLCA = minimal luminal cross-sectional area.

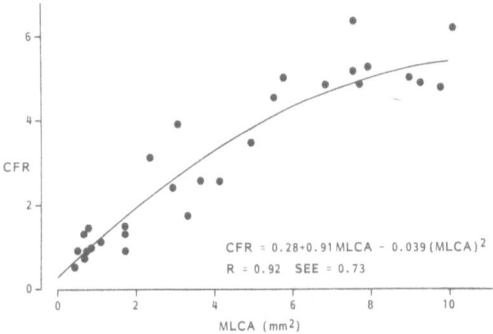

Fig. 6. Relation between coronary flow reserve and minimal luminal cross-sectional area MLCA.

$$CFR = 0.28 + 0.91 \, MLCA - 0.039 \, (MLCA)^2$$
$$(r = 0.92, \, SEE = 0.73),$$

as shown in Fig. 6. The relation between CFR and AS is also best described by a quadratic equation:

$$CFR = 5.0 - 3.3 \, (AS \times 10^{-2}) - 1.3 \, (AS \times 10^{-2})^2$$
$$(r = 0.92, \, SEE = 0.74),$$

as shown in Fig. 7. The CFR-values of the 12 normal coronary arteries were compared with those of the 6 coronary arteries with an AS between 50 and 70% and a MLCA between 2 and 4,5 mm² (moderate CAD), and with those of the 11 coronary arteries with an AS in excess of 70% and a MLCA less than 2 mm² (severe CAD); Table 2. The vessels with severe CAD had a mean CFR of 1.0 (s.d. = 0.3; range 0.5–1.5) and differed significantly (p = 0.001) from the CFR of the vessels with moderate CAD, that had a mean CFR of 2.6 (s.d. = 0.7; range 1.7–3.9). The difference between the normal vessels (CFR = 5.0 ± 0.8) and the vessels with moderate CAD was also significant ($p < 10^{-4}$).

Table 2. Relation between quantitatively assessed coronary artery dimensions and CFR.

	CAD		Normals
	Severe N = 11	Moderate N = 6	N = 12
MLCA (mm²)	< 2	2–4.5	> 4.5
AS (%)	> 70	50–70	0
CFR (mean ± s.d.)	1.0 ± 0.3	2.6 ± 0.7	5.0 ± 0.8
	⌐— p = 0.001 —⌐	⌐— $p < 10^{-4}$ —⌐	

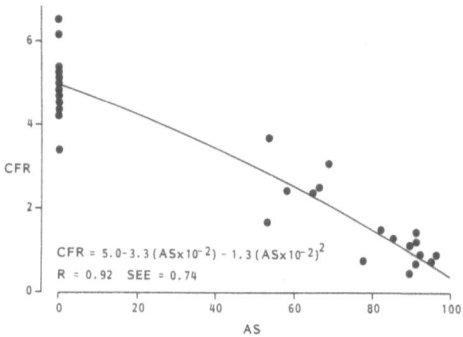

Fig. 7. Relation between coronary flow reserve and percent area stenosis AS.

By means of the hemodynamic equations that describe the pressure loss over a coronary stenosis for a given coronary flow the dimensional information from the quantitative analysis of the coronary angiogram, that is MLCA, length of the obstructive lesion and the normal distal area, is integrated into a single pressure gradient (Table 3), from which a theoretical coronary perfusion pressure-flow relation can be derived (Fig. 8). The pressure-flow relation of the 6 vessels with moderate CAD differs significantly ($p < 0.01$) from the vessels with severe CAD. Patients with severe CAD who have CFR values in the range 0.5–1.5 can be further subdivided into two groups: 6 patients with CFR ≤ 1 and 5 patients with CFR between 1 and 1.6 (Table 3); the theoretical pressure-flow relations of these two groups and the group of patients with moderate CAD are plotted in Fig. 8. The pressure-flow relation of coronary arteries with severe CAD and CFR ≤ 1 differs significantly from the pressure-flow relation of coronary arteries with a CFR > 1 ($p < 0.01$).

It is now of great interest to study whether the calculated distal coronary

Table 3. Calculated distal coronary perfusion pressure for theoretical coronary flows of 1 (P_1), 2 (P_2) and 3 (P_3) ml/sec for vessels with CAD subdivided according to CFR.

No. of patients	CFR threshold	CFR Mean	CFR Range	AS (%)	MLCA (mm²)	Ao (mmHg)	P1 (mmHg)	P2 (mmHg)	P3 (mmHg)
6	CFR>1.6	2.6	1.7–3.9	59	3.1	89	88	87	85
5	1<CFR<1.6	1.3	1.1–1.5	86	1.1	88	78	62	42
6	CFR≤1	0.8	0.5–1.0	87	0.8	86	68	40	−2.5

Abbreviations: AS (%) = mean percentage area stenosis; MLCA (mm²) = mean minimal luminal cross-sectional area, Ao = mean aortic pressure.

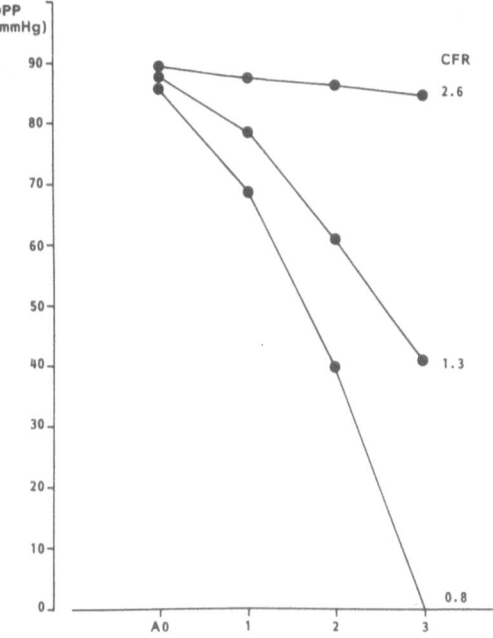

Fig. 8. Calculated distal coronary arterial pressure(P)-flow relation for theoretical flows of 1 (P1), 2 (P2) and 3 (P3) ml/sec for vessels with coronary artery disease, divided into three groups according to the coronary flow reserve: 6 patients with moderate CAD and CFR > 1.6, 5 patients with severe CAD and 1<CFR < 1.6 and 6 patients with severe CAD and CFR ≤ 1.

Table 4. Identification of coronary arteries with critical stenosis on the basis of calculated distal coronary perfusion pressure (DPP) at a coronary flow of 3 ml/sec.

DPP (mmHg)	CFR (mean ± s.d.)	No. of patients	
		CFR ≤ 1	CFR > 1
< 40	0.96 ± 0.3	5	2
	p = 0.01		
> 40	2.1 ± 0.9	1	9

Sens. $= \dfrac{5}{6} \times 100\% = 83\%$

Spec. $= \dfrac{9}{11} \times 100\% = 82\%$

perfusion pressure at a certain coronary flow has a predictive value in identifying patients with a critical coronary stenosis, defined as a coronary obstruction with a severity such that the CFR of that artery is less than or equal to 1. From the data it can be derived that a distal coronary perfusion pressure below 40 mmHg at a coronary flow of 3 ml/sec, identifies 5 out of 6 patients with a CFR ≤ 1 (sensitivity: 83%). Only 2 of 11 vessels with CAD and a CFR > 1 have a distal coronary perfusion pressure below 40 mmHg (specificity: 82%) (Table 4).

Discussion

In this study we have investigated the relation between the coronary arterial dimensions assessed quantitatively from 35 mm cineangiograms and the coronary flow reserve assessed from control and hyperemia induced myocardial perfusion images in a group of individuals with normal coronary arteries and a group of patients with single vessel coronary artery disease.

Bookstein and Higgins have shown in dogs that the coronary hyperemic response after a bolus injection of adenosine-triphosphate or papaverine into a coronary artery is of the same magnitude as after a 15 sec occlusion of the coronary artery [19]. The exact dosis of intracoronary papaverine which is needed to induce a maximal coronary vasodilation has recently been established. Wilson et al. compared the coronary hyperemic response after 4, 8, 12 and 16 mg intracoronary papaverine and reported a maximal hyperemic response after 8 or 12 mg in all coronary arteries [10]. Previous work from our own laboratory confirmed that 10 mg intracoronary papaverine is a safe and reproducible means of inducing a short-lasting and strong hyperemic response with a peak effect lasting from 24 until 37 sec, without alterations in systemic hemodynamics [11].

In our population the interpolated reference cross-sectional areas of the vessels with CAD was on average 7.0 mm^2 and the cross-sectional areas of the 12 normal coronary arteries was on average 7.6 mm^2, which indicates the isolated and focal character of their coronary artery disease. In these selected groups of patients, both AS and MLCA were curvilinearly related to the CFR, best described by quadratic equations. However, there was considerable scatter of the data about the relatively good overall correlation between the cross-sectional measures and the X-ray predicted coronary flow reserve. This relationship between AS and CFR confirms two essential points [20]. First, an AS in excess of 51% is associated with a diminished CFR, and second, a critical coronary stenosis defined as a coronary artery with a CFR of ≤ 1 exists when AS is $>90\%$.

However, in general, in patients with multivessel and/or diffuse coronary artery disease poor correlations between the absolute and relative minimal cross-sectional dimensions and the CFR can be expected [21, 22]. According to Gould and Kirkeeide, all angiographic dimensions of a coronary obstruction should be taken into consideration to obtain better correlations [22, 23].

A pressure-flow relationship that characterizes the severity of the coronary stenosis can be derived, by means of hemodynamic equations using MLCA, the length of the obstructive lesion and the expected normal cross-sectional area of the coronary artery. Kirkeeide et al. showed in dogs the good relation between such an angiographic approach and measured CFR [23]. In our patients, the pressure-flow relations calculated for individual coronary arteries from the angiographic dimensions have evident predictive value, not only by differentiating between patients with moderate and severe CAD, but also by indicating which patients with severe CAD had a critical coronary stenosis, defined as a vessel with a CFR $\leqslant 1$. When coronary perfusion pressure falls below 40 mmHg, the reactive hyperemic response to a 20 sec occlusion of the coronary artery has been found to be negligible [24]. We therefore postulate that a distal coronary perfusion pressure $\leqslant 40$ mmHg at a flow of 3 ml/sec might identify patients with a critical stenosis, defined as a vessel with a CFR $\leqslant 1$. Using this criterion, patients with severe CAD and a critical stenosis could be identified with a high sensitivity (83%) and specificity (82%).

From the relation between coronary perfusion pressure and coronary flow under conditions of maximal coronary vasodilation as described by Bache and Schwartz [25], and assuming a resting coronary flow velocity of 15 cm/sec, Kirkeeide et al. calculated a CFR from the angiographic data [23]. Whether this approach is used or distal coronary perfusion pressures are calculated for theoretical coronary flows, the major short-coming remains the fact that coronary flow is not actually measured. As regional coronary arterial beds will certainly differ in actual flow, this introduces a considerable uncertainty.

Values and limitations

Although we found a clear relation between AS, MLCA and CFR, individual coronary arteries, especially those with moderate CAD, may differ considerably in CFR. Because of the scatter in the relations, the CFR-value for an individual stenosis cannot be predicted accurately. Therefore, approaches that integrate all angiographic dimensions of the obstructions are conceptually attractive [22, 23], but should be combined with an angiographic or other technique to measure absolute coronary blood flow.

It must be clear that the findings described in this chapter which were obtained in a very selected group of patients, cannot be extrapolated to other patient subsets, for instance to patients with more diffuse CAD, collateral circulation or stenosis in more distal coronary arteries of smaller size.

The choice of a myocardial region of interest in the CMAP is also restricted. In the two-dimensional image there does not exist a one-to-one relation between a selected myocardial region and one particular coronary segment due to overprojection of myocardial regions in front of and behind the selected region of interest. At this stage, the functional significance of only proximal coronary obstructions can be assessed with reasonable accuracy; in these cases the perfusion of a large portion of the coronary bed is disturbed. In general, overprojections with other regions will occur. For some time, we as well as Onnasch et al. have been studying the possibilities of three-dimensional reconstruction of the myocardial perfusion from two orthogonal projections to overcome such problems [26, 27]. In the reconstructed myocardial slices the regions perfused by the individual coronary branches can be identified, leading hopefully to the assessment of the coronary flow reserve of proximally as well as centrally and distally localized obstructions. It is yet too early to indicate the possible success of such approach.

Conclusion

In conclusion, a technique for the assessment of relative regional coronary blood flow and coronary flow reserve from 35 mm cineangiograms has been implemented. By this approach the relation between the anatomic severity of a coronary obstruction and its functional significance can be studied in human beings during routine cardiac catheterization. From the results obtained sofar, it may be concluded that the reduction in CFR for a proximal stenosis in single vessel coronary artery disease can be predicted with reasonable accuracy by quantitative assessment of the coronary artery dimensions.

Further validation studies will be carried out to define exactly the value and limitations of the technique for the measurement of coronary flow reserve.

Summary

A rapid angiographic technique is described that allows the assessment of relative regional coronary blood flow in a user-defined myocardial region-of-interest (ROI) following the rapid administration of contrast agent in an atrially paced heart. The distribution of the contrast agent within the coronary vessels and myocardial muscle as a function of time can be determined in background-subtracted digitized end-diastolic cineframes. Functional parameters for the calculation of blood flow are presented in parametric images. From the sequence of background-subtracted cineframes a contrast medium appearance time picture is generated. A maximum intensity image provides information for the computation of regional vascular volume. From the mean intensity and the mean appearance time within a user-defined ROI, the regional coronary blood flow can be calculated. Acquiring and analyzing these image data at the control state and at maximal flow allows the measurement of coronary flow reserve to be a measure for the functional significance of an obstruction. The anatomic severity of the stenosis can be determined in an objective and reproducible manner using automated edge detection techniques.

To study the relation between the quantitatively assessed coronary artery dimensions with the regional coronary flow reserve as measured by digital subtraction cineangiography, 17 coronary arteries with a single discrete proximal stenosis and 12 normal coronary arteries, before and after intracoronary papaverine, were investigated. Coronary flow reserve was found to be curvilinearly related to minimal luminal cross-sectional area ($r = 0.92$, SEE $= 0.73$) and to percentage area stenosis ($r = 0.92$, SEE $= 0.74$). Normal coronary arteries have a coronary flow reserve of 5.0 (s.d. $= 0.8$), which differs significantly from the coronary flow reserve of the coronary arteries with obstructive disease, in which values ranging from 0.5 to 3.9 were found. Coronary arteries with a percentage area stenosis between 50 and 70% and a minimal luminal cross-sectional area between 2 and 4.5 mm^2 differ significantly ($p = 0.001$) with respect to the coronary flow reserve from coronary arteries with a percentage area stenosis in excess of 70% and a minimal luminal cross-sectional area less than 2 mm^2. Using hemodynamic equations that describe the pressure loss over a stenosis, a theoretical pressure-flow relation can be inferred which characterizes the severity of the stenosis. Based upon this theoretical pressure-flow relation, coronary arteries which have a limited coronary flow reserve and critical stenosis (distal coronary perfusion pressure below 40 mmHg at coronary flow of 3 ml/sec) can be identified with high sensitivity (83%) and specificity (82%). In conclusion, the consequent reduction in coronary flow reserve in coronary artery disease can be predicted with reasonable accuracy by quantitative assessment of coronary arterial dimensions.

Acknowledgments

The authors wish to thank Mrs S.M. Spierdijk, Mrs M.J. Kanters-Stam and Mrs E.F. van den Ende for their secretarial assistance in the preparation of this manuscript.

References

1. Reiber JHC: Morphologic and densitometric analysis of coronary arteries. In: Heintzen PH, Bürsch JH (eds) Progress in digital angiocardiography; pp 137–158. Kluwer Academic Publishers, Dordrecht, 1988.

2. Reiber JHC, Serruys PW, Slager CJ: Quantitative coronary and left ventricular cineangiography; methodology and clinical applications. Martinus Nijhoff, Boston/Dordrecht/Lancaster, 1986.

3. Reiber JHC, Kooijman CJ, Slager CJ, Gerbrands JJ, Schuurbiers JCH, Boer A den, Wijns W, Serruys PW: Computer assisted analysis of the severity of obstructions from coronary cineangiograms: a methodological review. Automedica 1984; 5: 219–238.

4. Smith HC, Robb RA, Ritman EL: Roentgen videodensitometric assessment of myocardial blood flow: clinical applications. In: Heintzen PH, Bürsch JH (eds) Roentgen-video-techniques for dynamic studies of structure: function of the heart and circulation; pp 39–48. Georg Thieme, Stuttgart, 1978.

5. Vogel R, LeFree M, Bates E, O'Neill W, Foster R, Kirlin P, Smith D, Pitt B: Application of digital techniques to selective coronary arteriography: use of myocardial contrast appearance time to measure coronary flow reserve. Am Heart J 1984; 107: 153–164.

6. Hodgson JMcB, LeGrand V, Bates ER, Mancini GBJ, Aueron FM, O'Neill WW, Simon SB, Beaumon GJ, LeFree MT, Vogel RA: Validation in dogs of a rapid digital angiographic technique to measure relative coronary blood flow during routine cardiac catheterization. Am J Cardiol 1985; 55: 188–193.

7. Hahne HJ: Time and flow parameter extraction in digital angiography: principles and methods. Herz 1985; 10: 220–227.

8. Bürsch JH: Densitometric studies in digital subtraction angiography: assessment of pulmonary and myocardial perfusion. Herz 1985; 10: 208–214.

9. Ratib O, Chappuis F, Rutishauser W: Digital angiographic technique for the quantitative assessment of myocardial perfusion. Annales Radiologie 1985; 28: 193–197.

10. Wilson RF, White CW: Intracoronary papaverine: an ideal coronary vasodilator for studies of the coronary circulation in conscious humans. Circulation 1986; 73: 444–451.

11. Zijlstra F, Serruys PW, Hugenholtz PG: Papaverine: the ideal coronary vasodilator for investigating CFR? A study of timing magnitude, reproducibility and safety of the coronary hyperemic response after intracoronary papaverine. Cath Cardiovasc Diagn 1986; 12: 298–303.

12. Zijlstra F, Ommeren J van, Reiber JHC, Serruys PW: Does the quantitative assessment of coronary artery dimensions predict the physiologic significance of a coronary stenosis? Circulation 1987; 75: 1154–1161.

13. Reiber JHC, Serruys PW, Kooijman CJ, Wijns W, Slager CJ, Gerbrands JJ, Schuurbiers JCH, Boer A den, Hugenholtz PG: Assessment of short-, medium- and long-term variations in arterial dimensions from computer-assisted quantitation of coronary cineangiograms. Circulation 1985; 71: 280–288.

14. Reiber JHC, Slager CJ, Schuurbiers JCH, Boer A den, Gerbrands JJ, Troost GJ, Scholts B, Kooijman CJ, Serruys PW: Transfer functions of the X-ray-cine-video chain applied to digital processing of coronary cineangiograms. In: Heintzen PH, Brennecke R (eds) Digital imaging in cardiovascular radiology; pp 89–104. Georg Thieme, Stuttgart, 1983.

15. Brown BG, Bolson E, Frimer M, Dodge HT: Quantitative coronary arteriography. Estimation of dimensions, hemodynamic resistance, and atheroma mass of coronary artery lesions using the arteriogram and digital computation. Circulation 1977; 55: 329–337.

16. Gould KL, Kelly KO, Bolson EL: Experimental validation of quantitative coronary arteriography for determining pressure-flow characteristics of coronary stenosis. Circulation 1982; 66: 930–937.

17. Serruys PW, Wijns W, Geuskens R, Feyter P de, Brand M van den, Reiber JHC: Pressure gradient, exercise thallium-201 scintigraphy, quantitative coronary cineangiography: in what sense are these measurements related? In: Reiber JHC, Serruys PW (eds) State of the art in quantitative coronary arteriography; pp 251–270. Martinus Nijhoff, Dordrecht/Boston/Lancaster, 1986.

18. Serruys PW, Wijns W, Reiber JHC, Feyter P de, Brand M van den, Piscione F, Hugenholtz PG: Values and limitations of transstenotic pressure gradients measured during percutaneous coronary angioplasty. Herz 1985; 10: 337–342.

19. Bookstein JJ, Higgins CB: Comparative efficacy of coronary vasodilatory methods. Invest Radiol 1977; 12: 121–127.

20. Gould KL, Lipscomb K, Hamilton GW: Physiological basis for assessing critical coronary stenosis: instantaneous flow response and regional distribution during coronary hyperemia as measures of CFR. Am J Cardiol 1984; 33: 87–94.

21. Harrison DG, White CW, Hiratzka LF, Doty DB, Barnes DH, Eastham CL, Marcus ML: The value of lesion cross-sectional area determined by quantitative coronary angiography in assessing the physiological significance of proximal left anterior descending coronary arterial stenoses. Circulation 1984; 69: 1111–1119.

22. Gould KL, Kirkeeide RL: Assessment of stenosis severity. In: Reiber JHC, Serruys PW (eds) State of the art in coronary arteriography; pp 209–228. Martinus Nijhoff, Dordrecht/Boston/Lancaster, 1986.

23. Kirkeeide RL, Gould KL, Parsel L: Assessment of a coronary stenosis by myocardial perfusion imaging during pharmacologic coronary vasodilation. VII. Validation of coronary flow reserve as a single integrated functional measure of stenosis severity reflecting all its geometric dimensions. JACC 1986; 7: 103–113.

24. Dole WP, Montville WJ, Bishop VS: Dependency of myocardial reactive hyperemia on coronary artery pressure in the dog. Am J Physiol 1981; 240: H709.

25. Bache RJ, Schwartz JS: Effect of perfusion pressure distal to coronary stenosis on transmural myocardial blood flow. Circulation 1982; 65: 928–935.

26. Dumay ACM: 3-D reconstruction from two orthogonal projections with linear programming techniques. Thesis. Information Theory Group, Delft University of Technology, June 1986 (in Dutch).

27. Onnasch DGW, Lindenau J, Bürsch JH, Heintzen PH: Reconstruction of the spatial distribution of the myocardial perfusion from multiple-view arteriography. In: Heintzen PH, Bürsch JH (eds) Progress in digital angiocardiography; pp 327–335. Kluwer Academic Publishers, Dordrecht, 1988.

27. Coronary Arteriography, Stress Test and Coronary Flow Reserve Measurements: Comparative Studies

G.B. JOHN MANCINI & ROBERT A. VOGEL

Cardiology Section, Veterans Administration Medical Center, Department of Internal Medicine, University of Michigan Medical School, Ann Arbor, MI, USA

Introduction

The determination of the functional significance of coronary stenoses is of central importance in clinical cardiology. The traditional methods of determining this have been through the use of coronary arteriography, and stress testing. A relative newcomer to this endeavor in clinical practice is that of measuring coronary flow reserve by various techniques. While the relation between flow reserve and coronary arteriography has been intensively studied, the relation between CFR and exercise test results and the interrelationship of all of these methodologies have not yet been extensively investigated. The purpose of this paper is to outline our results in attempting to put these various methodologies into a clinically relevant perspective through both animal and patient investigations.

Methods

Animal studies

Mongrel dogs were anesthetized with intravenous pentobarbital sodium and ventilated with room air using a Harvard respirator. A left thoracotomy was performed in the fifth intercostal space. The left anterior descending or the circumflex coronary artery was dissected free for a length of 1 to 2 cm and instrumented with a snare occluder, a hard plastic screw occluder or a rubber cuff occluder (R.E. Jones, Silver Spring, MD) and an electromagnetic flow probe (Carolina Medical Electronics, Inc.). Two pairs of subendocardial ultrasonic quartz crystals were implanted in the mid-equatorial region of the left ventricle and approximately parallel to the circumferential plane. One pair was implanted in the left anterior descending coronary artery distribution distal to the occluder and in the central area of the zone rendered dyskinetic

P.H. Heintzen and J.H. Bürsch (eds), Progress in Digital Angiocardiography. ISBN 978-94-010-7093-5
© 1988, Kluwer Academic Publishers, Dordrecht

and cyanotic during coronary occlusion (ischemic zone), and one pair was implanted in the left circumflex coronary artery region (nonischemic zone).

The severity of the stenoses was quantitated by the impairment of resting coronary flow reserve. Coronary flow reserve was determined at rest in the absence of a stenosis by the ratio of peak blood flow after a 20 second total occlusion to resting coronary blood flow. Dopamine (15 g/kg/min) [1] or isoproterenol (0.25 g/kg/min) [2] was then infused for three to five minutes in the absence of a stenosis. Or, the animals were subjected to maximal atrial pacing for 60 seconds [3]. After full recovery, the catecholamine or atrial pacing stress tests were repeated in the presence of graded impairments of coronary flow reserve. Stenoses that impaired resting coronary blood flow were excluded from analysis to constrain observations in the subcritical range. Percent systolic shortening was determined by calculating the ratio of end-diastolic segment length minus end-systolic segment length to end-diastolic segment length multiplied by 100.

The coronary flow reserve was expressed as a percent of the maximal coronary flow reserve obtained in the absence of a coronary stenosis. The percent of maximal coronary flow reserve was determined by:

$$\frac{CFR - 1}{CFRmax - 1} \times 100\%,$$

where CFR = measured coronary flow reserve associated with any lesion, and CFRmax = the maximal coronary flow reserve in the absence of a coronary stenosis.

Patient studies

Group A [4] included 19 patients without angiographic evidence of collateral vessels or previous myocardial infarction. Group B [4] included 20 patients with angiographically visible collateral vessels to a distal segment of an obstructed artery. Twelve had electrocardiographic and angiographic evidence of previous myocardial infarction (inferior in eight, lateral in two and anterior in two). A third group of 18 patients [5] was found to have angiographically normal coronary arteries. No patient had valvular heart disease, cardiomyopathy or a history of electrocardiographic evidence of myocardial infarction. Hypertension (blood pressure > 160/100 mmHg) or a history of hypertension controlled by medications was noted in 11 cases.

Radionuclide techniques

Exercise electrocardiography with thallium-201 perfusion imaging. Symptom-limited treadmill exercise was performed using the standard Bruce protocol with 12 lead electrocardiographic monitoring.

Thallium-201 (2.5 mCi) was injected intravenously 1 minute before discontinuation of exercise. Three myocardial scintigrams (40/ and 70/ anterior and left anterior oblique) were performed beginning approximately 8 minutes after cessation of exercise. Redistribution images were obtained 3 hours later using constant time of acquisition. Images were interpreted visually by the consensus of three experienced observers without knowledge of the patients' clinical status or the results of other tests. Semiquantitative grading of thallium uptake in each region in the rest and exercise images was based on a 3-point scoring method (0 = normal, 1 = mildly reduced, 2 = severely reduced). Fixed abnormalities were excluded from all statistical comparisons so that a difference in the regional exercise minus redistribution score of 1 or greater signified a positive test, reflecting exercise-induced ischemia. Quantitative analysis was used to substantiate the final interpretation. Once determined, myocardial regions were assigned to the coronary artery that provided the blood supply.

Radionuclide ventriculography. After in vivo labeling of red blood cells by technetium-99m (25 mCi), supine rest radionuclide ventriculography was performed in the left lateral and right and left anterior oblique views. With the camera in the left anterior oblique position, multistage exercise was begun at a workload of 200 kilopond-meters (kpm) and increased by 200 kpm every 3 minutes up to a symptom-limited maximal workload. Postpeak exercise right anterior oblique and left lateral views were also obtained while the patients continued to exercise at a reduced workload (200 or 300 kpm). Scintigraphy was performed in the left anterior oblique projection during the last 2 minutes of each stage.

Regional wall motion was assessed visually in three left ventricular segments in each view using a 3-point scoring method (0 = normal, 1 = hypokinesia, 2 = akinesia or dyskinesia). Regional exercise-induced dysfunction was defined as an increase in regional wall score of 1 or greater. Regions with abnormalities at rest that did not change with exercise were excluded from the statistical analyses. In the left anterior oblique view, one anteroseptal, one inferoapical and one posterolateral segment were analyzed. The left lateral and right anterior oblique views were used to substantiate the final interpretation and were each divided into three segments (anterior, apical, posterior and anterolateral, apical, inferior, respectively). Once determined, regional scintigraphic findings were assigned to the coronary artery that perfused the corresponding region.

Angiographic techniques

Cardiac catheterization. Selective coronary arteriography was performed in multiple projections by the Judkins technique; contrast left ventriculography was performed in the right anterior oblique projection. The maximal luminal narrowing of each of the three major coronary arteries was identified, and a fully automated quantitative program was used to determine percent diameter stenosis. In brief, an independent observer chose a circular region of interest encompassing the arterial lesion to be analyzed, after which computer software determined a centerline over the arterial segment. Background-corrected, linear density profiles perpendicular to this centerline were analyzed to determine the location of the first and second derivatives. Initial edge points were defined as those points falling at a value of 75% of the difference between the densities at these derivative extremes (that is, weighted toward the first derivative location). Edge continuity was ensured by excluding edge points lying greater than 4 pixels from contiguous edge points. These points were replaced by linear interpolation from the densities at neightboring valid edge points. Minimal percent diameter stenosis from the digitized cine film was then determined, and results from two orthogonal views were averaged. The anatomic distribution of the coronary circulation was noted so that perfusion of a given myocardial region was established from the angiographic data.

Digital image acquisition and coronary flow measurements. Coronary flow reserve was determined using a digital angiographic technique previously described [6]. Angiograms were acquired on a digital angiographic computer (DPS-4100C, ADAC Laboratories) interfaced to a standard cineangiographic system (Philips Optimus M200). The radiographic input signal was kept constant (fixed kV, mA and pulse width X-ray exposure). Video output signals were directly converted into digital images by logarithmic analog to digital conversion. One image per cardiac cycle was obtained during cardiac diastasis in 512×512 eight bit-mode matrices. Sodium meglumine diatrizoate (Renografin-76) was injected by means of an electrocardiographically triggered power injector (Medrad IV SYS 400), and the patient was instructed to maintain held inspiration for 10 to 15 seconds during image acquisition.

To determine coronary flow reserve, images during basal and hyperemic conditions were obtained. First, the passage of a single bolus of contrast medium was recorded at rest, at least 3 minutes after any preceding injection of contrast. In a second run, usually 2 or 5 minutes later, images during contrast-induced hyperemic flow were obtained by recording the passage of a bolus of contrast 10 to 15 seconds after a prior injection of contrast. The heart rate was kept constant during image acquisition by atrial pacing at a rate 5 beats/min higher than the basal heart rate.

Image processing was performed using standard mask-mode subtraction. The last single frame obtained before contrast administration was selected as the mask, and five to seven subsequent end-diastolic frames with contrast were selected as the image subset. A single contrast intensity and appearance time color-modulated functional image was then generated from each set of enhanced frames. On this functional image, the intensity value of each pixel corresponded to the cumulative contrast density reached during image acquisition. The appearance time of contrast was color-modulated, with a different color being assigned to each postcontrast injection cardiac cycle. Only pixels with an intensity above a preset threshold appeared on the final picture. This threshold was set at a level that excluded most of the background noise intensity. Acquisition and processing were identical for each paired basal and hyperemic image so that each set was technically comparable.

Mean myocardial appearance time and density for a region of interest, defined by the operator on the baseline and hyperemic images, was determined by automatic histographic analysis. Because contrast density is directly related to the volume of distribution in the myocardium and flow is inversely related to myocardial contrast appearance time, digital estimation of mean lesional coronary flow was calculated as:

$$Q \; \alpha \; \text{volume/time} \; \alpha \; kCD/AT,$$

where Q = mean regional coronary flow, CD = mean cumulative contrast density, AT = mean appearance time and k = radiographic constant. Because each pair was radiographically identical, coronary flow reserve, or the ratio of hyperemic (H) to basal (B) coronary flow, was given by:

$$\text{Coronary flow reserve} = Q_H/Q_B = (CD_H/AT_H)/CD_B/AT_B).$$

Results and conclusions

Animal studies

Fig. 1 shows that regional dysfunction during dopamine infusion was not consistently observed despite production of coronary stenoses resulting in total loss of reactive hyperemia at rest. Fig. 2 shows that relative regional function in response to isoproterenol infusion was maintained during the infusion until nearly total loss of coronary flow reserve. With this near-critical stenosis, function was lower than in the non-stenotic state but remained greater than resting control values. Moderate impairments of coronary flow reserve were not associated with isoproterenol-induced deterioration of regional function. Fig. 3 shows a curvilinear relation between pacing-induced deterioration of segment shortening and impairment in reactive hyperemia at rest with the most substantial decrease in regional function occurring when less than 20 to 40% of control reactive hyperemia remained. This corresponded to

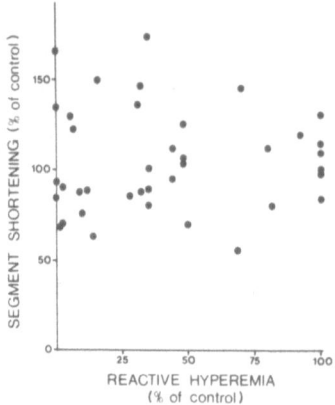

Fig. 1. The relation between graded impairments in coronary blood flow reserve at rest (reactive hyperemia) and regional function (segment shortening) (expressed as a percent of control) during dopamine infusion. (Reproduced with permission from [1].)

a reactive hyperemic ratio between 1.7 and 2.3. This nonlinear relation was paralleled by the relation between deterioration of regional function and the percent of control blood flow recorded at the time of regional postpacing dysfunction in the presence of coronary stenosis.

It is concluded that coronary flow reserve may be substantially reduced before regional dysfunction induced by atrial pacing or catecholamine stress becomes pronounced. The extent of regional dysfunction during these stresses differed due primarily to different alterations in subendocardial blood flow occurring during the stress in the presence of coronary stenosis.

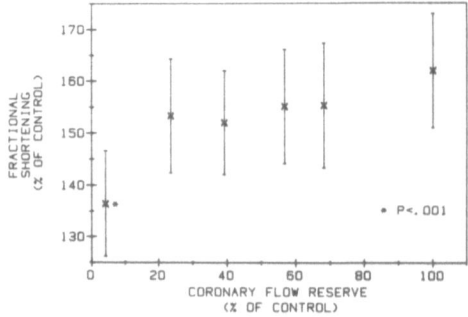

Fig. 2. The relation between coronary flow reserve and fractional shortening during isoproterenol infusion is shown. Significant deterioration occurred only in the face of near absence of coronary flow reserve. (Reproduced with permission from [2].)

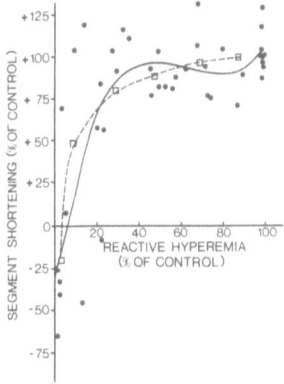

Fig. 3. Regional segment shortening expressed as a percent of rest control shortening decreased progressively as reactive hyperemia at rest was impaired. The *open squares* and *dotted line* represent the mean flow reserve and percent segment shortening values of six subgroups with increasing coronary stenosis. The *solid line* is the relation between impairment in reactive hyperemia and postpacing segment shortening that best fit the individual data points (*solid circles*). The shoulder of this curve occurs between 20 and 40% reactive hyperemia. (Reproduced with permission from [3].)

Patient studies

In Group A (Fig. 4), coronary flow reserve was inversely related to percent diameter stenosis ($r = -0.61$, $p < 0.001$), and scintigraphic abnormalities occurred only in vascular distributions with a coronary flow reserve of less than 2.00 (Figs 5, 6). There was a strong relation among abnormal regional exercise results, stenoses greater than 50% and reactive hyperemia of less than 2.00

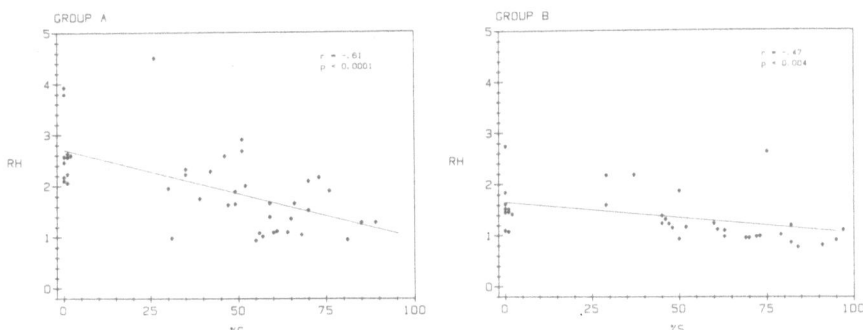

Fig. 4. Relation between quantitative percent diameter stenosis (%S) and reactive hyperemia (RH) in Group A (without collateral vessels) and Group B (with collateral vessels). (Reproduced with permission from [4].)

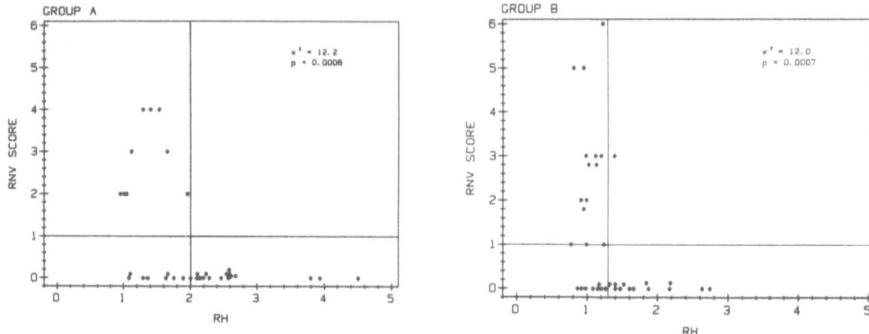

Fig. 5. Relation between reactive hyperemia (RH) and exercise radionuclide ventriculography (RNV). RNV score = the difference in radionuclide ventriculographic wall motion scores between exercise and rest evaluations, with a score of 1 or greater signifying a positive test; X^2 = the measured chi-squared value. (Adapted from [4].)

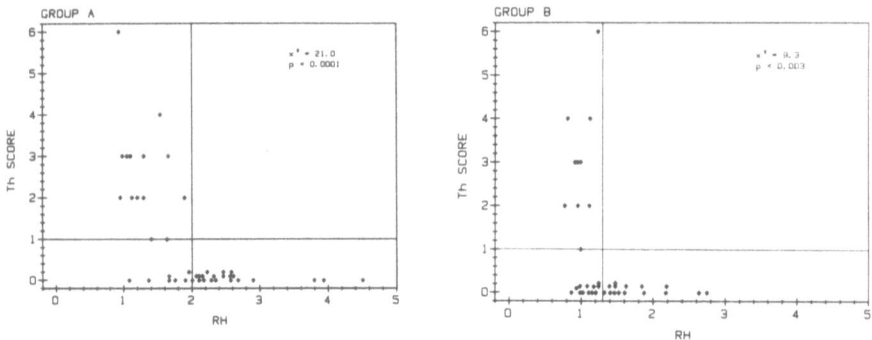

Fig. 6. Relation between reactive hyperemia (RH) and exercise thallium-201 (Th) scintigraphy. Th score = the difference in regional thallium scores between exercise and redistribution images, with a score of 1 or greater signifying a positive test; other abbreviations as in Fig. 5. (Adapted from [4].)

(Figs 7, 8). Patients with multivessel disease, however, often had normal exercise scintigrams in regions associated with greater than 50% stenosis and low coronary flow reserve when other regions in the same patient had a lower coronary flow reserve.

In Group B (Fig. 4) coronary flow reserve correlated less well with percent diameter stenosis than in Group A (r = −0.47, p < 0.004). As in Group A patients, there was a significant relation between abnormal exercise test results and stenoses greater than 50% (Figs 7, 8). However, reactive hyperemia values were generally lower than in Group A, and positive exercise stress results were strongly correlated only with highly impaired flow reserves of 1.3

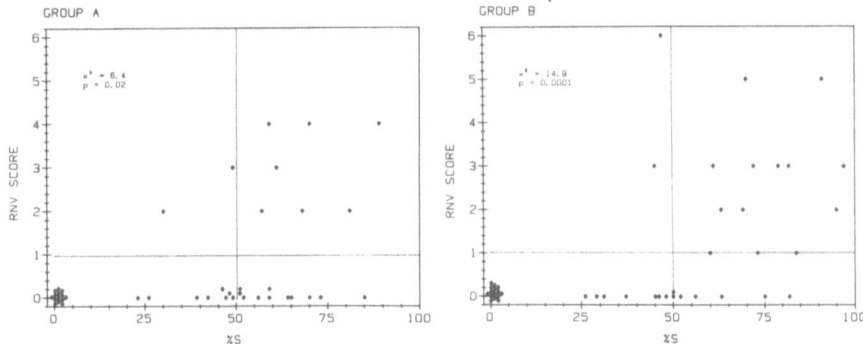

Fig. 7. Relation between exercise radionuclide venticulographic test results and quantitative percent diameter stenosis (%S) in Group A (without collateral vessels) and Group B (with collateral vessels). Format as in Fig. 5. (Reproduced with permission from [4].)

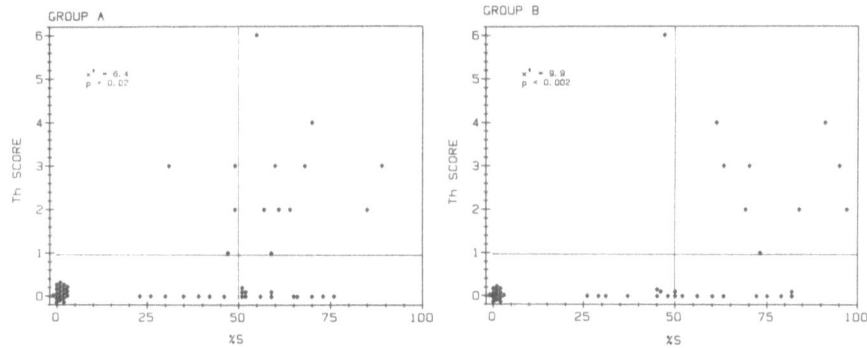

Fig. 8. Relation between exercise thallium-201 tests and quantitative percent diameter stenosis (%S) in Group A (without collateral vessels) and Group B (with collateral vessels). (Reproduced with permission from [4].)

or less (Figs 5, 6). In Group B patients, the coronary flow reserve of vessels with less than 50% stenosis was significantly lower than that of similar vessels in Group A patients (2.40 ± 0.79 versus 1.56 ± 0.43; $p < 0.0002$).

It is concluded that:

1. there is a general relation between quantitative percent diameter stenosis and reactive hyperemia that is not of sufficient precision to allow accurate prediction of coronary flow reserve in individual cases;

2. exercise scintigraphic abnormalities are usually associated with low coronary flow reserve, and the relation between these two functional tests is stronger than the relation between exercise test results and quantitative percent diameter stenosis;

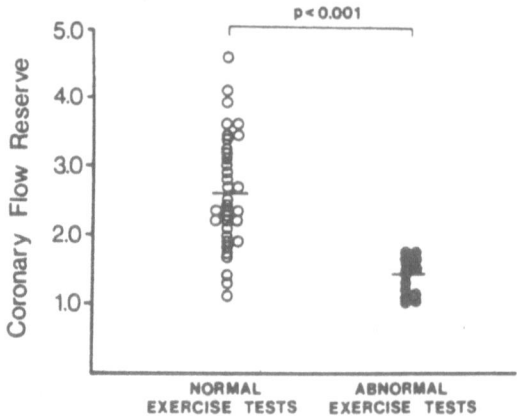

Fig. 9. Coronary flow reserve for arterial distributions without (*open circles*) and with (*closed circles*) radionuclide abnormalities (exercise thallium-201 scintigraphy or radionuclide ventriculography, or both), in patients with normal coronary arteriograms. (Reproduced with permission from [5].)

3. exercise scintigraphy underestimates the number of regions supplied by arteries with physiologically significant stenosis in patients with multivessel disease; and
4. in the presence of collateral vessels, profound alterations in coronary flow dynamics occur that preclude the use of coronary flow reserve as a reliable indicator of the functional significance of stenoses except when flow reserve is severely impaired.

In the patients with normal coronary arteries, the coronary flow reserve of arterial distributions with abnormal perfusion or regional dysfunction was significantly lower than that of distributions associated with normal radionuclide results (1.42 ± 0.23 versus 2.58 ± 0.83, $p < 0.001$) (Fig. 9).

All patients with abnormal scintigraphic results had low coronary flow reserve (< 2.00) in at least one distribution. Perfusion abnormalities appeared to be more localized in the arterial distributions with the lowest flow reserve. Only two patients had low flow reserve with normal scintigraphic results; both were hypertensive. These data suggest that abnormal exercise scintigraphic finding in patients with angiographically normal coronary arteries and chest pain are indicative of true blood flow or perfusion abnormalities and should not be considered false positive results.

Acknowledgment

These projects were supported in part by a grant from the Veterans Administration, Washington, D.C. entitled 'Correlation of ischemic dysfunction and impaired hyperemic reserve' (GBJM).

References

1. Hodgson JMcB, Mancini GBJ: Relation of coronary blood flow and reactive hyperemia to regional dysfunction induced by dopamine infusion in dogs: Limitations in detecting subcritical coronary stenoses. JACC 1985; 5: 664–671.
2. Mancini GBJ, Friedman HZ, Hramiec JE, Deboe SF: Relation between graded, subcritical impairments of coronary flow reserve and regional myocardial dysfunction induced by isoproterenol infusion in dogs. Am Heart J 1987; 113: 906–916.
3. Hodgson JMcB, Mancini GBJ: Relation between graded, subcritical impairments of coronary flow reserve and regional myocardial dysfunction induced by atrial pacing in dogs. JACC 1985; 5: 1116–1124.
4. Legrand V, Mancini GBJ, Bates ER, Hodgson JMcB, Aueron FM, Smith JS, Gross MD, Vogel RA: A comparative study of coronary flow reserve, coronary anatomy and the results of radionuclide exercise tests in patients with coronary artery disease. J Am Coll Cardiol 1986; 8: 1022–1032.
5. Legrand V, Hodgson JMcB, Bates ER, Aueron FM, Mancini GBJ, Smith JS, Gross MD, Vogel RA: Abnormal coronary flow reserve and abnormal radionuclide exercise tests in patients with normal coronary angiograms. J Am Coll Cardiol 1985; 1245–1253.
6. Hodgson JMcB, Legrand V, Bates ER, Mancini GBJ, Aueron FM, O'Neill WW, Simon SB, Beauman GJ, LeFree MT, Vogel RA: Validation in dogs of a rapid digital angiographic technique to measure relative coronary blood flow during routine cardiac catheterization. Am J Cardiol 1985; 55: 188–198.

28. Functional and Anatomic Assessment of Coronary Artery Stenoses

K. LANCE GOULD

Positron Diagnostic and Research Center, University of Texas Medical School at Houston, Houston, TX, USA

Introduction

Coronary heart disease remains the leading cause of death in the United States and most technologically advanced countries despite declining cardiovascular mortality since 1968. It is responsible for 640,000 deaths each year, including almost a third of all deaths between the ages of 35 and 64 years old [1].

Sixty per cent of patients with sudden death of myocardial infarction present with no prior symptoms [2–5]. Up to 13% of middle aged men in the general population have coronary artery disease [6, 7], apparently without symptoms. Silent ischemia is increasingly recognized in symptomatic and asymptomatic individals [8, 9] and may have a less favorable prognosis in the asymptomatic patient [10]. Finally, the community model of mass intervention for coronary atherosclerosis has been of questionable benefit compared to the medical model of intervention by risk factor control in specific individuals [11]. However, even assuming its effectiveness, the medical model of risk factor control is limited by the low sensitivity and specificity with which risk factors identify individuals who have significant coronary artery disease. For example, two thirds of healthy adult males, aged 40–55, who have the highest cholesterol and blood pressure risk factors remain well over the subsequent 25 years [12]. Consequently, a screening method for detection of early coronary artery disease (CAD) and a satisfactory way of objectively defining its severity in apparently healthy individuals would be useful for early therapy aimed at reversal or prevention of sequelae in specific individuals.

In the presence of clinically significant coronary artery disease, exercise frequently causes regional myocardial ischemia associated with angina, EKG abnormalities and defects on perfusion images. Therefore, diagnostic exercise stress has been a practical and useful procedure in evaluating coronary artery disease. However, current non-invasive diagnostic techniques have limited accuracy for detection of CAD in not only symptomatic, but particularly asymptomatic individuals. The exercise electrocardiogam may be diagnosti-

P.H. Heintzen and J.H. Bürsch (eds), Progress in Digital Angiocardiography. ISBN 978-94-010-7093-5
© 1988, Kluwer Academic Publishers, Dordrecht

cally and prognostically useful in patients with symptomatic ischemic heart disease but is limited in its specificity and sensitivity. For asymptomatic individuals, its sensitivity and specificity is so limited [13, 14] as to be nearly useless as a screening procedure. The technique of rest-exercise scintigraphy depends on imaging a radionuclide which is distributed to the myocardium in proportion to regional myocardial blood flow during stress. Abnormal stress images indicate sufficiently severe coronary artery disease to limit the blood flow increase in response to stress as compared to the normally greater flow increase through coronary arteries without significant disease. The sensitivity and specificity of exercise thallium imaging is about 80–90% in symptomatic patients but falls to unacceptably low levels in asymptomatic individuals.

Traditionally, the trigger for activating cardiovascular medicine has been symptoms, particularly of angina pectoris or myocardial infarction since coronary artery disease remains the dominant problem. Based on symptoms, appropriate non-invasive or invasive workup has been undertaken with medical or surgical treatment of symptoms or complications. Medical treatment by the cardiologist has been viewed as a stabilizing step. Surgery has been viewed as a definitive, albeit palliative step, carried out by the surgeon to whom the cardiologist refers his patients. The essence of this approach is reactive or passive, i.e., the treatment of symptoms or consequences of disease balanced against the risk of therapy, particularly for bypass surgery. Although saphenous vein bypass grafting undoubtedly prolongs life in certain subsets of patients with coronary artery disease, its greatest raison d'etre has been the treatment of angina pectoris.

The development of two technologies for routine clinical use, positron imaging and PTCA, has provided the technological basis for a profound change in this approach. Positron imaging is now routinely applicable for clinical cardiac applications with clinically oriented cameras available commercially and generator-produced Rb-82 as a positron tracer suitable for all cardiac studies without the cost of a cyclotron, thereby making cardiac PET economical. Cardiac PET provides sensitivity and specificity approaching 98% in asymptomatic or symptomatic man, an accuracy sufficient to use it for routine economical screening for CAD. No other non-invasive diagnostic modality, including other high-tech imaging methods, provides comparable information.

Current positron cameras have evolved through many design generations, and are clinically dedicated instruments with user-friendly, clinically validated software. For example, currently at the University of Texas, routine positron imaging is carried out for clinical diagnosis or assessment of stenosis severity by a nurse-technician team. A physician supervises the procedure without hands-on requirements by a physician. The rubidium-82 generator provides an economical source of positron radionuclide without the expense or complexity of a cyclotron. This single radionuclide is suitable for all current nuclear cardiac studies. The clinical value of positron imaging has been well documented, such as screening for coronary artery disease [15–21], assessment of physiologic severity of stenoses [15, 16, 34], myocardial infarct imaging [22–32], assessment of reperfusion and viability [23–28, 33], for assessing effects of interventions [27, 84], for identification of significant collateral function [35], and 3D imaging of LV performance [15, 36].

A formerly diagnostic procedure, cardiac catheterization, has become therapeutic and carried out by the cardiologist with potentially less risk than surgery. Furthermore, the goal of therapy has extended beyond relief of cardiac symptoms alone. It now involves the prevention of myocardial infarction and definitive restoration of coronary artery lumen with an overt goal of prolonging life. Although reactive treatment triggered by symptoms appropriately remains central to cardiovascular medicine, the widespread acceptance of more complex, ambitious goals for the patient at lower risk has been a major conceptual and technologic advance, bringing us to present-day practice. As a consequence of these epidemiologic observations and evolving imaging technology, this reviewer believes that another major step in the evolution of cardiovascular medicine has begun.

This next major step in our approach to cardiovascular medicine involves routine screening for coronary artery disease in asymptomatic as well as symptomatic patients by positron imaging. A variety of potent therapeutic algorithms may then be brought to bear on specific patients with known disease in order to prevent sudden death, acute myocardial infarction or other complications.

In the absence of symptoms, quantification of stenosis severity will be necessary both functionally and anatomically, since in these patients, therapeutic decisions will be required based on measured severity of lesions. Waiting for symptoms in patients with anatomically and functionally significant but silent coronary artery disease will place that individual at risk of sudden death or acute myocardial infarction, which is the presenting manifestation of disease in the majority of patients. Because of its highly selected population of the 'survivors' of existing disease, the benign course of patients with mildly symptomatic CAD cannot be extrapolated to the population with CAD identified by screening tests. Accurate quantitation of stenoses both functionally and anatomically thus becomes central to these advanced diagnostic and therapeutic technologies.

Consequently, we have proposed coronary flow reserve as a single measure of stenosis severity which is conceptually more physiologically oriented and more easily measured in the physiology lab by flow meter or radiolabeled microspheres [15, 16, 37–44]. With current development of positron emission tomography into a practical and affordable clinical method for assessing perfusion, the non-invasive determination of coronary flow reserve in man now also appears feasible. Although our initial studies beginning some years ago indicated the potential value of measuring coronary flow reserve, there has only recently been a rigorous, systematic theoretical or experimental proof to date that coronary flow reserve reflects the effects of all the combined, integrated dimensions of a tapering coronary artery stenosis in vivo [45–47].

Accordingly, the approach to this problem requires consideration of two different basic concepts about how stenosis severity is quantified: anatomically and functionally. The *anatomic* severity of a coronary lesion is measured in geometric terms, i.e., per cent narrowing, absolute diameter, length, and shape. Quantitative coronary arteriography delineates these dimensions which are then used to calculate the functional or pressure flow characteristics according to theoretical fluid dynamic equations. The *functional* severity of a stenosis is described in physiologic terms, i.e. by directly measured coronary blood flow, pressure gradient or distal perfusion pressure, and coronary flow reserve from which certain deductions about geometric severity can be made.

Both the anatomic and functional approaches to quantifying severity are derived from, or related to, fluid dynamics of flow in narrowed tubes. In theory, therefore, the two approaches should be interchangeable and equivalent both mathematically and experimentally. The purpose here is to provide an overview of functional and anatomic approaches for quantifying severity of coronary artery stenoses, to outline their validation in the literature and to indicate the remaining problems.

Anatomic imaging of the coronary arteries

Visual interpretations of coronary arteriograms are marked by such great interobserver and intraobserver variability that comparison of arteriograms from different subjects, or at different times in the same subject, are of limited value for assessing severity, changes in severity, or functional significance of coronary artery stenoses. The universal use of relative per cent diameter narrowing as a clinical measure of severity ignores other geometric characteristics of stenoses such as length, absolute diameter, multiple lesions in series or eccentric narrowings which may be worse in one view as compared to another view.

Quantitative coronary arteriography was originally proposed by Brown et al. [48] based on fluid dynamic studies by Young et al. [49] and Mates et al. [50] and subsequently validated in vivo by Gould et al. [45–47]. It requires high quality coronary arteriograms taken in two views angled at 90° to each other. Significant errors appear with deviation from orthogonal views [51]. The X-rays may then be processed in two different ways. In the first, the images are

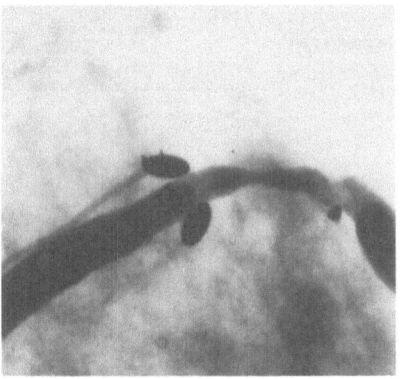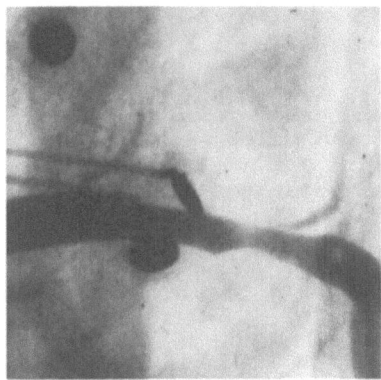

Fig. 1. Orthogonal arteriogram suitable for automated quantitation analysis.

optically magnified onto a digitizing tablet with the borders of the artery traced by hand and thereby digitized for computer processing [46–48, 52–54]. There is some subjectivity in tracing the arterial borders visually. In the second approach, the entire region of interest on the arteriogram is digitized with the borders of the artery identified automatically by computer software without visual interpretation [15, 45, 55, 56]. In our laboratory, this automated computer technique utilizes an edge detection method as well as analysis of the integrated optical density (gray scale) diametrically across the artery image. The cross-sectional areas measured by both techniques are automatically compared for each segment of the artery. Disagreements between the two methods may occur, especially for eccentric lesions in which the border recognition technique using orthogonal biplane views is not as accurate as the densitometry technique [45, 55], or in cases where other optically dense structures (catheters, other vessels, etc.) are superimposed on the arterial segment of interest. In the latter circumstance, the diameter is best determined by the automated border recognition approach. An example of the arteriogram is shown in Fig. 1 and of an automated analysis in Fig. 2 showing the arterial borders identified automatically. Also shown are the diameters of the artery measured at increments along the long axis of the stenosis for purposes of computing the various geometric dimensions of the lesion.

After the borders of the opacified artery on the arteriogram are identified, the stenosis is analyzed by quantitatively adding the exit losses to the integrated viscous losses along the length of the stenosis. The final computer print-out gives the measured dimensions and predicted pressure drop for a given coronary flow as well as the pressure gradient-flow relation [15–45]. It should be emphasized that quantitative arteriography above cannot predict the actual flow or the actual gradient unless flow is independently measured.

310

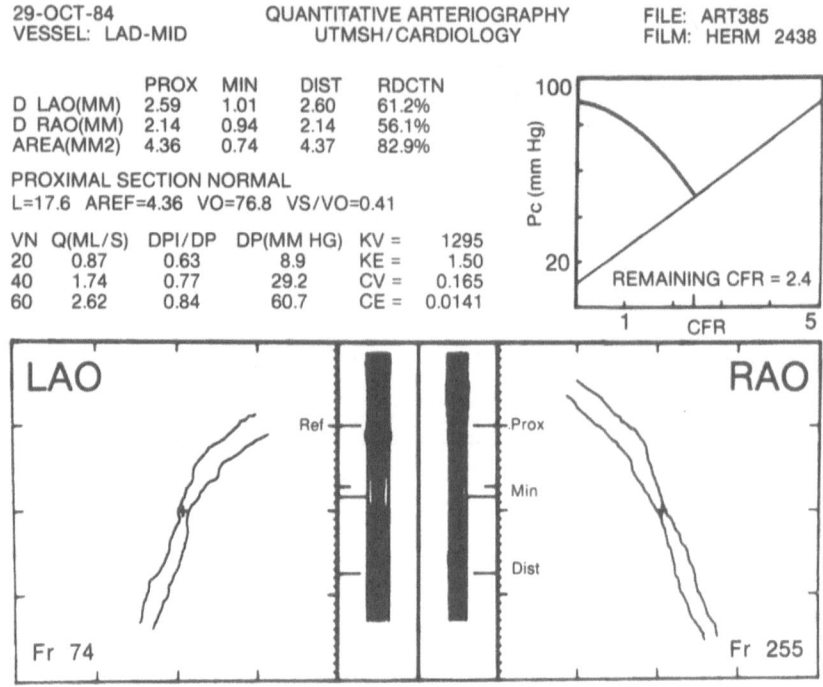

Fig. 2. Printout of automated quantitative analysis of coronary artery stenosis.

Since that is not possible in man, it predicts the pressure gradient-flow relations, i.e. the range of gradients, for a range of flows. The automated technique is accurate to 0.1 mm [15, 45, 55, 56] for absolute dimensions. The
reproducibility of any given dimension utilizing this approach is remarkably
good with approximately ± 2% to 3% variation on sequential repeated X-rays
of the same stenosis. As demonstrated by Brown et al. [54] such geometric
accuracy allows intervention studies using relatively small numbers of patients
in randomized therapeutic trials. Quantitative coronary arteriography is
therefore of great value in determining progression or regression of coronary
disease.

Functional analysis of coronary artery stenosis

Pressure gradient-flow relation

The functional severity of a coronary artery narrowing may also be defined by
the relation of pressure gradient to flow, measured directly by implanted

instruments without knowledge of anatomic geometry [39]. Coronary artery stenosis not only reduces the maximum increase in coronary flow but also causes a reduction in distal coronary perfusion pressure due to pressure losses across the stenosis. There is a direct correlation between the degree of flow increase and the increase in the pressure gradient across the stenosis. Coronary vascular bed vasodilatation may cause a modest increase in total arterial coronary flow, but it is associated with a large fall in distal coronary perfusion pressure [38, 39] with attendant fall in subendocardial perfusion [43, 57, 58]. This quantitative relation between coronary blood flow and the pressure gradient across the stenosis during diastole is a hemodynamic measure of stenosis severity. In the absence of a stenosis, there is a mild (5 to 8 mmHg) gradient at maximum flows following administration of a potent coronary vasodilator. In the presence of a stenosis, the pressure gradient-flow relation becomes much steeper, with a higher pressure gradient for any given flow. With a severe coronary stenosis, this relation becomes very steep, with a large increase in pressure gradient for a small increase in coronary flow caused by distal arteriolar vasodilation. This pressure gradient-flow relation acquired during diastole characterizes the functional severity of coronary artery stenoses in hemodynamic terms rather than in terms of anatomic geometry [15, 45–47].

For a fixed stenosis, the pressure gradient increases in a curvelinear relation to flow according to quadratic fluid dynamic equations accounting for viscous and inertial pressure losses. For anatomic analysis of angiograms, X-ray geometry is used to determine the viscous and inertial coefficients of the fluid dynamic equations from geometric dimensions [15, 45–47]. In functional or hemodynamic analysis, many simultaneous pressure gradients and coronary flows are directly measured over a wide range from low to high coronary flows. The values of the coefficients are then determined by an iterative process of finding the quadratic equation best fitting the directly measured pressure flow data [39, 46]. This approach is suitable only for experimental animals in which direct pressure flow measurements can be made by implanted instruments.

Coronary flow reserve

An essential concept relating stenosis anatomy to its functional effects is that of coronary flow reserve. It is defined as the ratio of maximum coronary flow after a maximal vasodilatory stimulus to resting flow, as first described experimentally by Gould et al. [37] and explained in fluid dynamic terms by Young et al. [49, 59–62] and Mates et al. [50]. Under resting conditions, coronary blood flow in an artery does not change until a relatively tight stenosis of 80–85% diameter narrowing. However, coronary flow reserve is impaired at 40–50% diameter narrowing, whereas flow in a normal artery increases three to four times in response to a vasodilatory stimulus such as pharmacologic coronary vasodilators, a brief coronary occlusion or physical stress. The normal three-to-four-fold relative increase after a vasodilatory stimulus identifies a coronary flow reserve of three to four. Coronary artery narrowing limits this coronary flow reserve to an extent that is proportional to the severity of the stenosis. This approach to evaluating coronary stenoses has been shown practical experimentally and clinically. For a stimulus which normally increases coronary flow to five or six times baseline levels, coronary flow reserve becomes impaired with mild stenoses 3 to 12 mm long of an approximately 30% to 40% diameter narrowing of a 3 mm diameter artery.

Isolated measurement of one dimension of a stenosis

Quantitation of arterial stenosis in vivo has been sufficiently complex and poorly understood in terms of basic theory, physiologic-hemodynamic effects, experimental preparation and imaging technology that a number of studies have utilized indices or approximate estimates of severity. The old issue of the relative value of per cent diameter narrowing versus absolute diameter narrowing is an example of controversy based upon approximations or incomplete analysis and lack of perspective into the multiple facets of the fluid dynamics or physiology involved.

The limitations of per cent diameter narrowing compared to absolute diameter was proposed as long as 20 years ago [63] with the discussion continuing to our own analysis integrating both approaches with fluid dynamic principles [45]. The issue frequently resurfaces, possibly in part due to lack of considering all the aspects of the problem based on complete fluid dynamic equations. For example, Collins et al. [64], White et al. [65], Harrison et al. [66] and Marcus et al. [67, 68] reconfirmed previous reports on the limitations of per cent diameter narrowing as a measure of stenosis severity by comparison to coronary flow reserve. They concluded that absolute diameter is a more important measure of severity. A generally applicable description of stenosis severity requires both absolute diameter and relative per cent narrowing in addition to length, absolute diameter of the normal artery and blood viscosity. In any given circumstance one of these factors may be the dominant contributor to total pressure loss. For example, for mild diffuse narrowing with no discrete stenosis, absolute diameter and length of the diffusely involved segment might be the most important geometry. On the other hand, for a short orifice like stenosis, per cent diameter narrowing might be most important. Most lesions are between these extremes. Their studies, however, do reemphasize the importance of functional assessment of stenosis severity using coronary flow reserve as we originally proposed.

Stenosis flow reserve bases on geometric stenosis dimensions by invasive QCA

Since our first introduction of the concept, we are evolving toward the viewpoint that maximum myocardial perfusion, or coronary flow reserve, may, per se, be the best integrated, single measure of stenosis severity reflecting all its combined geometric and fluid dynamic characteristics. The measurement of coronary flow reserve also reflects, or is affected by, diffuse narrowing where the entire artery is smaller than it would normally be relative to the size of its distal vascular bed.

We have previously documented the necessity of accounting for all stenosis dimensions which affect hemodynamic severity of stenoses. Per cent diameter narrowing correlates poorly with directly measured or arteriographically determined coronary flow reserve as described above, taking into account all stenosis dimensions of length, absolute diameter, relative per cent narrowing and asymmetry. Thus, per cent diameter narrowing is not very useful as a reference standard for measuring stenosis severity. For example, a 60% diameter narrowing is associated with a range of arteriographically determined coronary flow reserves from 1.5 to 4.5, based on all stenosis dimensions. Since the defects seen on perfusion images during pharmacologic stress are related to coronary flow reserve, those defects do not relate to per cent diameter narrowing. Therefore, we no longer utilize per cent diameter narrowing alone as the reference gold standard for determining physiologic significance or sensitivity and specificity of imaging techniques for diagnosing coronary artery disease.

Per cent area reduction also correlates poorly with arteriographically determined coronary flow reserve based on all dimensions. For example, an 80% area reduction is associated with an arteriographically determined coronary flow reserve ranging from 2 to 4.5, depending on the absolute dimensions. We therefore have also rejected area reduction alone as a reference gold standard. Minimum absolute cross-sectional lumen area of the stenosis has been previously suggested as a better measure of stenosis severity than per cent narrowing. However, minimum absolute lumen area of the stenosis also correlates poorly with arteriographically determined coronary flow reserve based on all stenosis dimensions. The correlation is poor because the effect of a given absolute minimum area will depend on the absolute diameter of the normal proximal artery and its length. A given stenosis cross-sectional area does not impair coronary flow reserve of a normally small vessel but will reduce coronary flow reserve of a large artery. For example, an absolute stenosis minimum area of 1 mm^2 may be associated with a coronary flow reserve ranging from 1.5 to 4.5 depending on the diameter of the normal artery as well as the length of the stenosis. We have therefore rejected absolute cross-sectional lumen area of the stenosis as a reference gold standard of stenosis severity. Thus, coronary flow reserve is a single integrated measurement of severity, accounting for all stenosis dimensions of length, absolute diameter, relative per cent narrowing and asymmetry [15, 45]. It may be directly measured or determined arteriographically based on all stenosis dimensions of absolute diameter, relative per cent narrowing, integrated length effects and asymmetry.

Arteriographically determined coronary flow reserve is theoretically and experimentally closely related to the relative distribution of a perfusion tracer in the heart during maximal coronary vasodilation. Accordingly, clinical coronary arteriograms in our laboratory are quantitatively analyzed by a completely automated technique utilizing simultaneously both border recognition algorithms and integrated, arterial cross-sectional densiometry to obtain all geometric dimensions of the stenosis with an accuracy of ± 0.1 mm for diameters less than 0.5 mm and a reproduceability of 2–3%. The program also predicts the pressure-flow characteristics [12, 22] and coronary flow reserve of the stenosis based on precise geometric dimensions as validated in vivo by direct flowmeter-pressure measurements in instrumented dogs. For comparison purposes, geometrically determined CFR by quantitative coronary arteriography has been compared to rest-stress positron imaging in patients with, or studied for, coronary artery disease. Signifcant coronary disease was defined as an arteriographically determined coronary flow reserve of less than 3.0 for any stenosis in one or more major proximal coronary arteries. For perfusion imaging by positron emission tomography, optimal coronary vasodilation was achieved using intravenous dipyridamole combined with hand grip stress [15, 40–44]. Since N-13 ammonia, previously described as a perfusion imaging agent [15, 16, 44] requires a cyclotron, a more readily obtainable radionuclide, Rb-82, from a ^{82}Sr-^{82}Rb generator has also been developed for intravenous injection as a perfusion indicator [15, 69–73] at rest and during coronary vasodilation. Simultaneous multislice tomography of the entire heart was carried out using the state-of-the-art University of Texas positron camera [15, 74–78].

The preliminary results of blinded reading of images indicate that our protocol, consisting of intravenous dipyridamole combined with hand grip stress, and positron tomography of the entire heart using the University of Texas positron camera, shows stress perfusion defects in 98% of patients with significant coronary artery disease, defined as a geometrically determined coronary flow reserve of less than 3. These results indicate that X-ray determined coronary flow reserve is a single measure of stenosis severity, taking into account all its geometric dimensions and correlates with perfusion defects seen by state-of-the-art positron imaging.

Functional imaging of coronary artery disease

Myocardial perfusion reserve by non-invasive positron imaging

In the past, positron emission tomography has been a complicated, expensive, imaging technology requiring a team of radiochemists, physicists, and physicians to carry out research studies providing important medical information, but limited in clinical application due to their complexity. The technology has now evolved into routinely applicable clinical equipment and procedures which provide information not previously obtainable with potentially significant impact on medical diagnosis and therapy. These technologic advances in positron emission tomography thus allow new approaches to management of cardiovascular disease including screening for coronary disease in asymptomatic individuals. More specific therapy not suitable for a general population without known disease may then be used aimed at preventing sudden death or myocardial infarction, reversing atheromatous progression, preventing coronary thrombosis, assessing thrombolysis or PTCA in patients undergoing acute myocardial infarction. Positron imaging therefore may provide the basis for specific therapeutic approaches toward preventing sequelae of CAD in specific individuals, thereby justifying the routine, clinical, economical use of positron emission tomography in cardiology.

Basic principles

Positron emission tomography utilizes coincidence counting of paired gamma photons produced by positron annihilation. Current positron cameras consist of up to 6 rings of rectangular, closely packed detectors providing multiple tomographic image planes for quantitation of a 3-dimensional reconstruction of activity in the field of view [15, 74–78]. The technology has been evolving for the past 15 years through multiple generations of cameras and radiochemistry techniques. It is, therefore, a mature technology suitable for major financial investment with little risk of rapid obsolescence.

Three characteristics of positron cameras are essential for all medical imaging, but particularly for cardiac imaging. The first is a camera design with overlapping image planes such that sampling is uniform between detector rings [15, 79]. If there is undersampling between image planes, artifactual defects may occur in images or real defect may be missed; three-dimensional imaging requires overlapping image planes. Most current positron cameras demonstrate undersampling between image planes. Consequently, anatomic structures lying parallel to the imaging plane may demonstrate significant artifactual defects, or real defects may be missed, because of undersampling between banks of detectors. Accordingly, we have developed a camera design in which there is significant overlap of the image planes to provide adequate sampling uniformly throughout the field of view. Recovery of activity data is also limited by the partial volume problem which affects all positron tomography. However, because our camera has comparable resolution in the X, Y, and Z axes, the partial volume problems are minimized compared to other cameras without these features. The greater sensitivity of positron emission tomography for perfusion imaging in the diagnosis of coronary artery disease would appear to be due to technically better 3-dimensional imaging and data recovery as compared to standard imaging.

The second important characteristic of a medical positron camera is high sensitivity in order to maximize patient throughput and to acquire high count rates necessary for measuring the arterial input function and first pass extraction of various radiotracers [70–72]. For example, this characteristic theoretically allows the quantitative measurement of myocardial perfusion in ml/min/g of myocardium using Rb-82 or N-13 ammonia without assuming fixed extraction, which is known to fall by 50% or more at high coronary flow rates seen in stress imaging for diagnosis of CAD [70–72, 80, 81].

The third characteristic essential for a clinical camera is complete, user friendly, clinically oriented software for data analysis that has been developed and validated in clinical applications. For example, the majority of patients move slightly between the transmission, rest, and stress images, thereby producing incorrect attenuation. Artifactual defects may result, particularly of the left lateral free wall of the left ventricle. However, by software which superimposes the transmission and emission images, we routinely recognize translation between the transmission, rest or stress images and are able to reconstruct corrected images allowing accurate interpretation. We have minimized the heavy technological support usually needed for positron tomography by designing clinical software transparent to the user and validated for routine applications. Currently, a nurse and technician carry out each study using the rubidium generator with the physician being available to oversee patient management and safety.

Finally, for widespread routine cardiac practice, a simple-to-use radionuclide source is essential, such as the rubidium-82 generator, which does not require a cyclotron but allows all of the major aspects of cardiac imaging for clinical purposes as outlined below.

Clinical applications

Of the high-tech imaging techniques, positron emission tomography provides the greatest range of functional imaging as compared to other methods which may have better anatomic resolution [82]. The images obtained are therefore highly specific for the physiologic process being measured, such as perfusion, metabolism, or function. Accordingly, the application and interpretation of positron tomographs require a physician addressing a specific physiologic question in a specific patient.

A total of over 600 patients have been studied from eight major centers [15–32]. The results of these clinical studies document the following current clinical indications for cardiac PET:

1. *Non-invasive diagnosis of coronary artery disease as a screening test in either symptomatic or asymptomatic patients.* The sensitivity of diagnosing coronary artery disease by positron emission tomography in comparison to coronary arteriography approximates 95–98% with a 99–100% specificity, even in asymptomatic individuals [15–21]. This application is particularly suitable for patients with high risk factors for CAD.

2. *Assessment of the physiologic severity of coronary artery stenosis.* The quantitative severity of perfusion defects under stress conditions reflects the anatomic severity of the coronary artery stenosis as determined by automated, quantitative coronary arteriography taking into account length, absolute dimensions, and per cent narrowing of the stenosis [15, 34]. Therefore, non-invasive positron emission tomography may be used to assess the physiologic severity of coronary stenoses as well as changes in severity after an intervention such as PTCA [84], vasodilator drugs,re-gimens for cholesterol control, etc., which may affect stenosis geometry.

3. *Imaging myocardial infarction and viability.* The location and extent of myocardial infarction may be imaged by 3-dimensional positron emission tomography utilizing rubidium-82, N-13 ammonia and/or F-18-deoxy-glu-cose, FDG [22–32]. Myocardial perfusion images utilizing Rb-82 or N-13 ammonia indicate the underperfused area at risk for myocardial infarction. In the presence of injured, ischemic but viable myocardial cells, myocardial metabolism is shifted toward anaerobic glycolysis. FDG uptake then increases relative to the rest of the myocardium, thereby identifying ischemic, viable tissue since necrotic myocardium does not extract FDG [23–26]. Viability may also be assessed by repeated sequential imaging of Rb-82 which, after initial extraction, leaks out of myocardium in the presence of irreversible injury [33]. By contrast, myocardium which is injured but viable retains rubidium with continuous redistribution or positive uptake during the period after i.v. injection. Accordingly, by assessing rubidium kinetics with two sequential PET images after a single i.v. injection of Rb-82, injured but viable myocardium may be identified and separated from necrotic myocardium. The advantages of Rb-82 for assessing viability are that a cyclotron is not required and only one injection of tracer is necessary with a standard 30 minute period for the entire study. The use of FDG/NH$_3$ for assessing viability requires two cyclotron produced radionu-clides in sequence with 3–4 hours required for a complete study.

4. *Left ventricular function and wall thickening.* By gating the positron emission tomographs with the EKG, left ventricular pumping function and wall thickening may be assessed regionally in 3 dimensions [15, 36].

5. *Identification and assessment of significant collateral function in man by imaging coronary steal during dipyridamole-handgrip stress.* Coronary steal occurs under conditions of near maximum coronary vasodilation if collaterals provide a significant proportion of resting myocardial perfusion. A fall in absolute myocardial uptake of activity after injection of a perfusion tracer during dipyridamole vasodilation as compared to rest then indicates coronary steal and the presence of significant collaterals [35].

Thus, positron emission tomography may substitute for current standard cardiac imaging utilizing thallium exercise perfusion imaging, pyrophosphate imaging of myocardial infarction and technetium gated blood pool imaging for left ventricular function. These three current cardiac imaging procedures may be replaced by a single generator produced radioisotope, rubidium-82, which allows these three standard studies to be carried out simultaneously by positron emission tomography. For those centers having a cyclotron, more complex metabolic studies may be carried out. Either asymptomatic or symptomatic patients may be studied on an outpatient or inpatient basis. A rest stress cardiac PET study for the diagnosis of coronary artery disease utilizing rubidium-82 and dipyridamole-hand grip stress requires approximately 45 minutes so that eight to ten patients may be studied per day.

Conclusions

Clinically silent coronary artery disease has been recognized as a major medical problem with fatal or life-threatening sequelae occurring without prior warning symptoms. A satisfactory medical approach to this problem requires an accurate non-invasive screening method for coronary artery disease and an objective quantitation of stenosis severity on arteriograms since decisions on intervention cannot be made on clinical grounds in the absence of symptoms. Technology for both routine screening and automated quantitation of stenosis severity on arteriograms is now available.

For accurate non-invasive diagnosis of coronary artery disease in asymptomatic or symptomatic individuals, cardiac positron imaging should be considered as one of the routine diagnostic tools of the clinician for the following reasons:

a) cardiac PET provides information not previously available for better diagnosis and management of cardiac disease. This new information includes the accurate, non-invasive screening for coronary artery disease in asymptomatic or symptomatic patients, the non-invasive assessment of functional coronary stenosis severity, myocardial infarct imaging, assessment of myocardial viability, and collateral function, none of which can be carried out as well or at all by other imaging techniques;

b) cardiac positron imaging may utilize a single tracer, generator-produced rubidium-82, to obtain better data on myocardial perfusion, function, and viability which now currently requires three separate procedures and radionuclides, i.e. thallium, technetium pyrophosphate, and technetium pyrophosphate labelled red cells;

c) cardiac positron imaging may be carried out economically at the same cost as other high-tech diagnostic imaging but provide functional information quantitatively.

For quantitation of stenosis severity on arteriograms, quantitative coronary arteriography should be routinely carried out because:

a) it provides an objective, automated anatomic or geometric analysis of stenosis severity combining all dimensions of relative per cent narrowing, absolute cross-sectional lumen area and integrated length effects into a single number, stenosis flow reserve, that is derived from basic fluid dynamic principles, related to accepted physiologic concepts and medical application and validated experimentally and clinically;

b) incomplete or partial descriptors of stenosis severity such as per cent narrowing or absolute cross-sectional lumen area alone are inadequate, incorrect and often clinically misleading or unrelated to functional or hemodynamic effects of stenoses or flow reserve or as determined by complete quantitative analysis of all dimensions;

c) in the absence of symptoms, automated quantitative analysis of coronary arteriograms provides the only objective analysis of stenosis severity suitable for widespread use for making decisions on prognosis or intervention.

Acknowledgments

This work was carried out in part as a joint collaborative project with the Clayton Foundation for Research, Houston, Texas, and was supported in part by grants ROLHL26862 and RO1HL26885 from the National Institutes of Health and DEFG05-84ER60210 from the Department of Energy.

References

1. National Institutes of Health: Exercise and your heart. Publication No 83–1677, Jan 1983.
2. Midwall J, Ambrose J, Picard A, Abedin Z, Herman MV: Angina pectoris before and after myocardial infarction. Chest 1982; 81: 681–686.

3. Reunanen A, Aromaa A, Pyörälä K, Punsar S, Maatela J, Knekt P: The Social Insurance Institution's coronary heart disease study: Baseline data and 5-year mortality experience. Acta Med Scand Suppl 1983; 673: 67–81.

4. Kannel WB, Abbott RD: Incidence and prognosis of unrecognized myocardial infarction. An update on the Framingham Study. N Engl J Med 1984; 311: 1144–1147.

5. Lown B: Sudden cardiac death: The major challenge confronting contemporary cardiology. Am J Cardiol 1979; 43: 313–328.

6. Langou RA, Huang EK, Kelley MJ, Cohen LS: Predictive accuracy of coronary artery calcification and abnormal exercise test for coronary artery disease in asymptomatic men. Circulation 1980; 62: 1196–1203.

7. Olofsson BO, Bjerle P, Aberg T, Osterman G, Jacobsson KA: Prevalence of coronary artery disease in patients with valvular heart disease. Acta Med Scand 1985; 218: 365–371.

8. Campbell S, Barry J, Rebecca GS et al.: Active transient myocardial ischemia during daily life in asymptomatic patients with positive exercise tests and coronary artery disease. Am J Cardiol 1986; 57: 1010–1016.

9. Resnekov L: Silent myocardial ischemia: therapeutic implications. Am J Med 1985; 79(3A): 30–34.

10. Gottlieb SO, Weisfeldt ML, Quyang P, Mellits ED, Gerstenblith G: Silent ischemia as a marker for early unfavorable outcomes in patients with unstable angina. N Engl J Med 1986; 314: 1214–1219.

11. Borhani NO: Prevention of coronary heart disease in practice. JAMA 1985; 254: 257–262.

12. Oliver MF: Strategies for preventing and screening for coronary heart disease. Br Heart J 1985; 54: 1–5.

13. Amsterdam E, Wilmore J, DeMaria A (eds): Exercise in cardiovascular health and disease. Yorke Medical Books, 1977.

14. James W, Amsterdam E (eds): Coronary heart disease, exercise testing and cardiac rehabilitation. Symposia Specialists Medical Books, 1977.

15. Gould KL, Goldstein RA, Mullani NA, Kirkeeide RL, Wong WH, Tewson TJ, Berridge MS, Bolomey LA, Hartz RK, Smalling RW, Fuentes F, Nishikawa A: Noninvasive assessment of coronary stenoses by myocardial perfusion imaging during pharmacologic coronary vasodilation. VIII. Clinical feasibility of positron cardiac imaging without a cyclotron using generator-produced rubidium-82. J Am Coll Cardiol 1986; 7: 775–789.

16. Schelbert HR, Wisenberg G, Phelps ME et al.: Noninvasive assessment of coronary stenosis by myocardial imaging during pharmacologic coronary vasodilation. VI. Detection of coronary artery disease in man with intravenous $^{13}NH_3$ and positron computed tomography. Am J Cardiol 1982; 49: 1197–1207.

17. Tamaki N, Yonekura Y, Senda M, Kureshi SA, Saji H, Kodama S, Konishi Y, Ban T, Kambara H, Kawai C, Torizuka K: Myocardial positron computed tomography with ^{13}N-ammonia at rest and during exercise. Eur J Nucl Med 1985; 11: 246–251.

18. Deanfield JE, Shea M, Ribiero P, Landsheere CM de, Wilson RA, Horlock P, Selwyn AP: Transient ST-segment depression as a marker of myocardial ischemia during daily life. Am J Cardiol 1984; 54: 1195–1200.

19. Deanfield JE, Kensett M, Wilson RA, Shea M, Horlock P, Landsheere CM de, Selwyn AP: Silent myocardial ischaemia due to mental stress. Lancet 1984; ii: 1001–1004.

20. Deanfield JE, Shea MJ, Wilson RA, Horlock P, Landsheere CM de, Selwyn AP: Direct effects of smoking on the heart: silent ischemic disturbances of coronary flow. Am J Cardiol 1986; 57: 1005–1009.

21. Selwyn AP, Allan RM, L'Abbate AL, Horlock P, Camici P, Clark J, O'Brien HA, Grant PM: Relation between regional myocardial uptake of rubidium-82 and perfusion: absolute reduction of cation uptake in ischemia. Am J Cardiol 1982; 50: 112–121.

22. Goldstein RA, Mullani NA, Wong WH, Hartz RK, Hicks CH, Fuentes F, Smalling RW, Gould KL: Positron imaging of myocardial infarction with rubidium-82. J Nucl Med, in press.
23. Marshal RC, Tillisch JH, Phelps ME, Huang SC, Carson R, Henze E, Schelbert HR: Identification and differentiation of resting myocardial ischemia and infarction in man with positron computed tomography, ^{18}F-labeled fluorodeoxyglucose and N-13 ammonia. Circulation 1983; 67: 766–778.
24. Tillisch J, Brunken R. Marshall R, Schwaiger M, Mandelkern M, Phelps M, Schelbert H: Reversibility of cardiac wall-motion abnormalities predicted by positron tomography. New Engl J Med 1986; 314: 884–888.
25. Brunken R, Tillisch J, Schwaiger M, Cild JS, Marshall R, Mandelkern M, Phelps ME, Schelbert HR: Regional perfusion, glucose metabolism, and wall motion in patients with chronic electrocardiographic Q wave infarctions: evidence for persistence of viable tissue in some infarct regions by positron emission tomography. Circulation 1986; 73: 951–963.
26. Schelbert HR, Henze E, Phelps ME, Kuhl DE: Assessment of regional myocardial ischemia by positron-emission computed tomography. Am Heart J 1982; 103: 588–597.
27. Sobel BE, Geltman EM, Tiefenbrunn AJ, Jaffee AS, Spadaro JJ, Ter-Pogossian MM, Collen D, Ludbrook PA: Improvement of regional myocardial metabolism after coronary thrombolysis induced with tissue-type plasminogen activator or streptokinase. Circulation 1984; 69: 983–990.
28. Ter-Pogossian MM, Klein MS, Markham J, Roberts R, Sobel BE: Regional assessment of myocardial metabolic integrity in vivo by positron-emission tomography with ^{11}C-labeled palmitate. Circulation 1980; 61: 242–255.
29. Sobel BE, Weiss ES, Welch MJ, SiegelBA, Ter-Pogossian MM: Detection of remote myocardial infarction in patients with positron emission transaxial tomography and intravenous ^{11}C-palmitate. Circultion 1977; 55: 853–857.
30. Geltman EM, Smith JL, Beecher D, Ludbrook PA, Ter-Pogossian MM, Sobel BE: Altered regional myocardial metabolism in congestive cardiomyopathy detected by positron tomography. Am J Med 1983; 74: 773–785.
31. Walsh WF, Harper PV, Resnekov L, Fill H: Noninvasive evaluation of regional myocardial perfusion in 112 patients using a mobile scintillation camera and intravenous nitrogen-13 labelled ammonia. Circulation 1976; 54: 266–275.
32. Harper PV, Schwartz J, Beck RN, Lathrop KA, Lembares N, Krizek H, Gloria I, Dinwoodie R, McLaughlin A, Stark VJ, Bekerman C, Hoffer PB, Gottschalk A, Resnekov L, Al-Sadir J, Mayorga A, Brooks HL: Clinical myocardial imaging with nitrogen-13 ammonia. Radiology 1973; 108: 613–617.
33. Goldstein RA: Kinetics of rubidium-82 after coronary occlusion and reperfusion. J Clin Invest 1985; 75: 1131–1137.
34. Goldstein RA, Kirkeeide R, Demer L, Merhige M, Nishikawa A, Fuentes F, Smalling RW, Mullani NA, Gould KL: Assessment of coronary flow reserve with positron tomography: A comparison with quantitative coronary arteriography (Abstract). J Nucl Med 1986; 27: 943.
35. Demer LL, Goldstein R, Mullani N, Kirkeeide R, Smalling R, Nishikawa A, Fuentes F, Gould KL: Coronary steal by noninvasive PET identifies collateralized myocardium (Abstract). J Nucl Med 1986; 27: 977.
36. Kehtarnavaz N, Philippe EA, DeFigueiredo RJP: A novel surface reconstruction and display method for cardiac PET imaging. IEEE Trans on Medical Imaging 1984; MI-3: 108–115.
37. Gould KL, Lipscomb K, Hamilton GW: Physiologic basis for assessing critical coronary stenosis. Am J Cardiol 1974; 33: 87–94.
38. Gould KL, Lipscomb K, Calvert C: Compensatory changes of the distal coronary vascular bed during progressive coronary constriction. Circulation 1975; 51: 1085–1094.
39. Gould KL: Pressure-flow characteristics of coronary stenoses in unsedated dogs at rest and during coronary vasodilation. Circ Res 1978; 43: 242–253.

40. Gould KL: Noninvasive assessment of coronary stenoses by myocardial perfusion imaging during pharmacologic coronary vasodilation. I. Am J Cardiol 1978; 41: 279–287.

41. Gould KL, Westcott RJ, Albro PC, Hamilton GW: Noninvasive assessment of coronary stenoses by myocardial imaging during pharmacologic coronary vasodilation. II. Clinical Methodology and Feasibility. Am J Cardiol 1978; 41: 279–287.

42. Albro PC, Gould KL, Westcott RJ, Hamilton GW, Ritchie JL, Williams DL: Noninvasive assessment of coronary stenoses by myocardial imaging during pharmacologic coronary vasodilation. III. Clinical trial. Am J Cardiol 1978; 42: 751–760.

43. Gould KL: Assessment of coronary stenoses with myocardial perfusion imaging during pharmacologic coronary vasodilation. IV. Limits of detection of stenosis with idealized experimental cross-sectional myocardial imaging. Am J Cardiol 1978; 42: 761–768.

44. Gould KL, Schelbert HR, Phelps ME, Hoffman EJ: Noninvasive assessment of coronary stenoses with myocardial perfusion imaging during pharmacologic coronary vasodilation. V. Detection of 47% diameter stenosis coronary stenosis with intravenous N-13 ammonia and positron emission tomography in intact dogs. Am J Cardiol 1979; 43: 200–208.

45. Kirkeeide R, Gould KL, Parsel L: Assessment of coronary stenoses by myocardial imaging during coronary vasodilation. VII. Validation of coronary flow reserve as a single integrated measure of stenosis severity accounting for all its geometric dimensions. J Am Coll Cardiol 1986; 7: 103–113.

46. Gould KL, Kelley KO: Physiological significance of coronary flow velocity and changing stenosis geometry during coronary vasodilation in awake dogs. Circ Res 1982; 50: 695–704.

47. Gould KL, Kelley KO, Bolson EL: Experimental validation of quantitative coronary arteriography for determining pressure-flow characteristics of coronary stenosi. Circulation 1982; 66: 930–937.

48. Brown BG, Bolson E, Frimer M, Dodge HT: Quantitative coronary arteriography. Estimation of dimensions, hemodynamic resistance, and atheroma mass of coronary artery lesions using the arteriogram and digital computation. Circulation 1977; 55: 329–337.

49. Young DF, Cholvin NR, Kirkeeide RL, Roth AC: Hemodynamics of arterial stenoses at elevated flow rates. Circ Res 1977; 41: 99–107.

50. Mates RE, Gupta RL, Bell AC, Klocke FJ: Fluid dynamics of coronary artery stenosis. Circ Res 1978; 42: 152–162.

51. Spears JR, Sandor T, Baim DS, Paulin S: The minimum error in estimating coronary luminal cross-sectional area from cineangiographic diameter measurements. Cathet Cardiovasc Diagn 1983; 9: 119–128.

52. McMahon MM, Brown BG, Cukingnan R, Rolett EL, Bolson E, Frimer M, Dodge HT: Quantitative coronary angiography: Measurement of the 'critical' stenosis in patients with unstable angina and single-vessel disease without collaterals. Circulation 1979; 60: 106–113.

53. Brown BG, Lee B, Bolson EL, Dodge HT: Reflex constriction of significant coronary stenosis as a mechanism contributing to ischemic left ventricular dysfunction during isometric exercise. Circulation 1984; 70: 18–24.

54. Brown BG, Bolson EL, Dodge HT: Arteriographic assessment of coronary atherosclerosis. Review of current methods, their limitations, and clinical applications. Arteriosclerosis 1982; 2: 2–15.

55. Kirkeeide RL, Smalling RW, Gould KL: Automated measurement of artery diameter from arteriograms. Circulation 1982; 66: II–325.

56. Kirkeeide RL, Fung P, Smalling RW, Gould KL: Automated evaluation of vessel diameter from arteriograms. Comp Cardiol 1982; 215–218.

57. Weintraub WS, Hattori S, Agarwal JB, Bodenheimer MM, Banka VS, Helfant RH: The relationship between myocardial blood flow and contraction by myocardial layer in the canine left ventricle during ischemia. Circ Res 1981; 48: 430–438.

58. Bache RJ, Schwartz JS: Effect of perfusion pressure distal to coronary stenosis on transmural myocardial blood flow. Circulation 1982; 65: 928–932.

59. Young DF, Cholvin NR, Roth AC: Pressure drop across artificially induced stenoses in the femoral arteries of dogs. Circ Res 1975; 36: 735–743.

60. Young DF, Tsai FY: Flow characteristics in models of arterial stenoses – I. Steady flow. J Biomechanics 1973; 6: 395–410.

61. Young DF, Tsai FY: Flow characteristics in models of arterial stenoses – II. Unsteady flow. J Biomechanics 1973; 6: 547–559.

62. Seeley BD, Young DF: Effects of geometry on pressure losses across models of arterial stenoses. J Biomechanics 1976; 9: 439–448.

63. Fiddian RV, Byar D, Edwards EA: Factors affecting flow through a stenosed vessel. Arch Surg 1964; 88: 105–112.

64. Collins SM, Skorton DJ, Harrison DG, White CW, Eastham CL, Hiratazka LF, Doty DB, Marcus ML: Quantitative computer-based videodensitometry and the physiological significance of a coronary stenosis. Comp Cardiol 1982; 215–218.

65. White CW, Wright CB, Doty DB, Hiratzka LF, Eastham CL, Harrison DG, Marcus ML: Does visual interpretation of the coronary arteriogram predict the physiologic importance of a coronary stenosis? New Engl J Med 1984; 310: 819–824.

66. Harrison DG, White CW, Hiratzka LF, Doty DB, Barnes DH, Eastham CL, Marcus ML: The value of lesion cross-sectional area determined by quantitative coronary angiography in assessing the physiologic significance of proximal left anterior descending coronary arterial stenoses. Circulation 1984; 69: 1111–1119.

67. Marcus ML, Armstrong ML, Heistad DD, Eastham CL, Mark AL: Comparison of three methods of evaluating coronary obstructive lesions: Postmortem arteriography, pathologic examination and measurement of regional myocardial perfusion during maximal vasodilation. Am J Cardiol 1982; 49: 1699–1706.

68. Marcus M, Wright C, Doty D, Eastham C, Laughlin D, Krumm P, Fastenow C, Brody M: Measurements of coronary flow velocity and reactive hyperemia in the coronary circulation of humans. Circ Res 1981; 49: 877–891.

69. Yano Y, Budinger TF, Chiang G et al.: Evaluation and application of alumina-based Rb-82 generators charged with high levels of Sr-82/85. J Nucl Med 1979; 20: 961–966.

70. Mullani NA, Gould KL: First pass regional blood flow measurement with external detectors. J Nucl Med 1983; 24: 577–581.

71. Mullani NA, Goldstein RA, Gould KL, Fisher DJ, Marani SK, O'Brien HA, Loberg MD: Myocardial perfusion with rubidium-82: I. Measurement of extraction fraction and flow with external detectors. J Nucl Med 1983; 24: 808–906.

72. Goldstein RA, Mullani NA, Fisher DJ, Marani SK, Gould KL, O'Brien HA: Perfusion imaging with rubidium-82: II. Effects of pharmacologic interventions on flow and extraction. J Nucl Med 1983; 24: 907–915.

73. Mullani NA: Myocardial perfusion with rubidium-82: III. Theory relating severity of coronary stenosis to perfusion deficit. J Nucl Med 1984; 25: 1190–1196.

74. Philippe EA, Mullani N, Wong W, Hartz R: Real-time image reconstruction for time-of-flight positron emission tomography (TOFPET). IEEE Trans Nucl Sci 1982; NS-29 (1): 524–528.

75. Mullani N, Wong W, Hartz R, Philippe E, Yerian K: Sensitivity improvement of TOFPET by the utilization of the interslice coincidences. IEEE Trans Nucl Sci 1982; NS-29 (1): 479–483.

76. Wong WH, Mullani NA, Phillipe EA, Hartz R, Gould KL: Image improvement and design optimization of the time-of-flight PET. J Nucl 1983; 24: 52–60.

77. Mullani NA, Gaeta J, Yerian K, Wong WH, Hartz RK, Phillipe EA, Bristow D, Gould KL: Dynamic imaging with high resolution time-of-flight PET camera – TOFPET I. IEEE Trans Nucl Sci 1984; NS-31 (1): 609–613.

324

78. Wong WH, Mullani NA, Wardworth G, Hartz RK, Bristow D: Characteristics of small barium fluoride (BaF$_2$) scintillator for high intrinsic resolution time-of-flight positron emission tomography. IEEE Trans Nucl Sci 1984; NS-31 (1): 381–386.
79. Senda M, Yonekura Y, Tamaki N, Tanaka Y, Komori M, Minato K, Konishi Y, Torizuka K: Axial resolution and the value of interpolating scan in multislice positron computed tomography. IEEE Trans on Medical Imaging 1985; MI-4 (1): 44–51.
80. Schelbert HR et al.: Regional myocardial perfusion assessed with N-13 labeled ammonia and positron emission computerized axial tomography. Am J Cardiol 1979; 43: 209–218.
81. Schelbert HR, Phelps ME, Huang SC, MacDonald NS, Hansen H, Selin C, Kuhl DE: N-13 ammonia as an indicator of myocardial blood flow. Circulation 1981; 63: 1259–1272.
82. Paans AMJ, Vaalburg W, Woldring MG: A comparison of the sensitivity of PET and NMR for in vivo quantitative metabolic imaging. Eur J Nucl Med 1985; 11: 73–75.
83. Goldstein RA, Kirkeeide R, Demer L, Merhige M, Nishikawa A, Fuentes F, Smalling RW, Mullani NA, Gould KL: Assessment of coronary flow reserve with positron tomography: A comparison with quantitative coronary arteriography (Abstract). J Nucl Med 1986; 27: 943.
84. Goldstein RA, Kirkeeide R, Nishikawa A, Smaller RW, Demer L, Merhige M, Mullani NA, Gould KL: Improvement in coronary flow reserve after coronary angioplasty as assessed with positron tomography (Abstract). J Nucl Med 1986; 27: 977.

Part IV: Technical Considerations on Digital Systems

29. Reconstruction of the Spatial Distribution of the Myocardial Perfusion from Multiple-View Arteriography

DIETRICH G.W. ONNASCH, JÖRG LINDENAU,[1]
JOACHIM H. BÜRSCH & PAUL H. HEINTZEN
Department of Pediatric Cardiology and Bioengineering; [1] Institute for Informatics and Practical Mathematics, University of Kiel, Kiel, FRG

Introduction

Digital image processing techniques allow to visualize the coronary microcirculation by enhancing the capillary phase opacification of selective arteriograms. However, the spatial distribution and local extent of the myocardial perfusion is difficult to judge from only one X-ray projection. The planar technique is limited by the fact that angiographic images are projections of three-dimensional structures potentially yielding significant overlap of normal, ischemic and infarcted myocardial areas.

Consequently, tomographic approaches have been proposed to calculate the shape and mass of the left ventricular myocardium as well as the location and extent of hypoperfused regions. However, these methods make use of large and expensive equipments [1, 2]. If it were possible to obtain relevant clinical data from the three-dimensional distribution of myocardial perfusion with the aid of a conventional angiocardiographic X-ray unit, and at the same cardiac catheterization that is performed for routine diagnostic purpose, this would be of great benefit.

Increasingly, new X-ray equipment is supplied with multidirectional double C-arm units allowing freely selectable beam projections and biplane digital imaging capabilities. These developments provide new possibilities for the realization of the spatial reconstruction of myocardial perfusion. The goal of our study was to investigate how the geometric and densitometric information inherent in two or more projection images can be combined and how many projections are required to arrive at reliable clinical data.

To develop these methods we performed experimental studies using plexiglas phantoms and pigs. Additional results have recently been published [3, 4].

P.H. Heintzen and J.H. Bürsch (eds), Progress in Digital Angiocardiography. ISBN 978-94-010-7093-5

Experiments

The plexiglas phantom consisted of two concentric cylinders, 60 and 100 mm in diameter, 200 mm long. The space between the cylinders was subdivided in eight sectors. This test object was used to simulate the non-homogeneously perfused myocardium by filling the sectors with contrast medium of different concentrations. While seven sectors were filled with 5ppm Urografin® (76%), the eighth sector and the central chamber were filled with pure water. The whole test object was put into a water basin ($20 \times 20 \times 25$ cm) in order to simulate the conditions of imaging the heart in the thorax.

Pigs (20 kg) were anesthetized with chloralose and pancuronium and intubated for controlled respiration, which was suspended during the time course of angiocardiography. Non-ionic contrast medium (Solutrast® 370) was injected into the three main branches of the coronary arteries or into the left ventricle using an ECG-triggered power injector.

Image acquisition and preprocessing

The angiocardiograms were taken in biplane orthogonal projection mode with the X-ray tubes being pulsed alternatively with a rate of 50 frames/s. Both TV-images were mixed on a split screen in a side-by-side fashion. The radiographic data were as follows: 20 μR per frame at 17 cm input screen behind a grid, 73 kV X-ray voltage, 2 ms pulse length. The X-ray equipment consisted of the generator Pandoros Optimatic, image intensifier Optilux 27/17 HN, saticon cameras Videomed N, and the multidirectional biplane positioning system Bicor (Siemens, FRG).

The biplane unit with the two image intensifiers perpendicular to each other was rotated clockwise in 6 steps of 15/ around the supine pig resulting totally 12 images with angulations between 120/ left posterior oblique and 45/ right anterior oblique (Fig. 1). In each of the 6 positions 2 ml contrast medium was injected.

End-diastolic images were digitized in $256 \times 256 \times 8$ bit format and stored on digital disk of a PDP 11. They were selected shortly after the washout of contrast medium from the coronary arteries and before venous opacification became visible. These images were taken at the 6th to 9th beat after onset of contrast injection. Background structures were removed by logarithmic subtraction of pre-injection end-diastolic images. These 'density images' representing the quasi-stationary phase of the left ventricular myocardial perfusion were evaluated slice by slice from the lower boundary of the mitral valve to the apex (Fig. 2).

The density images were evaluated not only densitometrically but also

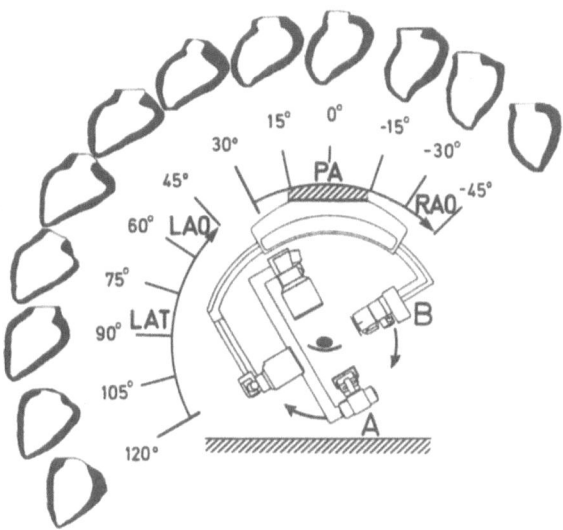

Fig. 1. Twelve end-diastolic projections of the myocardial shell of the left ventricle of a pig traced from the capillary phase of six biplane coronary arteriograms taken by the BICOR unit rotating stepwise from left posterior oblique to left anterior oblique (LAO) (system B) and from LAO to right anterior oblique (RAO) (system A) around the head to foot axis of a supine pig.

videometrically by tracing the endo- and epicardial contours of the left ventricular myocardium manually in each projection. In case of non-reliable border recognition the myocardial region was traced somewhat too large rather than too small. Resulting silhouettes are depicted in Fig. 1. These contours were used to define restrictive conditions to be considered when the density distribution is reconstructed within the muscular ring.

Ideally, all density profiles of a particular slice should have the same area – corresponding to the total amount of contrast medium in the projected cross-section. However, due to different radiation paths, different X-ray hardening and scattering effects, and the use of two imaging chains with slightly different image transfer functions, this is not true in reality. Therefore, the total densities were normalized for each cross-section.

To verify the results of the 3D reconstruction, we tried to identify the territories supplied by the left and right coronary arteries in the pig's heart anatomically. Immediately postmortem blue ink was injected into the right coronary artery. After removing the great vessels, the left and right atrium, and the right ventricle, the myocardium was cut into slices. Pictures were taken, which clearly disclosed the blue and red opacified myocardial regions supplied by the right and left coronary artery branches, respectively.

330

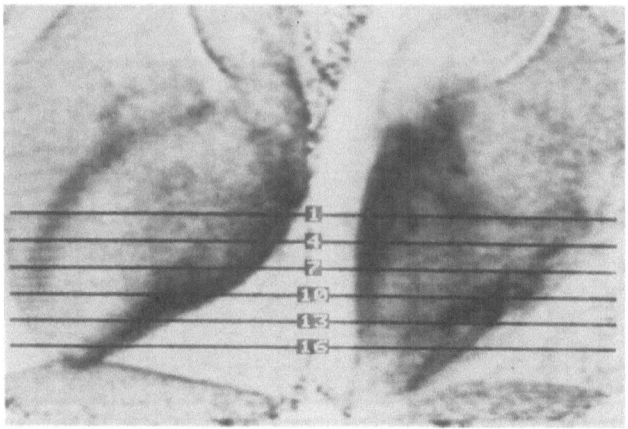

Fig. 2. An end-diastolic biplane density image of the myocardium seven beats after injection of 2 ml contrast medium into the left coronary artery, left seen from 15° left anterior oblique right from 105° left posterior oblique. Evaluations were made for the slices 1 to 16 from the lower level of the mitral valve to the apex.

Reconstruction methods

Two methods were developed to evaluate the density images: the biplane and the multiplane approach. The biplane approach has interesting aspects related to the combined densitometric and geometric evaluation of orthogonal images and is able to locate relatively less or strongly perfused sectors by simple logical reasoning. The results published elsewhere [4], however, suffer from a coarse resolution.

More than two views were combined by applying standard CT reconstruction techniques. Aiming at the reduction of the needed number of views we started to modify the CT reconstruction algorithm. The so-called projection difference method [3, 5] was used, which considers geometric a priori knowledge of the object. This was achieved by reconstructing only the difference between the measured projections and pseudo projections, which were derived from geometrically correct model cross-sections (Fig. 3). For each slice the cross-section was interpolated from the points given by the traced myocardial silhouettes. Fig. 7 presents an example.

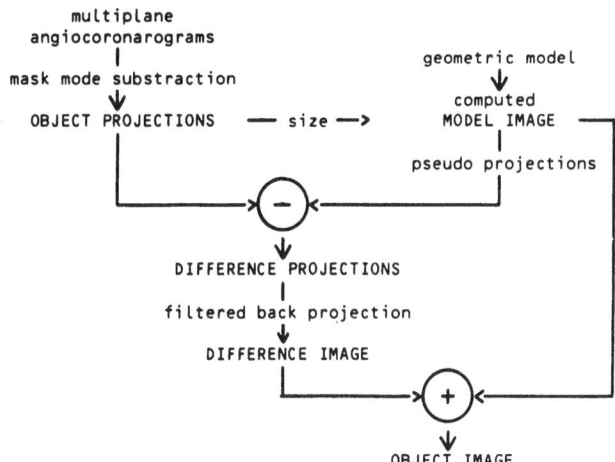

Fig. 3. Schema of the projection difference method.

Results and discussion

In principle there are two modes to get multiple-view myocardial images:
1. by combining mono- or biplane images taken after *several* separate selective coronary arteriograms taken at differently angulated X-ray planes, or
2. from the biplane image sequence recorded while the system is rotating around the patient, using only *one* coronary contrast injection, and by evaluating the images of those two or three end-diastolic beats obtained during the phase of the homogeneous myocardial opacification.

For this study the images were taken by the first mode.

One important feature to evaluate these images and to conceive the spatial distribution of perfusion of the myocardium is to rearrange the processed density images such that they can be displayed in a movie fashion on the TV monitor as if the rotating heart is projected in a stationary state. The motion facilitates to differentiate between frontal and rearward opacified areas remarkably. This display mode is also adequate to select the best projection image for an integrated densitometric evaluation of those myocardial compartments which are supplied only by certain branches of the coronary tree, as suggested by Bürsch [6].

The transfer from many projection images to a true 3D representation can be performed by CT-reconstruction techniques. Fig. 4 presents the result of standard fan beam filtered back projection technique applied to the 12 projections from a slice at mid-papillary level. In agreement with the postmortem

332

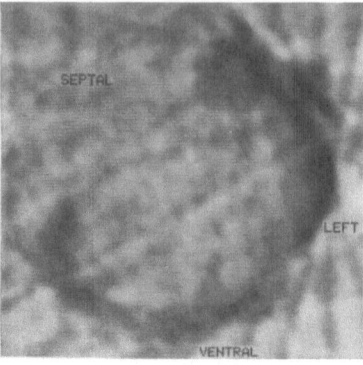

Fig. 4. Result of standard filtered back projection technique of slice 7 (Fig. 2) from 12 myocardial density images of the 8th beat after contrast injection into the left coronary artery.

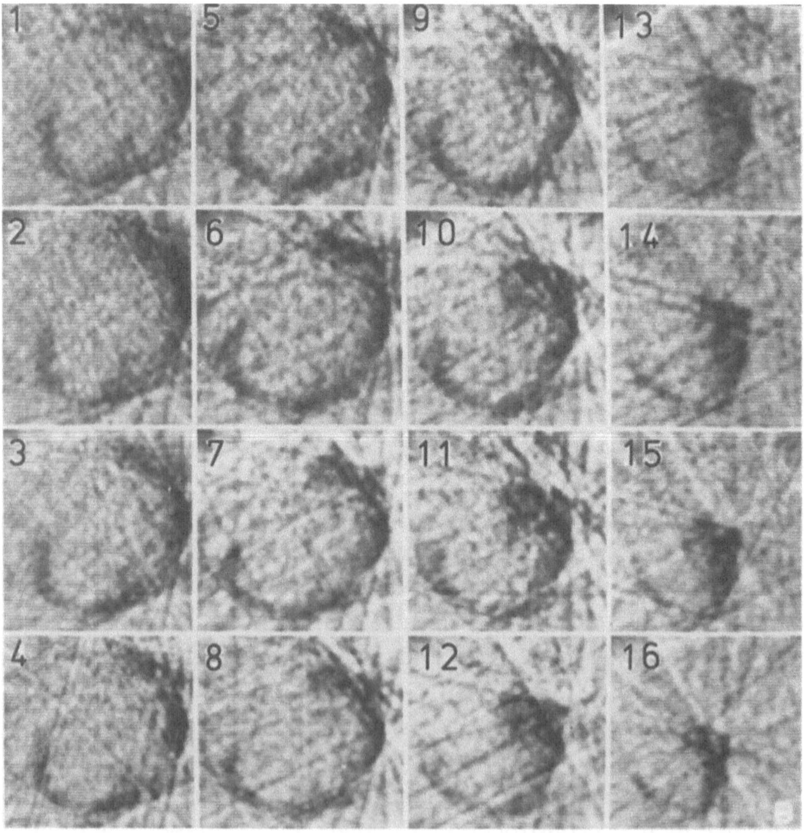

Fig. 5. Sixteen cross-sectional images at the levels indicated in Fig. 2, reconstructed by standard fan beam filtered back projection from 12 views (Fig. 1) from the 7th beat after contrast injection into the left coronary artery.

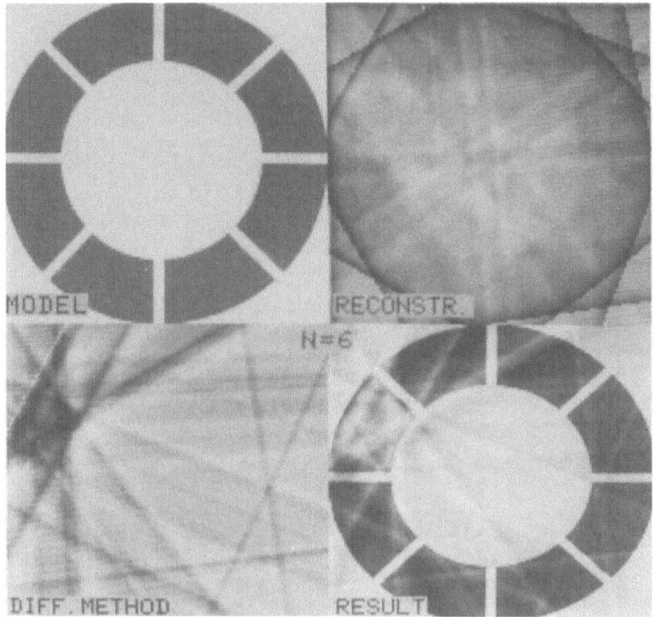

Fig. 6. The projection difference method (Fig. 3) applied to plexiglas phantom. The geometric model approximates the plexiglas ring filled with contrast medium (upper left panel). The result of standard reconstruction technique from 6 views shows a clearing up of the sector at 10 o'clock, which was filled with pure water (upper right panel). Reconstructing the differences of the density profiles yields the image presented in the lower left panel. In the last panel this difference image and the model cross-section are combined.

slices, the septal region is not opacified. Even the onset of the right ventricular free wall can be recognized. Fig. 5 presents 16 slices of the 7th end-diastole after injection, from the lower limit of the mitral valve down to the apex. They are 5 TV lines, that are 4 mm apart from each other. These cross-sections were reconstructed for the 6th to 9th end-diastole with nearly no differences. Only the images of the 6th beat had some more artefacts, produced by the still opacified coronary arteries.

Therefore we think that it is possible to acquire three biplane images, consequently six myocardial projections from only one contrast injection. The quality of the cross-sectional images reconstructed from 12 projections was unexpectedly good, so that one can expect that comparable good images can be reconstructed from only 6 or 8 projections, prerequisite a priori knowledge about the geometry of the cross section is considered in addition to its density profiles in order to reduce the ambiguity of the reconstruction process. For the clinical realization the following technical requirements have to be met:

1. use of a biplane, multidirectional X-ray system rotating synchronously

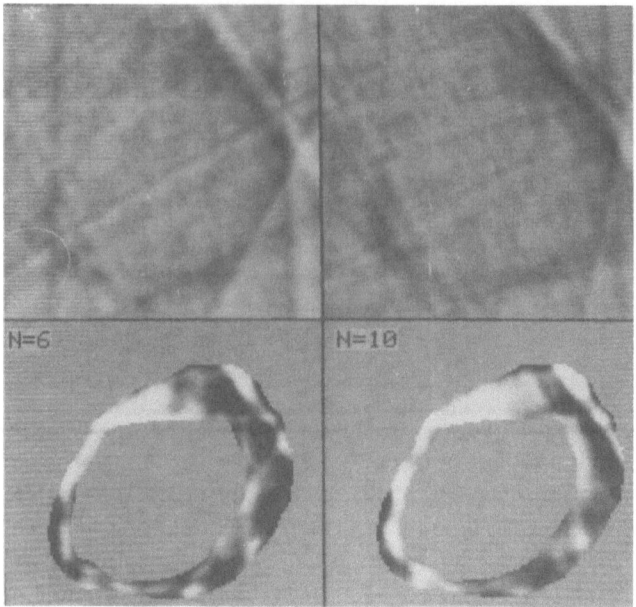

Fig. 7. Results of the difference method applied to myocardial images of a pig for slice 7 (Fig. 2) reconstructed from 6 and 10 views (lower panels) compared to the standard reconstruction technique (upper panels).

around the heart that has been positioned in the isocenter;

2. installation of a biplane digital system adopted to the television cameras of both planes for on-line ECG-gated image acquisition;

3. transfer of the actual spatial angles of the X-ray system to the image acquisition system and storage of those data in connection with the biplane images;

4. high versatility of the image processing system;

5. adequate solution of the problem for reconstructing the density distribution within ring-shaped areas, thus considering the anatomical knowledge about the myocardial structure in its spatial context.

This knowledge base can be derived by videometric evaluations of the projection images as depicted in Fig. 3. Results for a simple ring-shaped plexiglas phantom are given in Fig. 6. In this phantom seven sectors were filled with contrast medium, whereas one sector (at 10 o'clock) was only filled with water. While this can hardly be recognized in the standard reconstructed image in the upper right panel, it is clearly distinguished in the lower panels. Based on the videometrically traced contours this method was also applied to the density images of the animal experiment. Fig. 7 compares the result to the standard reconstruction technique for six and ten projections.

The sectional images generated by the projection difference method profit by the geometric information extracted from the projections. They are easier to understand even when there are only six projections taken. We think that these first results are promising and demonstrate the value of combined densito- and videometric evaluations of multiple-view arteriography aiming at regional myocardial perfusion, even though the algorithm has to be improved further.

References

1. Marcus ML, Rumberger JA, Reiter SJ, Stanford W, Stark CA, Feiring AJ: Clinical applications of cine computed tomography. In this volume.
2. Koiwa Y, Bahn RC, Ritman EL: Regional myocardial volume perfused by coronary artery branch: estimation in vivo. Circulation 1986; 74: 157–163.
3. Lindenau J, Onnasch DGW, Bürsch JH, Heintzen PH: Spatial reconstruction of the opacified myocardium from a small number of projections. Comp Cardiol 1985; 351–354.
4. Onnasch DGW, Lindenau J, Brossmann J, Rooseboom D, Heintzen PH: Steps towards three-dimensional reconstruction of myocardial perfusion from multiple-view arteriography. Comp Cardiol 1986; 265–268.
5. Heffernan PB, Robb RA: Difference image reconstruction from a few projections for non-destructive materials inspection. Appl Opt 1985; 24: 4105–4110.
6. Bürsch JH: Densitometric studies in digital subtraction angiography: assessment of pulmonary and myocardial perfusion. Herz 1985; 10: 208–214.

30. A Bottleneck Model of Imaging Systems for Digital Angiocardiography

R. BRENNECKE
2. Medical Clinic, Johannes Gutenberg University, Mainz, FRG

Introduction

Some ten years ago, the performance of real-time digital subtraction angiocardiography was demonstrated for the first time [1]. Subtraction became in the years after 1980 nearly synonymous with digital angiography [2–4]. This image enhancement technique was certainly very efficient in paving the way for the digital approach to imaging. Relatively simple processors and memory structures could perform subtraction methods with some degree of success. However, even in that early stage, it was clear to many of those involved in the technical developments and in early clinical evaluations that subtraction was only one of many features that would motivate the change from traditional film techniques to digital techniques of angiographic imaging so that digital angiocardiography could become the standard procedure in a large part of the angiocardiographic laboratories [5].

The following is a more complete list of features that could be integrated into a more advanced digital imaging system:

1. Dynamic image acquisition with a high signal-to-noise ratio and with instant availability of the recorded image sequence [5–8] for real-time display in original and modified form (e.g. for unsharp masking [9] and roadmapping [10]).
2. Integration of interactive and of automatic system tests and system optimization procedures for the optimum adaptation of system parameters to the geometry of the patient [6, 11–13].
3. Management of image sequences using a data base architecture for the retrieval of images from an electronic archive [14–16].
4. Image enhancement including subtraction, temporal filtering, and spatial filtering [2–4, 9, 17, 18].
5. Image restoration for compensation of errors in the imaging chain [11, 19–21].
6. Image analysis. Here, the integration of videometric [19, 20, 44, 49, 50] and

P.H. Heintzen and J.H. Bürsch (eds), *Progress in Digital Angiocardiography.* ISBN 978-94-010-7093-5
© 1988, Kluwer Academic Publishers, Dordrecht

videodensitometric techniques [5, 11, 22–25] known for a long time with the high quality and ease of management of image data provided by the steps 1 to 3 should be relatively simple. More importantly, parametric imaging [22, 26–30] as known in principle from nuclear imaging and newly developed image segmentation methods based on the principles of dye dilution techniques could be added for an extended functional analysis of the heart and the great vessels.

It is certainly difficult to state which of the above points is the most important besides image enhancement by subtraction. To many of the workers in this field mostly engaged in clinical work (including interventional procedures) the basic, but by no means primitive feature of getting high fidelity images that are instantly available and that can be easily retrieved is of primary importance. In the following, therefore, the most important features in system design for digital imaging will be primarily discussed. Additional points of current interest such as improved algorithms for image enhancement and analysis, and especially the progress in myocardial perfusion analysis, are discussed in much more detail in other contributions to this book.

The most important goal in system design as described here is to provide high quality image data (see 1–5 above) and provisions for incorporating new image analysis techniques as they evolve from research into practical tools supporting clinical decisions. Although much progress has been made in the design of industrial imaging systems as compared with the state of the art reported at the time of the previous Kiel conference [5] held in 1982, there are still many bottlenecks of system performance. The following article will not go into details of different systems available, but will stress the limitations that still have to be overcome generally before a widespread routine application of digital systems in angiocardiography can be expected.

Definition of the model

It is useful to consider the components of the digital imaging system as elements of a chain. The chain is not stronger than its weakest link, and so it does not make much sense to strengthen a single component without taking into consideration the quality of all other components of the imaging system. If, for instance, there are principal limitations in the X-ray dose or the digital storage capacity at one end of the chain or the other, then it is more economical to match the capacity of the other stages in the chain to the data flow in this principal bottleneck than to optimize them without giving attention to this bottleneck. Therefore, this paper describes a bottleneck model of the flow of energy and information that analyzes the digital imaging chain as an entity.

Traditionally, the foremost interest concentrates on the spatial resolution of the imaging chain [8, 31–38]. Some studies concerning the minimum temporal resolution are also known [11, 13, 36, 39, 40]. Recently, the analysis of subtraction imaging has increased the interest in the determinants of density resolution [3, 4, 6, 8, 11, 41, 42]. The three bottlenecks just mentioned – limitations in the spatial, temporal and density resolution – are interdependent due to basic physical laws although each of them, viewed separately, is of course also determined by the choice of technical factors in a given imaging system. In the digital part of the imaging system, physical limitations are of no concern, but cost considerations limit the performance achievable.

This short overview on the definitions and contents of the bottleneck model reminds us of the wide spectrum of problems involved. The following paragraphs will center in more depth on the questions just mentioned. The first goal will be to pinpoint bottlenecks in the flow of energy and information and the second goal is to match performance in the different stages of the system to each other.

The components of the imaging chain

Analog imaging components

Fig. 1 gives an overview on all stages of the imaging chain that will be discussed in the following paragraphs. The bottleneck model starts with some points of principal nature. The tube load and therefore the density of radiation energy are limited [36]. Thus, integration of energy is always necessary at the receiver end (film or video camera) of the chain [4]. Some elegant schemes of scatter reduction using moving slits for collimating radiation or similar devices [21, 43, 44] are thereby probably ruled out, at least for angiocardiographic applications, as is discussed in more detail below.

The total radiation dose applied is primarily limited by the patient exposure we are willing to accept and it depends also to some extent on the contrast material dose applied. The rule applicable here is very general. It says that for each diagnostic question we have to minimize both the X-ray dose and the contrast material dose as long as we do not lose in certainty of diagnostic decision. In subtraction imaging, radiation dose D and contrast material dose C are combined in a simple formula describing contrast or density resolution R:

$$R \sim C \sqrt{D}.$$

Thus, the reduction of contrast material dose by a factor of 2 has to be compensated for by an increase of X-ray dose by a factor of 4 to keep image contrast (noise contrast) constant.

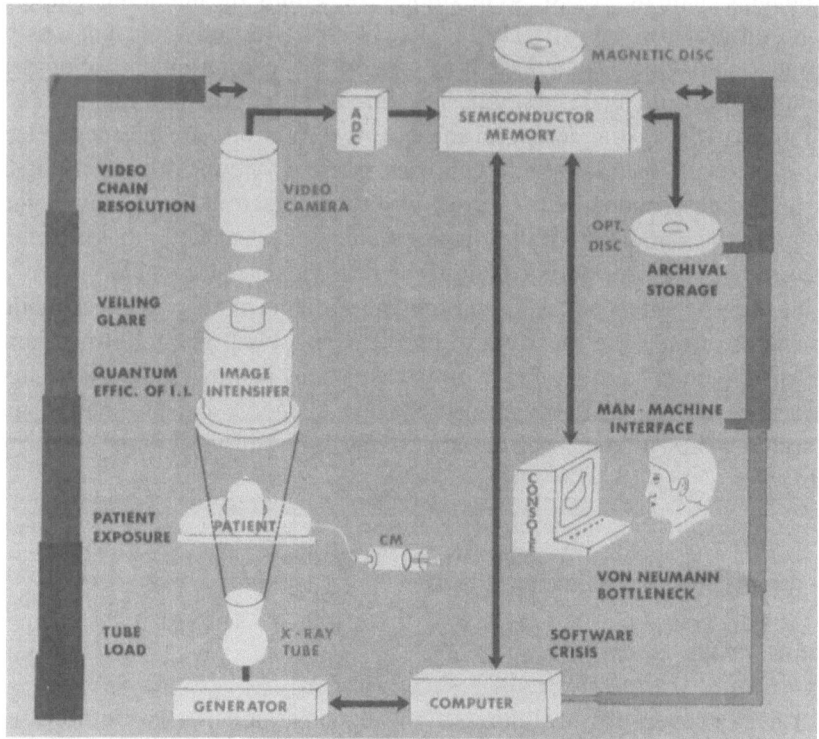

Fig. 1. Bottleneck model of the digital imaging chain. The components constituting critical regions or bottlenecks in the flow of energy or information are marked in this overview and they are discussed in the text.

The next critical point is the detective quantum efficiency (DQE, percentage of converted X-ray photons) of the X-ray intensifier. For a typical X-ray spectrum (ICRU), this number varies between 40 and more than 70 per cent [34]. A high DQE and a high spatial resolution (measured, as is usually done with a high contrast phantom) are presently conflicting requirements. In digital angiography, there is a trend to stress the importance of a high DQE more than a high spatial resolution, since the perceptibility of low contrast details depends on the noise structure and this is, at a fixed patient dose, a function of the DQE.

At the output screen of the image intensifier, the effect known as veiling glare limits the contrast of small details and, at the same time, the accuracy of densometric measurements. Scatter produced in the patient adds to this type of image degradation [19–21, 34, 44]. Veiling glare is reduced by improvements in the design of the output screen of the image intensifier. Scattered radiation can to some part be filtered out by grids mounted in front of the entrance screen of the image intensifier. However, these grids also absorb some of the primary photons. Progress in new imaging techniques using moving collimators such as narrow slits [6, 21, 44] is difficult to obtain due to the limitations of tube load already mentioned and the requirements of very short image exposure typical for angiographic imaging of the heart and the coronaries. Methods of image restoration operating on the digitized image sequences are being developed but they will invariably increase to some extent image noise [19, 20].

The limitations of the optical system between the output window of the image intensifier and the entrance window of the video camera are not marked in Fig. 1. The optical inhomogenity of the lens system could be reduced by a direct fiber link between these components. This type of direct coupling should also reduce the veiling glare effects just mentioned. The idea of a digital image intensifier converting an X-ray image directly into a stream of digital data seems still far from a practical realization.

The video camera is the first component in the imaging chain that can be considered as an electronic device. Together with the analog-to-digital converter, the technical parameters of the video camera determine the spatial resolution or matrix size of the imaging chain [32, 33, 35, 38, 42]. There are, however, other important factors determining spatial resolution. The distance between the object and the entrance screen of the image intensifier, the zooming factor or field of view and the focal spot size of the X-ray tube all contribute to the usable resolution of the total system. Even if all the other factors are optimized for matching it, the digital matrix size of 512 by 512 pixels in use today means a degradation in usable spatial resolution. Model computations lead to matrix size requirements of about 1024×1024 pixels to match under all circumstances the resolution provided by a modern image intensifier (4 line pairs per mm) at a field of view of 25 cm. However, we doubt that model calculations based on objects with a high contrast (lead test pattern) can describe adequately the performance of the imaging chain under the low contrast conditions typical for imaging contrast material distributions in the heart, the great vessels and especially in the coronary arteries. Preliminary results indicate that a resolution between 512×512 and 1024×1024 should be adequate for all of these fields of application including coronary angiography [8, 32, 33, 35]. The change from the interlaced to the progressive mode of scanning the video image [4, 38] improved video imaging to a large extent.

There are two other aspects that play a role in the discussion of the resolution of a digital system. The increase in spatial (and temporal) resolution also increases the data rate and the data capacity to be handled. Moreover, we can only make use of an increased matrix size if we increase, at the same time, the X-ray dose or the contrast material dose (or both) applied to the patient. Otherwise, an increase of noise variance due to the smaller matrix size will interfere. A rule of thumb (not to be read as a mathematical formula) connecting all of these physical parameters is:

Dose = S ∗ T ∗ SNR,

where S is proportional to spatial resolution, T to temporal resolution and SNR to signal-to-noise ratio (ratio of mean signal to its standard deviation (RMS noise)). The SNR thus describes an important parameter of density resolution.

Considering this relationship between cost (dose) and gain (resolution) of the imaging process, it becomes important to clarify still further the question, which resolution is necessary for a given decision, be it the decision to perform a coronary angioplasty or the operative correction of a congenital malformation of the heart.

If we just matched the performance of the digital image acquisition components to the technical specifications of the analog components of the system, we might end up with a large amount of overhead in our data and we might find that we have to increase the load to the patient (contrast and X-ray dose). Therefore, a bottleneck of some of the parameters just mentioned may be advantageous at the interface between analog and digital system. Of course, careful design is necessary to transform e.g. an overhead in resolution provided by the image intensifier into an increase of the signal-to-noise ratio of the total system.

Digital imaging components

The transformation of the analog (video) image into a digital image is primarily the function of the analog-to-digital converter (ADC) [45]. However, the vertical (line) sampling, a prerequisite for digitization of the two-dimensional image data, takes place in the video camera. Since the X-ray image is stored or 'frozen-in' as a charge distribution on the target of the video camera, the line and the pixel sampling rates can be defined separately without reference to the frame rate (which in turn is determined by the rate of X-ray pulses). In other words, an increase in the matrix size by a factor of 4 (e.g. from 512×512 to 1024×1024) must not automatically lead to an increase in data rate by the same factor. If the pulse rate is reduced accordingly, then we can read the image on the target of the video camera with the same rate in both cases. Thus, in a digital system, data rate and data capacity can stay the same while the temporal resolution provided by the lower number of pictures per second becomes lower. Of course, the usable resolution of the digital image depends not only on these parameters of the digitization (or sampling) process but also on parameters of the video camera. Here, the MTF (modulation transfer function) of the scanning system contributes to the spatial and the lag of the target material contributes to the temporal resolution obtainable.

A technical limitation of data rate is provided by the interface between the analog and the digital world, the ADC. Here, rates higher than about 30 MHz with 9 bit density resolution (equivalent to a 1024 × 1024 matrix at 25 frames/s, aspect ratio 1 : 1) are extremely costly to achieve. After this bottleneck, however, techniques such as spatial multiplexing can be used to match slower devices to the primary data rate provided by the ADC. In spatial multiplexing, the primary data stream is distributed into several parallel streams the rate of each stream being a fraction of the original rate. An example is the use of parallel disc magnetic drives. Although each single disc is too slow for image storage at the data rate provided by the ADC, the real-time distribution of ADC data to four or eight of these devices operating in parallel (at a rate only 1/4 of 1/8 of the original rate) solves the problem of real-time image sequence storage. For display, the data streams from the group of parallel discs are, of course, merged again. Image processing also can be speeded up by the implementation of parallel processors as will be discussed in the next paragraph.

Therefore, real-time data acquisition (or data rate) is not primarily the limiting step in digital imaging. The real bottleneck of the digital portion of the overall system is the size of the archival storage (or data capacity) required by the digital data acquired. Conventional magnetic tape and magnetic disc technology were not able to solve the problem of storage of the large amount of data involved in angiocardiographic examinations [5]. In some digital systems, a matrix camera was provided with a cine camera to record original images and processed images again on film. The advent of optical disc technology using a laser beam to store up to 2 Gigabytes per disc has changed this situation to some degree [16, 46]. An image sequence of 10 seconds with 25 frames/s and a matrix size of 512 × 512 is equivalent to more than 60 MByte of digital data. If 4 of these sequences are archived per patient and if the catheterization laboratory performs 1200 examinations per year, we end up wit 300 Gigabyte of data per year requiring 150 large (12 inch) optical discs. Digital magnetic tape technology is also making progress and we expect within 2 years digital tape recorders with a capacity of 15 Gigabytes per tape with a form factor similar to the VHS-standard as it is used in home video equipment. For this amount of data, eight 12 inch optical discs would be required. Larger tape cassettes will store up to 120 Gigabytes. If the philosophy of using one data carrier (film or video cassette) per patient is followed, small magnetic video cassettes could be applied. However, a transfer rate of only a few minutes per patient data is necessary requiring data tranfer rates of several MBytes per second. A critical point about magnetic media is the stability of storage. There is, of course, no experience yet concerning the durability of these media in terms of 15 or 30 years of storage time, a question of utmost concern in image archiving.

The problems discussed bring us again to the question: what is really relevant in the data acquired? This question was discussed in the previous paragraph in the context of the bottleneck in information flow provided by the video camera. In digital systems, we have, besides the irrelevancy reduction discussed previously, a further degree of freedom. By statistical analysis of image data, it is possible to detect which part of the image data can be derived from data already transferred. These data are 'redundant'. On the basis of this analysis it is possible to transfer only new or 'non-redundant' data. These require a lower data rate and a smaller storage capacity. Of course, we can reconstruct the original data from the non-redundant data without error (reversible coding). Under real-time conditions, today the statistical analysis is limited to relatively simple algorithms. Still 'compression factors' of $2:1$ to $3:1$ are achievable in typical imagery. In a typical system, for each pixel one transfers not the original code (10 bit) but only the difference between the code and the weighted sum of the codes of the three nearest neighbors of this pixel requiring a mean (Huffman) code length of only 4 or 5 bits per pixel in the non-redundant data.

In summary, we do not see the archival problem as a long-term bottleneck of digital angiocardiography. The flexibility provided by digital systems will help to reduce the amount of data by irrelevancy reduction and redundancy reduction. Irrelevancy reduction will, at the same time, help to reduce the X-ray dose applied to the patient and the doctor during the examination.

Digital processing architectures

Digital processing of images has much in common with computing in general. Digital storage devices (memories) are interconnected with digital processing devices (adders etc.) and this network is dynamically modified by a stored program. Indeed, one of the early terms for what we call today subtraction angiography or digital angiography was computer angiography. However, it soon became clear that it was extremely difficult to achieve in one system the universal flexibility of the typical general purpose computer and the high speed performance required in real-time and near real-time imaging applications. Still, it was possible to construct specialized computers that are more adequately called image processors being able to perform a narrow range of tasks at the speed required [47].

In this field of applications, the essential limitation of the general purpose computer structures applied today is the sequential nature of processing. The central processing unit of the general purpose computer performs essentially one task at a time. Thus, each computer operation has to pass through this bottleneck that is called 'Von Neumann bottleneck', since Von Neumann devised the otherwise very successful theory underlying the structure of the sequential computer.

The image processors described above were designed for real-time image sequence storage, logarithmic subtraction and time-interval differencing (TID). They could also perform at the same time image averaging for noise reduction. These goals could be fulfilled only by providing a number of processor units, each one specialized for a single task, and several semiconductor memory structures operating in parallel. All of these devices were connected into a rigid structure or 'hardwired'. The main limitation of this approach was that it is not possible to reconfigure the structure of the processor by program to match it to new classes of problems such as parametric imaging. This means, that very costly resources such as large digital memories are connected in a way that they cannot be universally applied. This problem turns up not only in computing applications, but also when thinking about ways to connect an image review station to the system that has access to image series digitized previously and that makes at least some use of the costly resources implemented in the central, real-time system.

The problem of performing image analysis could be alleviated by connecting a (slow) general purpose computer to the special purpose image processor so that complex image analysis tasks could be handled by the former. In some of these designs, the transfer of information between the real-time processor and the general purpose computer is, however, rather slow.

A more general approach to the problem will be the implementation of parallel computers, a network of many universal and specialized processors operating in parallel. The coordination (or programming) of the operations performed by structures like this is still under development. When working on details of this problems one becomes aware of the fact that an image processor for angiocardiography has to have many features of a communication system and that computing may be of secondary concern. Gilbert et al. [23] coined the word 'digital data interchange' for this type of processor structure. For a structure merging computing and communication tasks in the way described, probably one has not only to redesign the hardware (change from the sequential von Neumann computer to the parallel machines) but also needs new programming languages. Replacing sequential, command-driven programming by data-driven architectures is one of the ways to be explored. The ISAAC system designed at Kiel university in the years from 1979 to 1983 belongs to this class of image processor architectures [47].

The problem of image processor architecture becomes even more complex and more specialized when one considers the necessity to give the user and the programmer not only access to image data, but also to the physiological data (ECG, pressures) acquired by the catheterization laboratory system.

Progress into this direction is slow because of reasons discussed at the end of this paper. Here we mention only the extremely high complexity and cost of redesigning a large programming package. This problem is also called the 'software crisis', a term also mentioned in the bottleneck model shown in the figure.

Human-computer interface

The user has to have access to many groups of data with quite different scales of data capacity and structural complexity:

a) Image sequences (angiocardiographic, possibly also echo data):
– raw data to be acquired synchronously with physiological data (see point c below);
– processed data derived from the raw data and to be possibly shown in combination with these data for comparison.

b) Regions of interest (ROI)
– to be set in the time domain (gating, cine loops etc.), often with reference to events in the physiological data;
– to be defined in the spatial domain (ventricular outlines, densometric windows etc.).

c) Signals:
– raw data: ECG, pressure curves, dye injector pulse;
– processed data: densograms.

d) Parameters:
– per cent stenosis as derived from geometric or densometric models;
– enddiastolic/endsystolic volumes;
– regional wall motion.

e) Patient data:
– patient history;
– patient management data.

The integration of these data into a single framework and the development of well designed user interfaces for the access to these data and to certain subgroups of them constituting a functional context is of primary importance for the progress in routine applications of digital angiocardiography. This process can also be characterized as the development from an imaging system to a decision support system [48].

There is not yet much experience concerning user interfaces for complex systems like this [14, 15]. Electronic warfare and the cockpit situation are comparisons sometimes made, not necessarily with an affirmative meaning. Probably, we have to wait for a gradual change in the general attitude towards computers until we can design convincing human computer interfaces for complex image sequence processors. Without doubt, the advent of the personal computer means a large progress in this indirect sense, since it brings flexible hardware and human-engineered software to many people which had not been involved in data processing before.

To make it rapidly adaptable to different groups of users and new trends in human computer interfaces, we designed our image processing software in a way that systematically separates the computing portions of the programs from interactive portions (input of control from the user and output of status information). A special shell program handles the interactive tasks [15]. We expect that this shell program can be easily changed if, for instance, all users or a certain user group should prefer a command-driven interaction stile over menu- driven interaction or vice versa. It can, however, not be overlooked that these shell programs also tend to become extremely complex. We have already mentioned the problem of the software crisis as one of the bottlenecks in the development of adequate systems for digital angiocardiography by industry. Making use of available advanced data base technology and the application of methods of object-oriented programming can probably reduce this bottle-neck.

Discussion

The overview given by the figure and the preceding paragraphs indicate that a number of bottlenecks of physical, but also of technological nature exist that have to be overcome in order to make efficient use (in the sense of decision support) of the potential of digital imaging in the heart catheterization laboratory and in interventional cardiology.

After digitization of the angiocardiographic image series, there are practically no physical limits to the fidelity of storage and transfer of image information. However, the cost of storage systems makes some compromises necessary. Data reduction can, however, also mean dose reduction. The speed and complexity of image data processing is also limited by cost considerations but, in addition, some basic problems in contemporary computer architecture play a role. We cannot expect that the industry producing medical imaging equipment will solve this problem without efforts in other fields with a wider market penetration.

The optimum system will not be obtained by waiting for technological advances. Careful research into the clinical requirements (e.g. temporal and spatial resolution) combined with a careful evaluation of technological developments will bring us systems that are not ideal, but that match the bottlenecks of different stages of the imaging chain in a way that real requirements are met at a minimum of cost and complexity. In this overview taken at the end of the year 1986, the largest discrepancy between obvious requirements and the state of the art of digital systems offered by industry is found in the design of the digital image processing hardware and software available from industry. It cannot be overlooked that high investments are necessary to change this

348

situation. However, much progress is necessary to improve the acceptance of digital imaging in cardiology after the successful implementation of digital systems in general angiography.

Acknowledgments

The support of the Deutsche Forschungsgemeinschaft and of the Robert Müller-Stiftung is gratefully acknowledged.

References

1. Brennecke R, Brown TK, Bürsch JH, Heintzen PH: Computerized video-image preprocessing. In: Nagel HH (ed) Digital image processing; pp 244–262. Springer, Berlin, 1977.
2. Brennecke R, Hahne HJ, Bürsch JH, Heintzen PH: Optimization of generalized subtraction operations. In: Heintzen PH, Brennecke R (eds) Digital imaging in cardiovascular radiology; pp 67–80. Thieme, Stuttgart/New York, 1983.
3. Kruger RA, Mistretta CA, Houk TL, Riederer SJ, Shaw CG, Goodsitt MM, Crummy AB, Zwiebel W, Lancaster JC, Rowe GG, Fleming D: Computer fluoroscopy in real time for noninvasive visualization of the cardiovascular system. Radiology 1979; 130: 49–57.
4. Nudelman S, Capp MP, Fisher HD, Frost MM, Roehrig H: Photoelectronic imaging for diagnostic radiology and the digital computer. SPIE 1978; 164: 138–146.
5. Heintzen PH, Brennecke R (eds): Digital imaging in cardiovascular radiology. Thieme, Stuttgart/New York, 1983.
6. Balter S, Ergun D, Tscholl E, Buchman F, Verhoeven L: Digital subtraction angiography: fundamental noise characteristics. Radiology 1984; 152: 195–198.
7. Chang R, Kaufman SL, Kadir S, Mitchell SE, White RI: Digital subtraction angiography in interventional radiology. AJR 1984; 142: 363–36.
8. Tobis J, Nalcioglu U, Isert L, Johnston WD, Roeck W, Castleman E, Bauer B, Montenelli B, Henry W: Detection and quantitation of coronary artery stenoses from DSA compared to 35 mm film cine angiograms. Am J Cardiol 1984; 54: 489–496.
9. Loo LD, Doi K, Metz CE: Effect of unsharp masking on the detectability of simple patterns. Med Phys 1985; 12: 209–214.
10. Tobis J, Johnston WD, Montelli S, Henderson E, Roeck W, Bauer B, Nalcioglu O, Henry W: Digital roadmapping as an aid for performing coronary angioplasty. Am J Cardiol 1985; 56: 237–241.
11. Brennecke R, Hahne J, Bürsch JH, Heintzen PH: Digital videodensitometry: some approaches to radiographic image restoration and analysis. In: Heuck FHW (ed) Radiological functional analysis; pp 79–88. Springer, Berlin/Heidelberg/New York, 1983.
12. Levin DC, Schapiro RM, Eoxt LM, Dunham L, Harrington DP, Ergun DL: Digital subtraction angiography: Principles and pitfalls of image improvement techniques. AJR 1984; 143: 447–454.
13. Shearer DR, Moore MM: Lag in radiographic imaging systems: a simple method for evaluation. Radiology 1986; 159: 259–263.
14. Böhm M, Obermöller U, Pfeiffer G, Höhne KH: Image management in the system CA/1. SPIE 1982; 318: 161–165.
15. Brennecke R, Jung D, Clas W, Erber R, Meyer J: TALISMAN: An interpreter language for

image sequence management in digital angiography and echocardiography. Comp Cardiol 1985; 363–367.

16. James AE, Carroll F, Pickens DR, Chapman JC, Robinson RR, Zaner R, Pendergrass HP: Medical image management. Radiology 1986; 160: 847–851.

17. Lupon-Roses J, Montana J, Martinez: Venous digital angio-radiography: an accurate and useful technique for assessing coronary bypass graft patency. Eur Heart J 1986; 7: 979–986.

18. Neeley JP, Vannier MW, Gutierrez FR, Spadaro JJ: Digital subtraction angiography of the coronary arteries. CRC Critical Rev Diagn Imaging 1985; 25 (1): 23–60.

19. Nalcioglu O, Roeck WW, Seibert JA, Lando AV, Tobis JM, Henry WL: Quantitative aspects of image intensifier-television based digital X-ray imaging. In: Kereiakes JG, Thomas SR, Orton CG (eds) Digital radiography. Plenum, New York, 1986.

20. Shaw CG, Ergun DL, Myerowitz PD, Van Lysel MS, Mistretta CA, Zarnstorff WC, Crummy AB: A technique for scatter and glare correction for videodensitometric studies in digital subtraction videoangiography. Radiology 1982; 142: 209–213.

21. Shaw CG, Plewes DB: Quantitative digital subtraction angiography: two scanning techniques for correction of scattered radiation and veiling glare. Radiology 1985; 157: 247–253.

22. Bürsch JH, Hahne JH, Beyer C, Seemann S, Meissner L, Brennecke R, Heintzen PH: Myocardial perfusion studies by digital angiography. Comp Cardiol 1984; 343–346.

23. Heintzen PH, Bürsch JH (eds): Roentgen video techniques. Thieme, Stuttgart/New York, 1978.

24. Reiber JHC, Serruys PW (eds): State of the art in quantitative coronary angiography. Martinus Nijhoff, Dordrecht/Boston/Lancaster, 1986.

25. Seibert JA, Link DP, Hines HH, Baltaxe HA: Videodensitometric quantitation of stenosis. Radiology 1985; 157: 807–811.

26. Bürsch JH, Hahne JH, Brennecke R, Grönemeyer D, Heintzen PH: Assessment of arterial blood flow measurements by digital angiography. Radiology 1985; 141: 39–47.

27. Cusma JT, Toggart EJ, Folts JD, Peppler WW, Hangriandreou NJ, Lee C, Mistretta CA: Digital subtraction angiographic imaging of coronary flow reserve. Circulation 1987; 75: 461–472.

28. Höhne KH (ed): Digital image processing in medicine. Springer, New York, 1981.

29. Vogel RA, LeFree M, Bates E: Application of digital techniques to selective coronary arteriography. Am Heart J 1984; 107: 153–164.

30. Vogel RA: Digital assessment of coronary flow reserve. In: Buda AJ, Delp EJ (eds) Digital cardiac imaging; pp 106–115. Martinus Nijhoff, Boston, 1985.

31. Fujita H, Doi K, Giger ML, Chan HP: Characteristic curves of II-TV systems. Med Phys 1985; 13: 13–18.

32. Gray JE, Wondrow MA, Smith HC, Holmes DR: Technical considerations for cardiac laboratory high- definition video systems. Cath Cardiovasc Diagn 1984; 10: 73–86.

33. Haendle J, Horbaschek H, Alexandresce M: High-resolution X-ray television and the high-resolution video recorder. Electromedica 1977; 3: 83–91.

34. Hoffmann FW: Image intensifiers. In: Just H, Heintzen PH (eds) Angiocardiography. Springer, New York, 1986.

35. Holmes DR, Smith HC, Gray JE, Wondrow MA: Clinical evaluation and application of cardiac laboratory high-definition video systems. Cath Cardiovasc Diagn 1984; 10: 63–71.

36. Leeuw P: Quality considerations on cine- imaging and PTCA-fluoroscopy anticipating a digital future. In: Reiber JHC, Serruys PW (eds) State of the art in quantitative coronary arteriography; pp 3–16. Martinus Nijhoff, Dordrecht/Boston/Lancaster, 1986.

37. Schultz E, Fischer P: Zum Auflösungsvermögen der digitalen Subtraktionsangiographie (DSA). RöFo 1983; 139: 296–299.

38. Seibert JA: Improved fluoroscopic and cine-radiographic display with pulsed exposures and progressive TV scan. Radiology 1986; 159: 277–278.

39. Enzmann PR, Djang WT, Riederer SJ, Collins WP, Hall A, Keyes GS, Brody WR: Low-dose, high frame rate versus regular-dose, low- frame- rate digital subtraction angiography. Radiology 1983; 146: 669–676.
40. Ritman EL: Quantitative transaxial imaging of the heart. Eur J Cardiol 1977; 5: 203–220.
41. Revesz G: Conspicuity and uncertainty in the radiographic detection of lesions. Radiology 1985; 154: 625–628.
42. Roehrig H, Nudelman S, Fisher HD, Frost MM, Capp MP: Photoelectronic imaging for radiology. IEEE Trans Nucl Sci 1981; 28: 190–204.
43. Barnes GT, Cleare HM, Brezovich IA: Reduction of scatter in diagnostic radiology by means of a scanning multiple slit assembly. Radiology 1976; 120: 691–697.
44. Wagner RF, Barnes GT, Askins BS: Effect of reduced scatter on radiographic information content and patient exposure. Med Phys 1980; 7: 13–17.
45. Steiglitz K: An introduction to disrete systems. Wiley, New York, 1974.
46. Hindel R: Review of optical storage technology for archiving digital medical images. Radiology 1986; 161: 257–262.
47. Brennecke R: Image processors for digital angiography. In: Kereiakes JG, Thomas SR, Orton CG (eds) Digital radiology; pp 13–33. Plenum, New York, 1986.
48. Benett JL: Building decision support systems. Addison-Wesley, Reading, 1983.
49. Eigler N, Pfaff JM, Whiting J, Nivatpumin T, Forrester JS: The role of digital angiography in the evaluation of coronary artery disease. Int J Cardiol 1986; 10: 3–13.
50. Sigwart U, Heintzen PH (eds): Ventricular wall motion. Thieme, Stuttgart/New York, 1984.

Index